ESSENTIALS OF
CLINICAL BIOCHEMISTRY

ESSENTIALS OF

CLINICAL

BIOCHEMISTRY

D. N. BARON

MD, DSc, FRCP, FRCPath
Professor of Chemical Pathology,
Royal Free Hospital School of Medicine, London

Elsevier Biomedical

New York · Amsterdam · Oxford

Cover illustration: showing an electron micrograph of a lingitudinal section through three vertebrate cardiac muscle cells. Courtesy of Y. Uehara, G. R. Campbell and G. Burnstock, Department of Anatomy, University College, London.

Sole distributors in the United States and Canada:
Elsevier Science Publishing Company, Inc.,
52 Vanderbilt Avenue, New York, NY 10017

First published in the United Kingdom in 1982
as *A Short Textbook of Chemical Pathology* 4th edition,
by Hodder and Stoughton Educational,
a division of Hodder and Stoughton Ltd.,
Mill Road, Dunton Green, Sevenoaks, Kent.

ISBN 0–444–00684–2

Manufactured in the United Kingdom

EDITOR'S FOREWORD

'Books must follow sciences, and not sciences books'

Eight years have elapsed since the last edition of this book and so swift has been the stream of research in chemical pathology that Professor Baron has now produced what is virtually a new book, and a considerably larger one than its predecessor.

In these days chemistry is the very stuff from which so many of medicine's advances are made and a thorough knowledge of physiological chemistry is a basic requirement for a proper understanding of the whole subject of medicine. Thus for the student this book is exactly what he needs. But it is more than that for it provides a splendid conspectus of the whole sweep of chemical pathology without all the detail which a laboratory manual of the subject must include. Thus it not only constitutes an excellent introduction to the subject but also a most useful guide in the approach to higher qualifications.

Professor Baron has that inimitable gift of clarity, so essential in a textbook which remains as concise and compact as this one. It will surely not be long before yet another edition will be called for.

Selwyn Taylor

PREFACE

There are two aims in teaching clinical biochemistry. The first is to provide an under standing of the biochemical basis of disease. The second is to provide guidance in the proper use of the laboratory in the diagnosis and management of patients. This book is designed to meet these needs for medical students and doctors in general, to convey an adequate knowledge of the present theory and practice of clinical biochemistry, and to provide the basics of the subject on a reasonable scale and within the scope of clinical chemists and clinical pathologists. The range and depth of coverage are therefore more extensive than needed just for the examination of the National Board of Medical Examiners of the United States of America. The book is planned to meet the requirements of the examinations of the National Registry in Clinical Chemistry and the American Board of Clinical Chemistry, as well as the primary and diploma examinations of the British Royal College of Pathologists. While it may meet many of the background requirements for the American Board examination in clinical pathology, it is not designed or executed on the scale (or at the cost) of a complete reference text for candidates for the American Board of Pathology subspecialty examination in chemical pathology; they will need, in addition, to consult appropriate monographs.

A medical student should embark on the general study of laboratory medicine in the clinical years with a good knowledge of the essentials of physiological chemistry. Most teachers of laboratory medicine find, alas, that this background is deficient; a necessary reminder has therefore been provided. Particulars of analytical methodology and laboratory management are not included.

The overlong period of eight years since the last British edition of this book (published as *A Short Textbook of Chemical Pathology*) has been marked by an increase in the range of tests that are performed and by further advances in our knowledge of fundamental laboratory medicine.

This book have therefore been rewritten, and necessarily enlarged, maintaining the general plan of previous editions. The former introductory chapter has been divided into one on the principles of laboratory diagnosis (with an important new section on test sensitivity) and one on overall metabolic changes. Chapters 3–8 discuss abnormal metabolism of single or related substances, Chapters 9–15 the special clinical biochemistry of disorders of organ function. Particular problems of pediatric clinical biochemistry are included where appropriate. Rare diseases are described when their abnormal biochemistry illustrates important general points. Outdated tests may be mentioned because of their historical importance, because they may be met in the literature, or because they may still be used in parts of the world lacking expensive investigative facilities. There are appendices on procedures for specimen collection; SI units; reference values, with conversion factors from traditional to SI units; and simple biochemical test procedures. There is considerable cross-referencing between chapters and an extensive index. A selected list of further reading has been provided, rather than detailed references.

SI units have been used throughout, with emphasis on the mole for plasma concentrations. To convert these to traditional units the reader may use the conversion factors included in Appendix III. Mass units are also quoted for dietary intake, in describing urine tests, and in the tables of adult reference values. Rounded-off conversion values are generally applied. The recommendations in *Enzyme Nomenclature* (1979) have been followed, unless a new name would be confusing.

There are many new figures, and the others have been redrawn: I thank June Cluett for her help in designing the artwork. Miss Jane Lytle provided both skilled typing and initial subediting. I am indebted once again to Dr. J. H. Barton who has read the whole book in manuscript and made very many corrections and criticisms. My colleagues Dr. D. G. Cramp and Dr. P. Dandona have been continually helpful and stimulating in many discussions throughout all the preparation. I am grateful to Dr. D. Freedman and Dr. D. Mikhailidis (registrars in chemical pathology) for their detailed checking of the manuscript, their assistance with many points, and their collaboration on the reading list. Very many friends and colleagues answered my questions on problems within their special experience, and in particular Professor A. V. Hoffbrand provided much help cancerning the Haemopoietic system. It has been a pleasure to continue my association with Hodder and Stoughton.

GENERAL BIBLIOGRAPHY

It is generally useful to consult the text, and reading list of appropriate chapters in detailed multiauthor works such as:

Bondy PK, Rosenberg LE, eds. *Metabolic Control and Disease.* 8th ed. Philadelphia: W. B. Saunders, 1980.

Brown SS, Mitchell FL, Young DS, eds. *Chemical Diagnosis of Disease.* Amsterdam: Elsevier/North Holland, 1979.

Stanbury JB, Wyngaarden JB, Fredrickson DS, eds. *The Metabolic Basis of Inherited Disease.* 4th ed. New York: McGraw–Hill, 1978.

CONTENTS

CHAPTER 1

INTRODUCTION

Clinical biochemistry is the study of the changes that occur in disease in the chemical constitution and biochemical mechanisms of the body. These changes may be either the cause of a disease or its effect. As a fundamental science, clinical biochemistry applies physiology and biochemistry to the elucidation of the nature and cause of disease. As an applied science, it seeks by analysis of body fluids and tissues to aid the clinician in diagnosis and treatment. This branch of laboratory medicine, when the emphasis is on analysis is frequently called clinical chemistry; 'chemical pathology' may be used to emphasize the study of disease processes. Clinical biochemistry can have either meaning but is probably the best single descriptor for the discipline. It is a relatively new science and has therefore been mainly concerned with specific problems. An attempt can be made to determine whether any general principles of clinical biochemistry exist that are applicable to a wide range of special topics.

HISTORICAL DEVELOPMENT

The advance of Chemical Pathology has followed the development of medicine, of biochemical knowledge, and of chemical analytical techniques.

By the middle of the nineteenth century physicians could measure the concentration of hydrochloric acid in gastric juice; and analyse urine for sugar by Fehling's test, for protein by boiling with acidification, and for bile by nitric acid. The classical *Lectures on Chemical Pathology* of 1847 by Bence Jones, and many similar books of the time, were based on quantitative analyses of urine. Sugar, uric acid, and urea had been demonstrated in blood in diabetes mellitus, in gout, and in chronic renal disease respectively, but there were no methods for their easy estimation, especially in small quantities of blood. There were no important developments during the nineteenth century in the general application of chemical knowledge to medicine by the performance of biochemical analyses on patients, although many pioneers, of whom perhaps Thudicum and Garrod were the best known in Britain, were laying the foundations of the subject. In the first edition (1913) of Panton's textbook *Clinical Pathology*, which represented standard practice at that time, no satisfactory chemical tests on blood (except for spectroscopy) were described.

The first phase of modern chemical pathology was from 1910 to 1920, when important advances in methodology were made, notable pioneers being Bang in Sweden, and Folin and Van Slyke in the USA. By the early 1920s venepuncture had become routine practice, visual colorimeters were widely available, and analytical methods requiring only 1 ml of blood were generally adopted. This led to the second phase. By 1927, when the second edition of Panton's book appeared, he had had to add a chemical pathologist (Marrack) as co-author, and 20 blood analyses were included with the implication that 10 were in constant use. Because of this general acceptance of analyses of blood from patients, over the period 1920 to 1925 hospital laboratories that performed biochemical analyses had a five-fold increase in the number of investigations. Such tests had been transferred from being performed by physicians in ward side-rooms to being done by chemically trained staff in special laboratories.

From then until the late 1940s there was a steady and slow increase in the investigative work of biochemical laboratories, and this played its part in the increase in knowledge of biochemical changes in disease. The next major methodological developments were flame photometers which permitted easy analysis of sodium and potassium; photoelectric colorimeters which afforded greater speed and precision than did visual colorimeters; and 'micro' techniques for 0.1 ml samples, developed in Britain by King, which allowed more analyses to be done on single venous samples and permitted the use of capillary blood. These brought in the third phase. Because of these methodological advances, the greater knowledge of biochemistry applied by more scientifically minded clinicians, and the need for much greater biochemical control of potent therapy, a new steep increase in biochemical analytical work on patients began. The rate of increase in demand since 1950 in most large laboratories has been 10–15 per cent per year. As appreciation of the meaning of the results has led to more knowledge, and this to more tests, the rate of increase has been continuous. Gradually more complex analytical procedures moved into the clinical laboratories from the basic sciences – electrophoresis, chromatography, enzyme rate reactions, and isotopic and immunological procedures. Analytical procedures became possible on ultramicro samples (0.01 ml), thus allowing a more intensive biochemical study of paediatric and neonatal disease.

The fourth phase has been the introduction of automatic analytical equipment by continuous flow or discrete systems, of which the pioneer has been the Technicon AutoAnalyzer. Many manufacturers have further developed multichannel analysers (or 'plasma-crunchers'), by which more than 20 simultaneous analyses may be done on a single plasma sample, and 200 or more of these samples processed per hour. With this type of equipment we are progressing to the fifth phase, when in large laboratories computers are becoming necessary to maintain the identification of the sample, to control the analytical machinery, and to calculate, store, and deliver the results. Simple-to-operate machines, for performing analyses at the bedside, are being developed as well.

When pathology, in any of its disciplines, is concerned with patient care (and may then be called *Clinical Pathology*), finance, efficacy, and priorities, as well as medical science, become involved. Considerations of cost, and the problems of allocation of resources, are forcing control of hitherto unrestricted demands for analyses: one patient investigated at too great a cost may have to mean another patient under-investigated. The sixth phase will have to be much improved selectivity in the choice and frequency of biochemical investigations. Laboratory tests are justified only when the clinician determines *beforehand* how the results will assist in diagnosis or management.

THE INVESTIGATION OF POSSIBLE ABNORMALITIES

Reasons for investigations

Discretionary tests

There are two main types:

Discriminating. The usual biochemical investigation of a patient can be put into a logical sequence, and more information is obtained by testing in series than in parallel:

1 Decide what information is needed: you cannot get an answer unless you ask a question.
2 Choose the test(s) most likely to provide the information.
3 Use the analytical procedure(s) that best combines speed and quality.
4 Correlate the result(s), which strictly are relevant only at the time of testing, with the existing information.
5 Decide, in the light of these results, whether further, different, tests are needed.
6 Decide if and when to repeat the test(s).

A test that asks a specific question of an individual patient can be considered as one of five types.

(a) *Is anything wrong?* implies that a biochemical investigation is being used as the extension of a clinical examination to determine the presence or absence of an abnormality, under circumstances when the biochemical test is more sensitive than the clinical approach.
(b) *What is wrong?* implies that a general clinical abnormality has been identified, but the specific diagnosis is not known. A discriminating biochemical test (or preferably and more usually a particular combination of tests) can then be chosen which will give a different pattern of results in each of the several diseases of possible diagnosis.
(c) *How badly is it wrong?* implies that the specific diagnosis has been established, but it is necessary to use a biochemical test to assess progression or regression (perhaps after treatment) more sen-

sitively than can clinical observation. On the whole, biochemical tests are probably more important for monitoring progress and treatment than for diagnosis.

(d) *What else is wrong?* implies that a biochemical test is being used to detect a complication of the disease, or an expected or unexpected side-effect of treatment, before it becomes evident clinically.

(e) *Why is it wrong?* implies that the investigation is for research, to learn more about the chemical pathology of the disease. The patient being tested may not benefit, and informed consent, and the approval of the local Ethics Committee, may be necessary. Investigations whose results are required only for teaching come into this category.

Base-line. It is desirable to know the initial values for biochemical components before a patient undergoes a procedure that may alter them significantly, e.g. plasma electrolyte concentrations before major surgery or before diuretic therapy, or liver function tests before receiving possibly hepatotoxic drugs.

Screening tests

There are two main types:

Population screening. It is feasible to examine a whole apparently healthy population for a particular disease or toxic effect which is present at low frequency, and which can be detected at a sub-clinical phase by a specific biochemical (or other) test. The population may be selected geographically as in a town, or by occupation, or by age or sex, or by choosing only members of affected families. There must be an advantage in treatment, or prevention of further toxic effects, by early detection of the disease being sought: if not, instead of giving the patient, say, an extra year forward of life, he is being given an extra year backwards of disease. The most widely used biochemical population screening test of generally accepted value is that of blood phenylalanine, done on week-old infants for diagnosis of phenylketonuria (p. 101). Neonatal biochemical screening for congenital hypothyroidism (p. 152), and antenatal screening for neural tube defects (p. 165), are now accepted. An example of a screening test of negligible value, because there is no sharp boundary between normal and abnormal, and because of doubts about the advantage of treating asymptomatic patients, is random blood glucose analysis for detection of sub-clinical diabetes mellitus in the general population.

Admission screening. This implies testing all hospital inpatient admissions, or perhaps outpatient referrals, or even 'check-ups' in a clinic just to see if there is 'anything wrong', for a large number (10–20) of biochemical variables on plasma at the same time. This screening is done irrespective of whether all these investigations are warranted by the patients' presenting condition. Such screening is made possible, and encouraged, by the above-mentioned availability of multichannel automatic equipment, and of computers. It had been hoped that such screening would be economical and provide a 'data-base' as many of the tests might eventually be requested anyway, and the patient's stay in hospital be shortened. It is also hoped that unexpected biochemical abnormalities will provide important diagnostic information. These hopes have generally not been fulfilled. Also the clinician may find it troublesome because the result he-wanted, or an unexpected abnormal result, may be swamped by 'noise' from unwanted results. Much effort is often spent in working up biochemical 'abnormalities' of no clinical importance: a healthy person is one who has not been sufficiently investigated! Such multiphasic screening is not cost-effective.

Profiles, namely performance of an initial set small group of tests related to a specific organ or system, such as four or five tests in the investigation of jaundice (p. 205), are generally worthwhile.

Types of test

In general, biochemical investigations of function are first performed in the resting state as the patient presents clinically. This applies whether the function is of an excretory organ such as the renal glomerulus, of a secretory organ such as the pancreatic acinar cells or the adrenal cortex, or of a system such as the blood buffers. Gross changes are detected by such investigations, but a minor abnormality may well be covered by compensatory mechanisms. So for the investigation of minimal changes it is often necessary to test the function when stressed, and this may sometimes be helpful in determining the physiological level of an abnormality. One type of stress is an extreme load of a normal metabolite, such as using a large dose of ammonium chloride to test the ability of the renal tubules to acidify the urine: a small loss of function may be insufficient to destroy the ability to compensate for the acidity of a normal diet. Another type of stress test is to measure the reserve ability of a target organ to respond to a hormonal stimulus, such as the gastric acid response to pentagastrin to assess parietal cell function. The response measured may itself be hormonal, such as the increase in plasma cortisol concentration, after injection of adrenocorticotrophic hormone, to measure adrenal function (p. 159). The converse stress is a suppressant usually via a negative feedback mechanism. This is usually hormonal, and tests both the integrity of feedback and the response of the target organ, such as changes in plasma cortisol after dexamethasone, which test the suppression of adrenocorticotrophic hormone and assume the capability of the adrenal cortex to produce corticosteroids (p. 160).

The meaning of diagnostic test results

Some of the reasons why clinicians overemphasise the value of a test and have too much faith in laboratory diagnosis are lack of understanding of the possibility of laboratory variation and error (p. 256), and of important concepts related to the efficacy of a test which should influence their decisions.

True positives (TP) are those ill patients who have that illness correctly diagnosed by the test relevant to their disease

True negatives (TN) are those without the disease, who are correctly identified by the test as unaffected

False positives (FP) are those unaffected subjects who are wrongly diagnosed by the test as having the disease

False negatives (FN) are those affected patients who are wrongly identified by the test as free from the disease

Sensitivity and specificity

Sensitivity of a test is the percentage of all ill patients classified as positive for their disease

$$= \frac{TP}{TP + FN} \times 100$$

The higher the sensitivity of a test, the less likely it is to fail to diagnose a patient as having the disease for which that test is relevant.

Specificity of a test is the percentage of negative results in subjects without that disease

$$= \frac{TN}{TN + FP} \times 100$$

The higher the specificity of a test, the less likely it is to misclassify an unaffected subject as having the relevant disease. Sensitivity and specificity do not depend on the prevalence of the disease for which the test is being made.

Predictive values

These take account of the prevalence of the disease in the population. Predictive value of a positive test is the percentage, in a mixed population, with and without the disease, of positive results that are true positives

$$= \frac{TP}{TP + FP} \times 100$$

Predictive value of a negative test is the percentage, in a mixed population, of negative results that are true negatives

$$= \frac{TN}{TN + FN} \times 100$$

The higher the predictive value of a test, the higher the likelihood, in any population, that a positive test means disease, or that a negative test means absence of disease. Most tests were developed in hospitals where a high proportion of patients had the relevant disease, so the tests would then have a high predictive value. If a disease has a low prevalence in the population being tested, such as an ambulatory population in the community, then because of the higher proportion of non-diseased subjects there will be a higher likelihood of false positives. A positive result then has a lower predictive value, that is a lower chance of being a true positive.

As an example, the parameters of Fig. 1.2 can be taken for a single test. Assuming a prevalence of the disease in the population tested of 1/3, then the predictive value of a positive test is 97 per cent, namely only 3 per cent of positive results will not be from patients with the disease. However if the prevalence were 1/100, then the predictive value would be only 30 per cent, namely 70 per cent of positive results would not be from diseased patients.

REFERENCE VALUES, NORMAL RANGES, AND ABNORMAL RESULTS

The normal range for any analysed body constituent is a convenient but artificial concept. A statement such as 'normal plasma sodium 136–148 mmol/l' implies that there is strict boundary between normal and abnormal. This means that all normal subjects ('normal' is indefinable but implies the general population) have plasma sodium values within that range, and that it is abnormal to have a plasma sodium less than 136 mmol/l or more than 148 mmol/l. Because these assumptions are not true, the term has been replaced by 'reference values', or reference interval, meaning a range of results to which the result in question can be compared, without making any assumptions about the meaning of 'normal'. It is fair to say that if a value falls within the reference values, then with regard to that component the subject is much more likely not to be diseased than to be diseased, whilst the converse applies to a value outside the reference values – though 'diseased', like 'healthy' and 'unhealthy', is also indefinable (Fig. 1.1). In practice most analysed variables have either a roughly Gaussian or a log-normal distribution, and by convention the reference values are taken to be those which apply to 95 per cent of the population under study (Fig. 1.2), thus excluding 2.5 per cent at either extreme. They can usually be calculated as the mean ±2 standard deviations; and if the distribution is non-parametric, then the convention is even more artificial.

However for different circumstances different conventions may be used, and medical judgement is important. If reference values of mean ±3 s.d. (99.7 per cent of the population) are used, then this will virtually eliminate the risk of a healthy subject being counted as unhealthy should this be considered necessary, as in measuring α-fetoprotein as an indication for therapeutic abortion (p. 165); but a greater number of unhealthy subjects will be missed (Fig. 1.3). Such a procedure will reduce

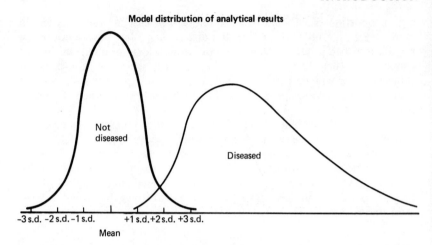

FIG. 1.1. Theoretical Gaussian curve for the distribution of a component (e.g. measurements of plasma concentration) in a non-diseased population, showing the range at different multiples of 1 standard deviation (s.d.) from the mean. This is compared with a positively skewed curve for the same component in a theoretical diseased population, showing overlap between the values found with and without disease.

the number of false positives, and operates the test at high specificity. If the risk may be the other way, and diseased patients must not be missed whilst occasional (perhaps temporary) misattribution of the unaffected is acceptable, as in screening for phenylketonuria (p. 101), then a narrower set of reference values than '95 per cent' could be chosen, such as mean ± 1 s.d., or 67 per cent of the population (Fig. 1.4). This procedure operates the test at high sensitivity, and reduces the number of false negatives.

The accepted convention leads to the apparent paradox that if a population group of 'normal' subjects each has 15 independent tests performed, by, say, a screening multichannel analyser, then more than half of the subjects will have at least one 'abnormal' result. A binary concept of health versus disease is not supported by biochemical evidence.

Problems of methods

Reference values are dependent on methodology, for this affects the absolute value of the results. A method is *accurate* if the results are close to the true concentration (or activity) of the substance being measured – which may be difficult to establish in a biological system. A method is *precise* if repeated analyses give very similar results – even though not necessarily accurate. For virtually all substances analysed no method is either absolutely precise, or absolutely accurate. A measurement of plasma concentration requires dividing the amount of substance present (as the numerator) by the volume of solution (as the denominator). There

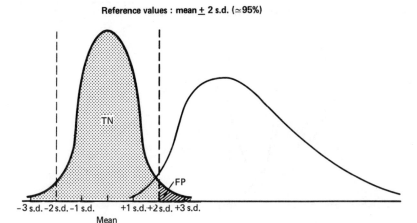

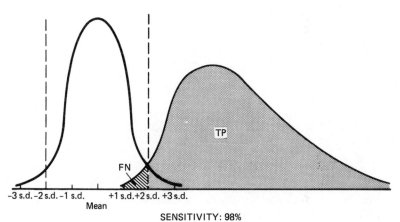

Fig. 1.2. The use of mean ±2 s.d. (≃95 per cent of population) as reference values, and its effect on the distribution of true and false positives (TP and FP) and of true and false negatives (TN and FN), and on specificity and sensitivity. The distributions are the same as in Fig. 1.1.

are reference methods available that can measure the numerator, sometimes called the analyte, with high precision, but the denominator (should it be whole plasma, or fat-free plasma, or plasma water?) cannot be known so exactly. In the interpretation of possible clinical significance of changes in results, consideration of variability due to the method is important, and the local laboratory can provide information. For example, flame photometry for plasma sodium is precise, so a 5 per cent change, say from 140 mmol/l to 147 mmol/l, is unlikely to be due to laboratory variation and represents a true change in the patient. Extraction and titration for faecal fat is an imprecise method, so the same 5 per cent change, say from

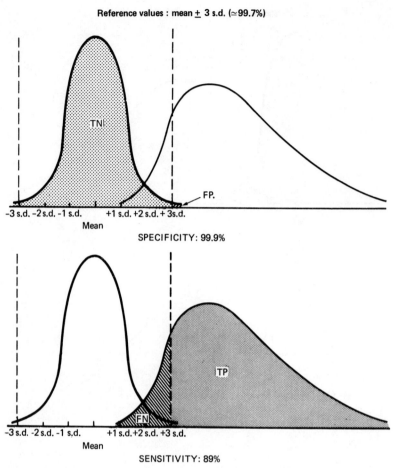

FIG. 1.3. The use of mean ± 3 s.d. ($\simeq 99.7$ per cent of population) as reference values.

14.0 g/24 h to 14.7 g/24 h, may well be due to laboratory or collection variation.

Limitations of measuring concentration

Most analyses in chemical pathology measure the concentration of the substance being studied, which means the total amount of that substance, or of similar substances detected by the analytical procedure, per unit volume of material analysed. However it is not only concentration that is important.

Concentration and activity. The effect of a substance on a biological process depends on its activity, which is not necessarily the same as its concentration. This applies in blood plasma, and even more in cells.

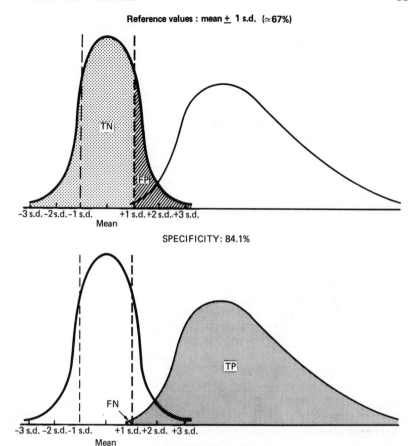

FIG. 1.4. The use of mean ±1 s.d. (≃67 per cent of population) as reference values.

Concentration in plasma water, though rarely determined, is a better reflection of activity than is concentration in whole plasma. An increase in the plasma concentration of other substances (p. 30) will lower the concentration in whole plasma of the substance studied without altering its true concentration in plasma water.

For electrolytes the presence of free (active) and bound (inactive) forms has to be taken into account (p. 17); ion-sensitive electrodes can measure activity directly (p. 22). Many non-peptide hormones are present in plasma in free and bound forms; measurement of the active component may be possible (p. 149). For polypeptide hormones it is possible that current immunoassay methods also detect inactive derivatives; bioassay procedures (p. 137) have the advantage of measuring hormone activity. For enzymes current methods generally measure activity, which depends on inhibitors and activators; sometimes measurement of the concentration of enzyme protein is useful and feasible (p. 119).

Concentration and content. When intake or output of a substance is studied, the importance of making the conversion from concentration to content, for example in a 24 hour urinary excretion, is rarely forgotten. Total blood loss does not alter concentrations in the blood until secondary fluid shifts develop, though the total content of all substances in the intravascular compartment is reduced. Loss or gain of water in blood plasma will affect the measured concentrations of substances in plasma, and such changes will mask any changes due to loss or gain of a substance in the plasma compartment (p. 28).

Measured changes in body constituents due to factors other than disease and drugs

Because of physiological variations, the concentration or excretion of a body component is affected by accountable factors such as time of day and of menstrual cycle (and pregnancy), exercise and recumbency, mental state, general diet, fluid balance, and specific meals. Body build will affect the amount of some substances that are excreted (e.g. creatinine, p. 100) but influences few plasma concentrations. The existence of seasonal variations is controlled by environmental temperature, sunlight, and probably an endogenous rhythm. The causes of racial variation are partly nutritional, partly environmental (including endemic disease), and possibly genetic (including blood groups). The main causes of variation in the reference values of a healthy population are age and sex: these are being established for all analytes, and the changes with ageing are not always the same for men and for women. Plasma concentrations usually (except for albumin and iron) tend to rise with age, probably because of diminution of renal clearance. In general, except for chloride and phosphate, and excluding the female sex hormones, plasma values in men are higher than those in women: this difference is hormone-mediated, as it tends to disappear after the menopause. If a drug, such as aspirin, ascorbic acid, alcohol, or the hormonal contraceptives, is taken regularly by a high proportion of healthy subjects, should these be counted as 'normal'? Slight differences in reference values from those found in the ambulant healthy population may be seen in 'hospital normals', which implies that measurements are made on inpatients who do not have any disease that is known to affect the measured constituent. The differences may then be due to hospital diet, recumbency, and the 'stress' non-specific effects of hospitalisation and of any illness. A severe illness may affect results for weeks after clinical cure.

To understand the full significance of serial changes in a single patient would depend on knowing that patient's own reference values, or inherent variability, to which analytical error may contribute significantly.

THE IDEAL DIAGNOSTIC TEST

Can be done at the bedside
Painless for the patient
Free of risk

Quick and easy
Does not need great skill
Inexpensive equipment
Low cost for reagents
Accurate and precise

Sensitive and specific
No false positives
No false negatives

High predictive values
Easy to interpret

It does not exist

Further Reading

Caraway WT. The scientific development of Clinical Chemistry to 1948. *Clin Chem* 1973; 19:373–383.
Williams RJ. *Biochemical Individuality*. New York: Wiley, 1965.
Young DS, Nipper H, Uddin D, Hicks J, eds. *Clinician and Chemist: The relationship of the laboratory to the physician*. Washington DC: American Association for Clinical Chemistry, 1979.

CHAPTER 2

GENERAL METABOLISM

STEADY-STATE

The body can be considered in some respects as a set of open steady-state systems whose composition varies regularly and irregularly with such factors as meals, exercise, and circadian rhythms. The body has many compartments, principally plasma, interstitial fluid, the differing intracellular fluids, and the transcellular fluids such as lymph or intestinal contents. Each compartment has a different and slightly variable composition, and movement between the compartments is not necessarily free.

The gut is the main site of intake and is also a site of excretion, and this includes excretion via the bile, which is derived from the liver cells. The lungs are similarly sites of intake and of excretion. The kidneys are a site of excretion and to a certain extent of synthesis. The sweat glands are only a site of excretion. The plasma compartment exchanges its components directly with the blood cells, and through the interstitial fluid with body cells. Some material in the body cells is readily exchangeable, and some may be in storage form. Within the cells metabolic processes of synthesis and degradation take place. The generally constant compositions of the various compartments are maintained by balances between inward and outward flows (Fig. 2.1).

Compartmental analysis

Measurement of only the plasma concentration of a body component in a disease (a *static* observation) therefore gives a very limited view of the *dynamic* changes of disturbed rates of flow of the component under study between the body compartments, and of any alterations in the size of the compartmental pool. All of these, as well as the altered concentrations usually measured, are part of the chemical pathology of the disease. For example, a low plasma albumin concentration may be due to diminished formation of albumin, or to increased loss or destruction, or to haemodilution. Only in occasional instances, by complex research procedures, is it possible to measure the actual exchanges between the compartments, and their pool sizes. Measurement of actual secretion or production rate, usually of a hormone, is also usually difficult. An alternative approach which is often useful is to measure input (food) and output (urinary and/or faecal) of the component under study by a balance technique (p. 94). Measurement of the urinary excretion of a substance is often a guide

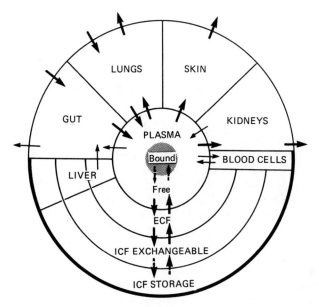

Fig. 2.1. A generalised picture of the exchanges between the exterior, the plasma, the extracellular fluid (ECF), and the intracellular fluid (ICF) that maintain the composition of the body compartments.

to the secretion or production rate of that substance or of its precursor. As long as inward and outward flow are equal, the plasma concentration of a component remains unchanged, unless there is also a change in plasma water volume, or metabolism of that component within the plasma compartment. The plasma concentration of a component in a sample analysed is the ratio, at a given instant, between its total content in the plasma compartment, and the total volume of the plasma compartment, assuming even distribution. This concentration will rise when the rate of entry of the component exceeds the rate of disposal, provided that there is no diminution of plasma water: the rise goes on until if possible a new steady state is set up in which inward and outward flow are again equal. The reverse arguments apply to a fall in concentration in plasma. For example, in non-progressive renal failure the increased plasma creatinine concentration will stabilise as, with the reduced clearance, there develops an excretion of creatinine once again equal to its production.

Cell assay. Analysis of particular cells, usually of skeletal muscle removed by biopsy, is done to obtain a view of the overall state of the intracellular compartment. This is a semi-research procedure but has been valuable particularly in elucidating disorders of water and electrolyte balance. The most obviously accessible cells, erythrocytes, are atypical. The most practical use of cell analysis is to demonstrate particular enzyme defects in inborn errors of metabolism, when fetal cells from amniotic fluid, or leucocytes, are the most useful.

Alterations of the steady state

One of the main subjects of study of chemical pathology is to determine how derangements of steady-state mechanisms can cause disorders of a biochemical nature. For example, in diabetes mellitus the effective primary derangement is lack of insulin activity, causing (amongst other abnormalities) continuing release of glucose from liver cells and failure of glucose to enter muscle cells. Because glucose continues to enter the plasma at a faster rate than it leaves, this disturbs the steady state primarily by increasing the concentration of plasma glucose. There results the secondary effect of increased filtration of glucose through the glomeruli, and so on. The steady state is disturbed also within the peripheral cells because of the decreased rate of formation of glucose-6-phosphate from lack of available intracellular glucose.

A similar pattern can occur even when the primary disturbance is not biochemical but anatomical. For example, the urinary loss of albumin is maintained in health at a very low value by a balance between glomerular filtration and tubular reabsorption. This normal albuminuria thus does not significantly affect the plasma albumin concentration, which is maintained by a balance between the rates of synthesis and degradation of albumin. In the nephrotic syndrome the increased glomerular filtration of albumin becomes much greater than the tubular reabsorptive capacity and there is massive albuminuria. This leads eventually to a fall in the plasma albumin because of the limited capacity to increase albumin synthesis. The plasma albumin would only remain unchanged, though with an increased turnover, if synthesis of albumin were increased in parallel with the increased loss.

In chronic disease a new steady state will be set up, with altered concentrations of the affected components in the different compartments, and often altered volumes of the compartments and of rates of transfer of the components between them. This can be considered as an application of Le Chatelier's principle to medicine. This steady state is not well maintained when there is the stress of an unphysiological load. In chronic non-progressive disorders this is handled more slowly and less efficiently then in normal subjects.

The disturbance of the biochemical steady state may be an effect of the disease, valuable for diagnosis or management but not part of the main metabolic disorder. For example, the normal level of activity of plasma aspartate transaminase, which is maintained by a balance between leakage from cells and disposal into the protein pool, is in chronic hepatitis set at a higher level because of increased leakage from the cells.

Disorders of transport

In many disturbances of the steady state there are alterations of active or passive transport across the cell membrane, and in the example of diabetes mellitus given above this is secondary to deficient insulin activity. There are many disorders where the disturbance is primarily that of the cellular transport mechanisms, and many of these primarily affect the main transport organs, namely the mucosa of the small intestine and the renal tubules.

Disorders of binding

Within a given compartment, apart from any exchange with other compartments, there is an internal steady-state mechanism for many components because of the existence of free and bound forms. A proportion of many components of the body is held in an inactive or storage form. In the plasma this is usually due to binding to proteins, which are specific for some hormones and for metals. The mechanism in the cells is not known, but is probably also of a protein nature. In plasma, where these factors are better understood, what is biologically significant is not the total concentration of a component but its free (unbound) or active concentration. The concentration or capacity of binding protein can be increased or decreased by disease or drugs, thus altering the amount of bound component. When this happens the total concentration of a component in the plasma changes in the same way, but the active fraction may remain unchanged. Free and bound forms for electrolytes are respectively in the ionised and non-ionised states: for hormones the mechanism is more complex. Some substances, especially drugs, may displace components from protein-binding, thus increasing the free fraction without change in the total concentration.

Feedback

One way in which the steady state is maintained is by *negative* feedback. A simple mechanism is when the concentration in the plasma or tissue compartment of a specific product (released from a body target cell) may be mainly controlled by a hormone through its influence on a metabolic process; and the secretion of that hormone be mainly controlled by the plasma concentration of the product (Fig. 2.2): this is applicable, for example, to the control of parathyroid hormone secretion by the plasma ionised calcium concentration (p. 175). Alternatively the concentration of this hormone, or its activity, will often itself be controlled by another hormone from the anterior pituitary gland. The secretion of this pituitary hormone will be controlled directly, or through a hypothalamic mechanism, by the concentration in plasma of the hormone, or other substance, which is the end-product of the various stimulant activities (p. 139). The steady-state mechanisms attempt to maintain the final product approximately constant, because any alteration in its concentration will

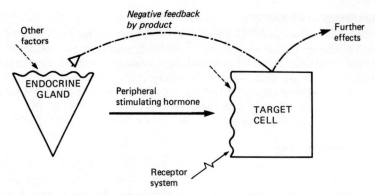

FIG. 2.2. Model of simple negative feedback system.

react back on the anterior pituitary or other hormonal stimulant. This in its turn regulates directly or indirectly the concentration of the final needed product. An abnormality at any stage of the process will disturb the steady state, and cause a biochemical abnormality – this is one of the fundamental disturbances of chemical pathology.

There can be a pathological vicious circle. A biochemical example may be found in gout. Hyperuricaemia can result in formation of uric acid calculi: these can damage renal function, which will further raise the plasma urate concentration.

Circadian rhythms

These are natural biological rhythms whose mean time is between 20 and 28 hours. They have very complex control mechanisms, and amongst the known factors causing circadian rhythms are light and dark, and social influences, including meals, sleep, rest and work – the causes have not been completely elucidated. Many of the circadian biochemical rhythms are mediated through a fundamental rhythm of adrenocorticotrophic hormone, which affects plasma cortisol, which itself affects many metabolic activities: this is largely driven by a central nervous system 'clock', though the pituitary and the adrenal cortex have endogenous rhythms. Various circadian rhythms throughout this book will be mentioned where relevant: the marked circadian variation of plasma cortisol, iron, and phosphate must be taken into account when collecting blood for their analysis. Failure of circadian rhythms can be an effect of a fundamental biochemical disturbance. As far as it is known such alterations do not in themselves cause disease.

INBORN ERRORS OF METABOLISM

A particular type of disturbance of the steady state occurs in the inborn errors of metabolism: important specific disorders are described under the appropriate system or organ elsewhere in this book. In these disorders the primary defect must be present from conception, though it may not manifest itself until adult life, as in gout (p. 97). A disorder may be dependent for its clinical manifestation on external factors, and these can be natural, as in galactosaemia (p. 73) or artificial, as in suxamethonium paralysis (p. 121). The disturbance caused by an inborn error of metabolism may be completely harmless, as in pentosuria (p. 74).

The course of many biochemical reactions can be expressed simply as:

$$A \rightsquigarrow A \xrightarrow{\nearrow X} B \longrightarrow C \longrightarrow D$$

Defects of a transport system

The reaction $A \rightsquigarrow A$ is transport across a membrane, believed to be mediated by a carrier protein system known as a 'permease'. One type of inborn error of metabolism occurs when the transport reaction $A \rightsquigarrow A$, in intestinal mucosa or renal tubules, is deficient as a genetic defect as in cystinuria (p. 225) – the deficiency of the common carrier system in the renal tubules for reabsorption of the basic amino acids cystine, ornithine, arginine and lysine, leads to their excretion in excess and the formation of cystine calculi.

Defects of a metabolic enzyme

The reactions $A \rightarrow B$, $B \rightarrow C$, $(B \rightarrow X)$, and $C \rightarrow D$ and so on, are controlled by specific enzymes. The concentration or the rate of formation of product D can control the rate of the earlier reaction $A \rightarrow B$ by a feedback mechanism.

A second major type of inborn error of metabolism develops if there is alteration in the gene which controls the formation of the enzyme which mediates the rate-limiting reaction $B \rightarrow C$ ('B:Case') and produces a variant or reduces the activity of that enzyme. This may manifest in a number of different ways:

Diminished rate of formation of product. This may be the immediate product, C, as in von Gierke's disease (p. 66) – the deficiency of glucose-6-phosphatase leads to diminished formation of glucose from glucose-6-phosphate. It may be a product at a remove, D, as in the adrenogenital syndrome (p. 157) the deficiency of 21-hydroxylase leads to diminished formation of cortisol which is the end-product of the synthetic sequence.

Diminished rate of removal of substrate. This may be the immediate substrate, B, as in alkaptonuria (p. 102) – the deficiency of homogentisic acid oxidase leads to retention (and urinary excretion) of homogentisic acid. It may be a substrate at a remove, A, as in von Gierke's disease

p. 66) – the deficiency of glucose-6-phosphatase leads to retention of glycogen which is the origin of the catabolic sequence. A common additional effect may be increased formation of by-product X, as in phenylketonuria (p. 101) – the deficiency of phenylalanine hydroxylase leads to retention of phenylalanine, which is converted in excess to phenylpyruvic acid and phenyllactic acid, both being excreted in the urine.

Altered feedback. An example is in the adrenogenital syndrome (p. 157) – the deficiency of 21-hydroxylase causes diminished formation of cortisol, which leads to increased secretion of adrenocorticotrophic hormone; this stimulates the earlier stages of the steroid synthetic pathway and excess androgens are produced.

Diagnosis of inborn errors of metabolism

It may be necessary to diagnose a homozygous case, or a heterozygote or carrier. The appropriate analysis to be used will depend on many factors, including the solubility of the relevant compounds (do they pass from cells to plasma to urine?) and the metabolic activities of other enzymes in the chain. Using the above convention, one may look for more A, B, or X, or for less C or D, or for less enzyme B:Case. Analysis may be on plasma, or urine, or blood cells, or organ biopsy; or prenatally by enzyme analysis on a culture of skin fibroblasts obtained by amniocentesis (p. 165).

Other inherited diseases

Other alterations of genes can cause altered production of proteins that are not transport or metabolic enzymes. These genetic disorders are by convention not included in inborn errors of metabolism. They include the haemoglobinopathies (p. 129), or defects of structural proteins such as muscular dystrophy (p. 121), or disorders of clotting such as haemophilia.

Further reading

Baron DN, Levin GE. Intracellular chemical pathology. In: Alberti KGMM, ed *Recent Advances in Clinical Biochemistry, 1*. Edinburgh: Churchill-Livingstone, 1977:153–174.

Harris H. *The Principles of Human Biochemical Genetics*. 2nd ed. Amsterdam: North Holland, 1975.

Riggs DS. *The Mathematical Approach to Physiological Problems*. Baltimore: Williams and Wilkins, 1963.

CHAPTER 3

WATER AND ELECTROLYTES

NORMAL DISTRIBUTION

Water makes up 50–60 per cent of the body of a healthy adult, to a total of about 45 litres in the average 70 kg man. Of this, 25–30 litres (30–40 per cent) is intracellular fluid (i.c.f.), and 13–16 litres (15–20 per cent) is extracellular fluid (e.c.f.) of which plasma takes up 3–3.5 litres (Fig. 3.1). About 1.5 litres is lymph, and another 1.5 litres is transcellular fluid – a term used to include alimentary secretions, cerebrospinal fluid, pleural and peritoneal fluid, aqueous humour, and synovial fluid. A sub-compartment of interstitial fluid, with a volume of about 4 litres, is the slowly exchanging fluid of connective tissue and bone. Solids comprise 40–50 per cent of the body. About a third of the solid is fat, but this is very variable; this adipose tissue contains less than 10 per cent of water and takes little part in exchange of water.

In infants a smaller proportion of the body is intracellular water. About 25 per cent of the mass of an infant is solid, 30 per cent i.c.f., and 45 per cent e.c.f.

Methods of measurement

No procedures for measuring the volume of the various body compartments in health or disease are entirely satisfactory, and many give conflicting results. The most accurate measure of total body water uses the distribution space of tritiated water, and for clinical purposes antipyrine is often used as it can be estimated chemically. The e.c.f. volume is usually measured as the distribution space of inulin, and of the many isotopic procedures the use of $^{82}Br^-$ gives most consistent (though slightly higher) results. The sodium space is larger than the true e.c.f. space because of diffusion of sodium into cells.

The plasma volume is measured by using a marker that is bound to albumin and does not diffuse into the tissue fluid, for example ^{125}I-labelled albumin. Alternatively, the total circulating erythrocyte volume can be measured by using isotopically labelled erythrocytes (^{32}P or ^{51}Cr). The total blood volume should be measured as the sum of the volumes (total plasma + erythrocyte); calculations employing haematocrit values are unsatisfactory because this varies in different parts of the circulation.

The i.c.f. volume is measured as the difference between the total body water and the e.c.f. volume. Isotopic methods can also be used to

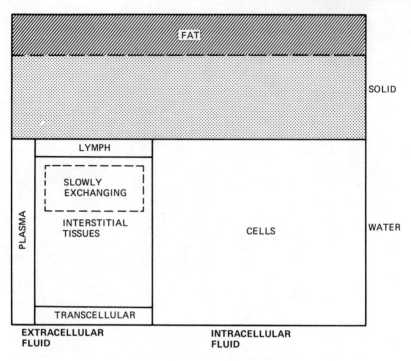

FIG. 3.1. Proportional distribution of solids and water in a healthy adult.

measure whole-body potassium, which gives an assessment of the mass of metabolising cells.

The total solute content of the body fluids (particularly plasma or urine) is best measured as the osmolality (per unit mass of solvent: osmolarity is per unit volume of solution), normally about 275–295 mmol/kg in plasma, of which about 50 per cent is due to sodium ions. Osmometers usually depend on depression of freezing point as the measure of solute content, there being a slight reduction of osmotic effect due to association of ions. Sodium and potassium concentrations are easily measured by flame photometry, and methods are available for assessing sodium and potassium ion *activity*, using special glass electrodes, in the same way as hydrogen-ion *activity* is measured: in plasma about 1 mmol/l of sodium, and 0.1 mmol/l of potassium, are protein-bound, and not ionically active. Chloride is measured chemically or electrometrically, and a special electrode is available. Changes in plasma water can be measured indirectly by considering either the haemoglobin or the total protein concentration – unless these components are themselves primarily altered by the disease: the packed cell volume is not a

reliable measure because of changes in the shape and volume of erythrocytes when the concentration of water in plasma is altered.

The contents of the body spaces

The e.c.f. cannot be considered to be a uniform compartment: water in
dense tissue, such as bone, is not readily available for exchange. The
boundary between the i.c.f. and the e.c.f. is normally permeable to water
and small organic molecules, selectively permeable to ions (active cell
metabolism maintains the sodium pump), and to a very limited degree
permeable to protein. The boundary between interstitial fluid and plasma
is freely permeable to water and ions, but only to a small extent to
protein or lipid. The protein content of interstitial fluid, a plasma
ultrafiltrate, is low (less than 200 mg/l) despite the high protein content
of plasma and of cells.

The movement of water is controlled by osmotic pressure, which is
normally about equal in all the body spaces, though most cells are
probably slightly hypertonic. Water moves freely from one compartment
to another to adjust any temporary imbalance of osmotic pressure. For
example, if hypertonic saline were ingested or infused, the e.c.f. would
become temporarily hypertonic; water then moves from the i.c.f. to the
e.c.f. to lower the osmotic pressure in the plasma and tissue fluid. There is
a dynamic not a static equilibrium; movement of water and of ions is
continuous, and this maintains osmotic and electrolyte equilibrium.

The water content of plasma is about 93 per cent and of most cells is
about 70 per cent. In plasma the dominant cation is sodium, and the
dominant anion is chloride. In cells the dominant cation is potassium
and there is little sodium or chloride: the dominant anions are protein,
organic acids, and organic phosphate. Because of the Gibbs-Donnan
equilibrium, diffusible cations are at higher concentration in plasma
water than in interstitial fluid, whilst the opposite is true for diffusible
anions (Fig. 3.2).

To measure body electrolytes plasma (or serum) is normally used
because it is easily available. Such assays measure only e.c.f. concentrations; assay of cell constituents, by using muscle biopsy or leucocytes, is difficult, and the easily available erythrocytes are atypical.
Some ions in cells are bound or polyvalent, therefore intracellular
osmotic pressure cannot be calculated from simple addition of ionic
concentrations.

Units of measurement

It is generally recognised that to express ions according to their mass/
volume concentration does not give a true picture of their activities,
which are proportional to the number of ions present. For convenience
in considering the ionic and osmotic relationships in the body fluids, the
concentrations of the important ionic components of the body fluids are

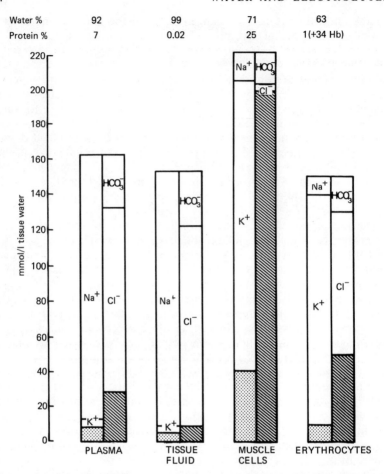

FIG. 3.2. Comparative composition of extracellular fluids and intracellular fluids, expressed as concentration of ion charges, and ignoring binding of ions. The shaded areas represent other cations (e.g. Ca^{2+}) and other anions (e.g. HPO_4^{2-}).

expressed in units which are proportional to their ionic concentrations (molarity, per unit volume of solution) and are according to the principles of the Système International d'Unités: this concept has now been extended to non-ionic substances (Appendix II). The subunit of most convenient size for clinical biochemistry is the millimole (mmol): this gives values numerically identical to those with the formerly familiar milli-equivalent (mEq) for monovalent ions.

The familiar *Gamble* diagrams can still be used if the components are expressed in terms of electrovalency, as the concentration of ion charges (Figs. 3.2, 3.3, 4.1).

Water balance

In a healthy subject water intake is equal to water output, and any minor short-term discrepancies are balanced by an alteration in the volume of the intracellular pool.

Intake		Water Pool		Output	
Moist food		Plasma	3 000 ml	Lungs	500 ml
and drink	2000 ml	Tissue fluid	12 000 ml	Insensible skin	400 ml
Water from		Cell fluid	30 000 ml	Urine	1300 ml
oxidation and dry				Faeces	200 ml
food	500 ml			Sweat	100 ml
	2500 ml		45 000 ml		2500 ml

This table shows an approximate typical daily water balance of a healthy 70 kg adult. The volume of urine which is required for excretion of waste products is at least 500 ml/24 h, and if to this minimal urine output is added the insensible fluid loss through the lungs and the skin, the daily obligatory water loss of a normal active adult in a temperate climate is seen to be 1500 ml – which is about 2 per cent of the body weight: the insensible loss is less from a patient at rest in bed. An adult patient who is completely deprived of fluid may lose, therefore, up to 2 per cent of his body weight per day. If there is no additional loss of fluid, the daily fluid intake, to prevent any risk of water depletion, should be 2000–2500 ml.

If the concentrating power of the kidneys is diminished through disease, or if the renal load of metabolic waste products is increased, then the minimum volume of urine which is required for excretion of the waste products will be higher. For example, if the urine cannot be concentrated to an osmolality greater than 750 mmol/kg then the obligatory minimal urinary output becomes about 1000 ml.

In hot climates or when there is severe fever considerable water loss can occur as sweat: even minimal obvious sweating may lose 1000 ml per day. In health the endogenous gastrointestinal tract water turnover is about 8000 ml/24 h – 1500 ml saliva, 2500 ml gastric juice, 500 ml bile, 500 ml pancreatic juice, 3000 ml intestinal secretions. In any disorder of the gut in which fluid is lost to the exterior enormous water losses can also occur.

Paediatric problems. Infants develop water deprivation more easily than do adults. An infant utilises about three times as much water per unit weight, has a relatively greater energy production, and a relatively larger surface area. This leads to relatively greater losses of fluid through the skin and lungs, and to a relatively greater load of metabolic waste products for the kidneys. The kidney of an infant has less concentrating power than that of an adult; the adult kidney needs less than a litre of water to excrete

1000 mmol of solid, whereas the infant kidney needs at least 2 litres for this purpose. The daily turnover of fluid in an infant is about one-half of its e.c.f. volume, compared to one-fifth in an adult. As a result of these factors an infant deprived of fluid may lose 4 per cent of its body weight per day.

Sodium (and chloride) balance

In a healthy subject sodium and chloride intake equals sodium and chloride output, and any minor discrepancies are balanced by an alteration of the sodium and chloride concentrations in the e.c.f. The reference values for plasma sodium concentration are 136–148 mmol/l, and for plasma chloride concentration are 95–105 mmol/l. The normal muscle cell sodium is about 10 mmol/kg wet weight (15 mmol/l cell water), and muscle chloride is about 3 mmol/kg wet weight (5 mmol/l cell water).

The table below shows an approximate typical daily sodium balance of a healthy adult in a temperate climate. Ample sodium is normally taken: if there are no extra losses, then an adequate intake of sodium, to prevent depletion, is probably about 20 mmol (i.e. about 1 g of sodium chloride). In health the endogenous gastrointestinal tract sodium turnover is about 1500 mmol. However, considerable losses can occur in disease; 200 mmol may be lost in the sweat in tropical fever, and more than 500 mmol in severe diarrhoea and vomiting.

When constructing sodium balance in patients, drugs given as salts must not be forgotten: for example, 20 g of Carbenicillin contains 94 mmol of sodium.

Intake		Sodium Pool		Output	
Food, drink and seasoning (10 g as sodium chloride)	170 mmol	Exchangeable Plasma	450 mmol	Insensible loss Urine Faeces	Nil 150 mmol 5 mmol
		Tissue fluid	1600 mmol	Sweat and Skin	10 mmol
		Rest of body soft tissue bone	330 mmol 500 mmol		
		Non-exchangeable Bone	1000 mmol		
	≃170 mmol		≃4000 mmol		≃170 mmol

Although it is customary to speak of salt deficiency and salt replacement, it is the sodium that is osmotically important. The body fluids do not however contain equal proportions of sodium and chloride, for example gastric juice contains much less sodium than chloride. Average anion and cation concentrations (compared to plasma) in those body

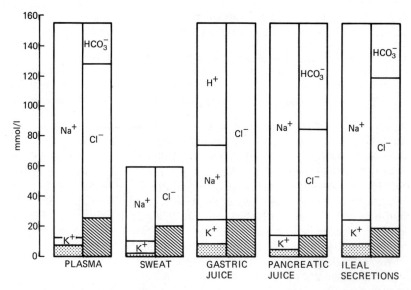

FIG. 3.3. Comparative electrolyte composition (expressed as ion charges, millimoles per litre of fluid) of plasma, and of body secretions that may be lost in disease.

fluids which may be lost in disease are shown in Fig. 3.3. The salt content of sweat may vary considerably, and falls on adaptation to a hot climate.

Because of their variable sodium/chloride content, losses of body fluid may result in disturbances of acid-base balance as well as causing water- or salt-depletion. The healthy kidney, by its power to excrete sodium and chloride differentially, can usually redress the imbalance when adequate saline treatment is given. The deficient ion is retained, the unwanted ion is excreted.

'DEHYDRATION' – WATER AND SODIUM DEPLETION

Clinical syndromes due to loss of water or sodium are common. The word 'dehydration' is commonly applied to all forms of water and sodium loss, but the word means loss of water and should not be used to describe conditions in which redistribution and loss of body water is secondary to loss of sodium. It is advisable to consider water depletion and sodium depletion separately as their causes, metabolic effects, and clinical courses are different, and appropriate replacement therapy depends on correct appreciation of the initial deficiencies and on experienced judgement of the patient's responses. Pure water depletion or pure sodium depletion are rare, but combined depletion usually favours one or the other component. It must be remembered that changes in the general body store of water or ions do not necessarily take place in the same direction as do changes in the plasma concentrations.

Water depletion

Causes

The syndrome of water depletion develops when fluid intake is insufficient due to neglect or unavailability, and there is continuing loss of water or of fluid of low sodium concentration. Water depletion may be seen post-operatively, when oral fluid intake has ceased because of surgical necessity, or because the patient is unconscious, or has severe dysphagia, or is old and feeble. Post-operatively, after the immediate oliguria and sodium retention of the first few days, there is a water and sodium diuresis and any tendency to water depletion is increased. Water depletion of renal origin may develop in primary or nephrogenic diabetes insipidus, in chronic nephritis and pyelonephritis, or in the diuretic phase of acute renal failure unless water intake is increased to match the water output. Excess water can be lost in sweat, or through hyperventilation as at high altitudes before acclimatisation. After brain injury, there may be a combination of hyperthermic sweating and diabetes insipidus.

When intake of water ceases the insensible fluid loss from lungs and skin, and obligatory secretion of urine, continues.

Metabolic aspects

In water depletion the concentrations of sodium and chloride in the e.c.f., and the osmotic pressure of the e.c.f., gradually rise. This promotes release of antidiuretic hormone. The plasma sodium may exceed 160 mmol/l. A rise in the plasma urea is late, and retention of nitrogenous waste products develops when the urine flow falls below about 30 ml/h. Effects tend to be more severe in infants and in old people, because of poor renal compensating capacity, and in infants also because of relatively smaller fluid reserves.

The primary loss of water from the e.c.f. (to urine, skin, and lungs) is replaced from the i.c.f., to maintain as far as possible the osmotic pressure of the plasma and tissue fluid. The concentrations of the ions in the plasma rise because there is a lag in water-electrolyte adjustment. The osmotic pressure of the i.c.f. rises. As replacement of the e.c.f. is not complete there is a fall in the plasma volume, and slowly progressive haemoconcentration and circulatory changes.

The diagram (Fig. 3.4) shows the state of the body fluid compartments in water depletion.

Clinical aspects

Symptoms begin to appear when about 2 litres of water has been lost. The main symptoms are apathy, thirst, and dryness of the mouth and tongue: there is a slight loss of skin turgor. The patient complains of general weakness and there is an oliguria with urine of high osmolality (and specific gravity). If renal function is unimpaired a daily urine

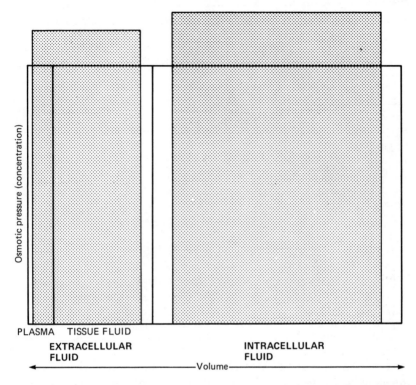

PLASMA   TISSUE FLUID

EXTRACELLULAR   **INTRACELLULAR**
FLUID   **FLUID**

←————————————————Volume————————————————→

Osmotic pressure (concentration)

FIG. 3.4. Changes in body fluid compartments due to water depletion, indicated by the shaded areas. The horizontal axis shows changes in volume, and the vertical axis shows changes in osmotic pressure (or concentration of solutes).

volume of less than 750 ml means that a patient has water depletion; a severely dehydrated patient may excrete in a day only 500 ml of urine at an osmolality of more than 1200 mmol/kg (specific gravity 1.040). Measurement of the fall in body weight is an important method of detecting the extent of loss of water. Death after coma, possibly due to a rise in intracellular osmotic pressure, occurs when about 15 per cent of the body weight has been lost: in adults this happens after about 10 days without water, and in infants after less than 7 days.

Therapy
The treatment of choice is water orally until the daily urine volume exceeds 1500 ml. Thirst is not necessarily a reliable index of water depletion. If the oral route is not possible or insufficient, water must be given intravenously, and 5.0 per cent w/v glucose (50 g/l, 280 mmol/l) is acceptably isotonic. Most pharmaceutical companies still label glucose

for intravenous use as 'dextrose': this can be confusing. The rectal route is a last choice because of its relatively limited absorptive capacity. Oral salt or intravenous saline must not be given unless there is also sodium depletion; any addition to the extracellular sodium will withdraw more water from the cells.

Sodium depletion

Causes

The syndrome of sodium depletion develops when there is a greatly diminished intake of sodium with normal water intake, or when there is general loss of both water and sodium which is replaced only by water. A low plasma sodium concentration may be due to sodium depletion or to haemodilution (p. 34). Pseudohyponatraemia, with normal plasma osmolality and normal sodium concentration in plasma *water*, is due to excess protein (p. 112) or lipid (p. 81) lowering the relative amount of water in the total plasma volume.

Loss of sodium-containing fluid results from burns, severe exudative skin lesions, or through massive sweating; 'heat exhaustion' is due to sodium loss in sweat. Large amounts of sodium and water can be lost in alimentary secretions, through fistulae, vomiting and diarrhoea (especially in cholera), steatorrhoea, and intestinal aspiration or high intestinal obstruction.

Many diuretics lead to excessive urinary sodium loss, as do Addison's disease, 'salt-losing' chronic nephritis, and diabetic ketoacidosis. In these conditions the urinary sodium exceeds the intake. A mild sodium depletion may develop when sodium intake is greatly diminished, and this can happen without excessive sodium loss in prolonged starvation, e.g., due to anorexia nervosa, and is seen in chronic alcoholism. Before an operation many patients are sodium deficient from a combination of these causes. In these conditions the urinary sodium is less than 10 mmol/l.

Sodium depletion, with or without oedema, generally causes secondary aldosteronism (p. 158) by activating the renin-angiotensin mechanism.

The *sick-cell syndrome* is part of many severe chronic illnesses, and is due to failure of the sodium pump. Sodium passes into the cells (which lose potassium) and the plasma sodium concentration falls, but the total body sodium is unaltered.

Considerable amounts of sodium may be lost from the general e.c.f. into the gut in paralytic ileus, into oedema, into interstitial fluid in an injured limb, or into pleural or ascitic fluid; these pools take only a limited part in the general ionic exchanges of the e.c.f. However, until this is withdrawn from the body by, for example, paracentesis, the whole body sodium will be high although water retention may lead to hyponatraemia.

Metabolic aspects

When sodium is lost from the body the e.c.f. becomes hypotonic. Water leaves the e.c.f. in an attempt to restore the plasma osmotic pressure. Rather more water is lost from the tissue fluid than from the plasma as the osmotic action of the proteins tends to hold water in the plasma. The e.c.f. volume change is therefore greater than that calculated from the change in plasma sodium, and the urine volume does not fall in the early stages. Some water passes into the i.c.f. The sodium in the bones forms a reserve which can be drawn on to maintain the osmotic pressure of the e.c.f. The kidneys can combat sodium deficiency by increasing tubular reabsorption, via aldosterone stimulation, more efficiently than they combat water deficiency.

The simple Fantus test for urinary chloride concentration has no place in clinical practice to assess chloride (and therefore sodium) deficiency unless, as in many parts of the world, facilities for flame photometry are not available.

The concentrations of sodium and chloride in the plasma are normal in the early stages of sodium depletion, and fall when depletion is severe: the loss of water from the e.c.f. leads to an early fall in the plasma volume and to haemoconcentration with high plasma proteins. The altered

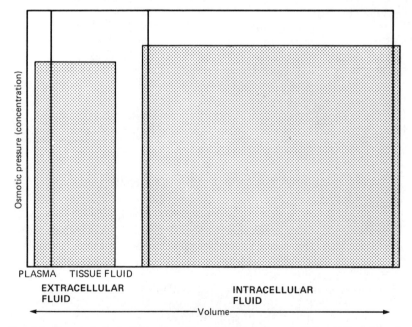

FIG. 3.5. Changes in body fluid compartments due to sodium depletion, indicated by the shaded areas. The horizontal axis shows changes in volume, and the vertical axis shows changes in osmotic pressure (or concentration of solutes).

circulation and the increased viscosity of the blood cause a fall in the renal plasma flow and glomerular filtration rate, secondary renal damage, and a fall in the urine volume. Once the kidney is affected homoeostatic control is lost. There is an early rise of plasma urea. The diagram (Fig. 3.5) shows the state of the body fluid compartments in sodium depletion.

Clinical aspects

Symptoms begin to appear when the patient has lost the sodium equivalent of 4 litres of isotonic (physiological) saline. The patient has vasoconstrictive shock. There is usually nausea, vomiting, cramps, and intestinal dilatation; and the latter often lead to further effective loss of sodium. The loss of extracellular water is manifest as visible 'dehydration': the patient may not be especially thirsty. The cause of death is circulatory failure.

Therapy

The treatment of choice is saline intravenously. For the usual post-operative salt-depleted patient, isotonic saline (155 mmol/l: 9 g/l, 0.9 per cent w/v) is suitable, and if there is severe sodium depletion with water excess, two or three times isotonic saline (e.g. 300 mmol/l:1.8 per cent w/v) may be used. Labelling as 'per cent', instead of as g/l, is still done on infusion fluids by many pharmaceutical companies. Also it is incorrect, and may be dangerous, to call this concentration of saline: Normal. The term Normal is used *chemically* for solutions of 1 equivalent per litre, i.e. for NaCl of 5.85 per cent w/v.

If large volumes of saline have to be given it may be advisable to add potassium chloride and sodium bicarbonate to the infusion to counteract the saline-engendered hyperchloraemic metabolic acidosis and hypokalaemia, because isotonic saline, when compared to plasma, contains excess chloride and is acid.

Combined water and sodium depletion

A combined depletion is the commonest clinical abnormality of water and sodium distribution. It results from loss of both water and sodium when there is an inadequate fluid intake. Water and sodium depletion is also seen when e.c.f. is removed from the general circulation in pools of fluid without being lost from the body, for example, in ascites, gross oedema, or paralytic ileus.

In combined depletion there is a combination of the thirst oliguria and lethargy of water loss (i.c.f. loss), with the circulatory symptoms and desiccation of sodium loss (e.c.f. loss). Plasma electrolyte values may be normal.

Therapy

Treatment must be based on the presenting disturbance and previous losses of the patient, and (as in all these disorders) a well-kept fluid balance chart is essential, and is the easiest method of assessing the patient's needs. If for a few days after an operation an adult patient requires fluid intravenously because he cannot take fluid by mouth, and if there is no renal functional impairment or additional loss of secretions, then combining 500 ml of isotonic saline solution and 2000 ml of isotonic glucose solution provide a suitable daily infusion. Unless oral feeding can begin within a few days, potassium should also be given intravenously as 50 mmol of potassium chloride included in the above infusion. In the first 24 hours following operation no potassium, and not more than 2000 ml of total fluid per day, should generally be given because of the oliguria. If intestinal secretions have been lost they should if possible be collected, analysed, filtered, and replaced: valuable enzymes and bile contents will not then be wasted. Two to three days (but no more) without energy from food or intravenous nutriment can be easily tolerated. Daily weighing of the patient helps assessment.

Oral glucose (or perhaps sucrose) and electrolytes may often be used together in water for the treatment of severe fluid loss in diarrhoea. This simpler procedure is important for infants in the tropics.

In the water and sodium depletion syndromes the total volume of the body fluids is decreased. The opposite occasionally occurs usually because of therapeutic mishandling. Primary water excess or sodium excess (or a mixed syndrome) causes an increase in the total volume of the body fluids.

Water excess

Causes

Water excess, usually called water intoxication, develops when the urine volume is low, especially if a patient is given large volumes of a salt-poor fluid and above all in chronic renal failure. Water intoxication does not result if renal function is normal. Retention of water is particularly likely to take place within 24 hours of a major trauma or operation, probably due to inappropriate over-secretion of antidiuretic hormone which implies continuing secretion of ADH with a low plasma sodium. Other causes of inappropriate ADH secretion (p. 169) causing water retention are carcinoma of the bronchus, encephalitis, and head injury; and sometimes lung infections, intracranial haemorrhage, and many drugs. Water intoxication may be produced if sodium depletion is misdiagnosed as water depletion and treated with water (e.g. as intravenous glucose), or in gross polydipsia, or from irrigation during prostatic resection.

Metabolic and clinical aspects

Dilution of i.c.f. and also e.c.f. develops, with reduced osmolality but there is no oedema (body sodium content is normal), and the plasma concentrations of sodium (sometimes less than 100 mmol/l) and chloride fall: the plasma urea and protein concentrations are low. The symptoms, less severe and later than in sodium deficiency, may be headache, anorexia, lethargy and bradycardia, and eventual convulsions and delirium, probably due to overhydration of brain cells.

Therapy

The treatment of excess water intake is to stop it and to give intravenous hypertonic (e.g. 850 mmol/l: 5 per cent w/v) saline. Water loss, as sweat (which is hypotonic), may be encouraged by hot cradles. Water excess due to ADH excess must not be treated by isotonic saline (as the sodium will be excreted) but by treating the primary cause, by moderate water deprivation or by drugs that inhibit ADH activity; severe hyponatraemia may require hypertonic saline.

Sodium excess

Causes

Sodium excess, often called sodium or salt intoxication, develops when there is excessive intake or deficient excretion of sodium. It is difficult to cause sodium intoxication by the excessive oral intake of sodium (e.g., drinking sea-water) as saline taken by mouth in large quantities will be vomited. However, high solute artificial milk is a danger in infants. Excess intravenous saline may, however, easily cause sodium overload, and this happens when water depletion is treated by saline.

Excess adrenocortical hormones, whether iatrogenic or in Conn's syndrome or Cushing's syndrome, may cause marked sodium (and therefore water) retention. Sodium retention, partly due to over-secretion of adrenocortical hormones, is particularly likely to develop in the few days following a major operation. Hypernatraemia may occur when there is head injury or intracranial lesions in association with water depletion due to diabetes insipidus (p. 169). In severe heart failure, partly because of secondary renal impairment, there may be retention of sodium and water, and a high plasma and e.c.f. volume. Sodium and water retention, often with secondary aldosteronism, are always more likely to be found in patients with heart failure, renal failure, or hypo-proteinaemia: during the development of ascites or in hypertensive renal failure the e.c.f. is retaining even more water than sodium, so there is hyponatraemia with increased total body sodium.

Metabolic aspects

The typical picture of sodium excess is found during over-infusion with saline. The maximum possible sodium concentration in urine even in a healthy adult is about 350 mmol/l; when the sodium intake exceeds the possible rate of excretion, sodium intoxication will develop. There is an increase in the e.c.f. volume, so the rise in plasma sodium and chloride concentrations is small. There may be a metabolic acidosis. Water passes from the i.c.f. to the e.c.f. in an attempt to maintain the plasma osmotic pressure.

Clinical aspects

There is a raised central venous pressure, peripheral oedema (which indicates a high body sodium and becomes apparent when the volume of the e.c.f. has increased by more than 10 per cent), and pulmonary oedema with eventual respiratory failure.

In the less usual picture of sodium retention without water retention, oedema is less common, and cerebral symptoms are associated with hyperosmolality of the plasma.

Therapy

The treatment is to stop the intake of salt, but the intake of water should not be reduced as this would throw an additional load on to the kidneys.

Oedema

As well as being a result of sodium retention, oedema may be caused by lowering of the plasma osmotic pressure due to hypoproteinaemia (p. 107), or by non-biochemical disturbances such as capillary damage. The oedema of heart failure is due to increased venous pressure and to sodium retention.

Summary

In the diagnosis of these disorders of sodium and water balance, estimations of the concentrations in the plasma of the various ions, or the plasma osmolality, indicate the concentrations or the osmotic pressure only in the e.c.f. Plasma water changes are estimated by the haemoglobin and total protein concentration. The changes in the distribution of sodium and water can usually be assessed from this information, from knowledge of the changes in body weight, and of fluid and electrolyte intake and output – although sweat volume is difficult to assess. Treatment must be based on knowledge both of concentrations (usually by daily or even twice-daily analyses) and of body contents. The table below gives a summary of the important changes in the body fluids in these disorders.

	Water Depletion	Sodium Depletion	Water Excess	Sodium Excess
Total body fluid volume	Decreased	Decreased	Increased	Increased
Osmotic pressure of e.c.f.	Increased	Decreased	Decreased	Increased

POTASSIUM

Potassium is the principal cation in the cells, and it is present in a relatively low concentration in the e.c.f. The reference interval for plasma potassium concentration is 3.8–5.0 mmol/l: the plasma must be removed from the cells within three hours of venepuncture, and serum values are about 0.4 mmol/l higher due to release of potassium from the clot. The potassium concentration in the erythrocyte is about 85 mmol/kg wet weight (160 mmol/l cell water). Potassium is freely filtered by the glomeruli and largely reabsorbed in the proximal tubules: urinary potassium is derived from distal tubular secretion under the influence of mineralocorticoids (p. 154), and linked with sodium transport. Renal mechanisms are more competent in excreting excess potassium than in conserving diminished potassium.

Potassium moves from the e.c.f. into the i.c.f. when either protein is being deposited or glucose is being taken in and metabolised; or during extracellular alkalosis. Potassium moves from the i.c.f. into the e.c.f., and can then be lost from the body into the urine, when body protein is being catabolised in starvation or after stress or trauma (about 2.5 mmol potassium per gram protein), in severe illness ('sick-cell syndrome'), during exercise, after loss of water sodium and chloride from the body, or during acidosis.

The body contains about 3500 mmol (150 g) of exchangeable potassium and about another 1000 mmol of slowly exchangable potassium. The average intake in an adult is about 100 mmol (4 g) per 24 hours, of which at least 80 per cent is excreted in the urine and less than 20 per cent in the faeces. Up to 10 mmol may be lost in shed skin and sweat. If there are no additional losses of potassium the daily potassium intake to prevent potassium depletion should be about 30 mmol (1.2 g): about 20 mmol/24 h is lost in urine even if there is no intake. In disease potassium may be lost in any body secretion, most of which contain potassium in higher concentration than in the plasma (Fig. 3.3). Intake of salts in drugs must not be forgotten: for example, 20 g of Penicillin G contains 52 mmol of potassium.

Assessment of abnormalities

It is important to realise that changes in the body store of potassium do not always take place in the same direction as changes in the plasma concentration of potassium. So by measuring the plasma potassium only a limited view is obtained of the changes in the total body potassium. In general a 1 mmol/l change in the plasma potassium implies a 200 mmol change in body potassium. In practice the clinical degree of abnormality of potassium balance is usually reflected fairly adequately by the plasma potassium concentration and measurement of cell potassium is not readily practicable: important exceptions such as diabetic coma are considered below. Neuro-muscular conduction and the electrocardiographic changes which are characteristic of abnormal plasma potassium levels possibly depend on the e.c.f./i.c.f. potassium gradient and not on the plasma concentration of potassium. These may be abnormal, with a normal plasma potassium level, when the cell potassium concentration is altered.

Hyperkalaemia and potassium retention

Causes

In clinical practice hyperkalaemia is not as common as hypokalaemia. A high plasma potassium level may occur when there is excessive intake, diminished excretion, or shift of potassium from the cells to the e.c.f., and is accentuated by acidosis when hydrogen ions displace potassium ions from the cells. An extracellular acidosis and intracellular alkalosis will be promoted. Because of the high potassium of cells, extravascular haemolysis or breakdown of leukaemic leucocytes (especially during treatment) will produce a falsely high plasma potassium.

Hyperkalaemia due to excessive intake may develop during treatment of hypokalaemia, especially if large doses of potassium are given intravenously when renal function is impaired: also the potassium content of the plasma of stored blood which is used for transfusion may be much higher than that of normal plasma, increasing by 1 mmol/l per day of storage. In severe renal failure, due to disease of the glomeruli or to a diminished renal plasma flow, potassium is retained, and the rise in the plasma potassium concentration can be correlated with the fall in the glomerular filtration rate – symptoms which are attributed to hyperkalaemia are part of the uraemia symptom complex. In adrenocortical deficiency, particularly in Addisonian crisis, and rarely in hypopituitarism, there may be hyperkalaemia, and this hyperkalaemia is due to alteration of renal tubular function by deficient mineralocorticoid activity: potassium-retaining diuretics such as spironolactone (an aldosterone antagonist) may have a similar effect. Potassium is released from cells when there is increased cellular catabolism such as after crush injury, burns, or in the early post-operative phase; or whenever much sodium is lost from the e.c.f. There may be then a raised plasma potassium level – but urinary excretion eliminates most of the cellular potassium and the body as a whole is potassium-deficient.

Metabolic and clinical aspects

The chief toxic effect of hyperkalaemia is on neuromuscular conduction, especially in the heart, and signs develop at a plasma potassium level of about 7.5 mmol/l. Bradycardia develops with distinctive electrocardiographic changes of an absent P wave, broad QRS complex, and particularly high T waves. At high plasma levels (9 mmol/l), a-v block and cardiac arrest can develop.

Therapy

Treatment is required in all severe cases. The cause of the hyper-kalaemia can often be remedied by stopping the excessive intake, or by correcting the acidosis and any water and salt depletion. Reversal of toxic effects on the heart may require intravenous calcium. Hyper-kalaemia of renal origin is difficult to treat. Insulin (with glucose) may be given to transfer potassium to the cells. Potassium may be withdrawn from the e.c.f. into the gut and thence excreted by the use of a suitable ion-exchange resin that binds potassium. Peritoneal dialysis and haemo-dialysis will correct hyperkalaemia as well as the other abnormalities of uraemia.

Hypokalaemia and potassium deficiency

Causes

Hypokalaemia, which is commonly seen, is usually associated with general cellular deficiency of potassium.

All foods that contain cells contain potassium, and deprivation of food, with inadequate intravenous replacement, is an additional reason for the potassium deficiency that may develop in a severe illness or after an operation. Protein malnutrition such as kwashiorkor leads to severe potassium depletion though hypokalaemia may be masked by water depletion. Potassium-binding resins may remove enough potassium from the gut to cause clinical deficiency.

Hypokalaemia is most commonly seen in patients with disease of the gastrointestinal tract, especially when this is associated with diarrhoea (or steatorrhoea) and vomiting, and may be marked in children; it often occurs after gastrointestinal surgery, especially with ileostomy, or after prolonged use of purgatives. In these conditions potassium intake is often also reduced. It is commoner in old people because of long-standing poor intake. There is increased catabolism of protein post-operatively, and potassium is lost from the cells to be eventually excreted in the urine. Patients with chronic gastrointestinal disease who require surgery are usually potassium-deficient even before operation. The resultant body potassium deficiency and hypokalaemia are an important cause of post-operative 'weakness', morbidity, and mortality.

In diabetic coma there may be considerable loss of body potassium into the urine. Because of dehydration, the initial plasma potassium may be normal or raised. Insulin treatment halts the loss of potassium because restoration of intracellular glucose metabolism with correction of acidosis fixes potassium in the cells, but the shift to the cells and fluid replacement lowers the plasma potassium level. Prolonged treatment with intravenous glucose likewise shifts potassium from plasma to cells.

There may be excessive urinary loss of potassium due to prolonged diuresis from any cause, including the diuretic recovery phase of acute renal failure, and excessive potassium will be excreted in any prolonged acidosis. Many drugs, including liquorice derivatives (with aldosterone effects), and diuretics, such as the thiazides and especially frusemide, can cause hypokalaemia, and necessitate monitoring of plasma electrolytes. Excessive potassium loss may occur in chronic pyelonephritis with mainly tubular disease, and in the Fanconi syndrome and other renal tubular disorders, and is the probable cause of the hypokalaemia of acute myeloid leukaemia; there is a rare potassium-*losing* nephritis. Because of the alterations in tubular function there is urinary loss of potassium (causing hypokalaemia) in Cushing's syndrome, primary or secondary aldoste-ronism, or from overdosage with ACTH or adrenocortical hormones. A urinary potassium of more than 20 mmol/24 h when there is hypokalaemia suggests that this is due to urinary loss.

In the rare disease, *familial periodic paralysis*, attacks of paralysis are associated with temporary hypokalaemia due to passage of potassium from the e.c.f. to the cells, although there is no change in the total body potassium.

Alkalosis accentuates hypokalaemia, and chronic potassium deficiency is a frequent cause of metabolic alkalosis (p. 50).

Metabolic and clinical aspects
The ill-effects of potassium deficiency depend both on the plasma level and on the total loss of potassium from the body: symptoms appear after about 500 mmol have been lost. Potassium deficiency affects principally the neuro-muscular system; the presenting symptoms are lethargy, mus-cular weakness, and ileus. If the diaphragm is affected there will be respiratory weakness and dyspnoea. The heart may be affected, and there are distinctive electrocardiographic changes with depression of the ST segment and a low or inverted T wave, and prominent U wave; arrhyth-mias, such as paroxysmal fibrillation, may develop, and hypotension is common. Prolonged hypokalaemia can lead to renal tubular damage, loss of concentrating power, and further loss of potassium (pathological vicious circle, p. 18). At first losses of potassium from the e.c.f. are replaced from the cells; thus mild potassium deficiency may exist with a normal plasma potassium level. The plasma level falls when the rate of loss from the plasma exceeds the rate of potassium transference from the cells to the plasma. If a patient has, as well as potassium deficiency, sodium depletion which has caused loss of extracellular water, this haemoconcentration will cause renal functional impairment and a second-ary rise of the plasma potassium *concentration*. When the e.c.f. volume is restored the plasma potassium concentration falls to its appropriate low value. Hypokalaemia may develop during recovery from intracell-ular potassium deficiency.

It has been suggested that, in the absence of anaemia (which alters the electrolyte values), erythrocyte potassium changes are a guide to whole body changes.

A plasma potassium concentration below 1.5 mmol/l is often fatal. It is not fully known why potassium depletion causes death, but respiratory depression and cardiac arrhythmias play a part.

Therapy

Treatment is required if there is a history indicative of potassium loss from the body, electrocardiographic changes of potassium deficiency, or if the plasma potassium level falls below 3.0 mmol/l. If the 24 h urinary potassium is less than 10 mmol, then urinary loss is unlikely to be the cause of the hypokalaemia. Potassium should be given orally if possible, as slow-release potassium chloride. The intravenous route is indicated if this is not possible or if the need is urgent, but must be used with great care if there is oliguria, renal damage, or heart failure. A daily input of 120 mmol of potassium chloride in divided doses is generally suitable for the treatment of the potassium deficiency of diabetic ketosis (after insulin therapy), or of moderate secretion loss.

A variety of intravenous potassium solutions have been recommended. Except in emergency, solutions stronger than 60 mmol of K^+/l should not be used. Potassium (as the chloride, generally 40 mmol/l) is nowadays usually given to adults by addition to isotonic glucose or saline.

Unless for emergency treatment of dangerous hypokalaemia not more than 20 mmol of potassium may be infused in an hour, and not more than 120 mmol should be given in a day. Great care must be taken, by serial plasma potassium estimations or electrocardiograms, to avoid hyperkalaemia.

MAGNESIUM

Magnesium balance in health and disease has been studied less extensively than has potassium balance. Atomic absorption spectrophotometry is the usual analytical method. The reference values for plasma magnesium are 0.7–1.0 mmol/l: about 80 per cent of this is diffusible, and the remainder is probably protein-bound in the same manner as calcium. Almost all of the 750 mmol of magnesium of the body is in the cells (about half in the bones), where its concentration is about ten times as great as in the plasma. The minimal daily intake of magnesium to maintain long-term balance may be about 10 mmol. About one-third of the usual intake (at least 12 mmol, 300 mg) is absorbed and excreted in the urine.

Although changes in magnesium ions affect neuromuscular irritability in a way similar to that of changes in calcium ions, alterations of clinical significance do not often occur. Raised plasma magnesium levels may be found in chronic renal failure, particularly in patients who have been given magnesium sulphate. Because magnesium is largely intracellular, magnesium depletion (which presents as mental confusion and twitches) accompanies loss of cell potassium. It may be seen in the malabsorption syndrome, or due to prolonged post-operative gastrointestinal excretion loss, for this is usually treated by intravenous fluids that lack magnesium. Magnesium deficiency is occasionally seen in primary aldosteronism and in alcoholism. It takes many weeks to develop, as renal conservation is good. A low plasma magnesium (with lowering of the plasma calcium) can occur after removal of a parathyroid tumour when the bones are avid for divalent cations. Magnesium may be bound as soaps, causing hypomagnesaemia, in acute pancreatitis (p. 235).

LITHIUM

This monovalent cation, normally absent from all body fluids, is administered as lithium carbonate in the treatment of manic-depressive patients. Consequent changes in water and sodium distribution are controversial. Plasma lithium is measured by flame photometry for the monitoring of therapy, being maintained usually within the range of 0.7–1.4 mmol/l.

ZINC

Knowledge of zinc balance in health and disease is relatively recent. Zinc deficiency is a result of malnutrition, whether due to a poor diet (often also high in phytate), or to intestinal malabsorption, or to prolonged intravenous feeding. It may also be an effect of alcoholic cirrhosis. Zinc deficiency can present as failure to thrive, hypogonadism, rashes, and infantile diarrhoea. It can lead to impaired wound healing.

Estimation of tissue zinc concentration is impracticable though hair analysis has been suggested; and urinary zinc excretion may reflect body stores. In the investigation of a possible cause of post-operative delay in wound healing, plasma zinc analysis (by atomic absorption spectrophotometry) may be helpful. Reference values for plasma zinc concentration are 12–17 μmol/l.

Further reading

Pitts RF. Volume and composition of the body fluids. In: *Physiology of the Kidney and Body Fluids.* 3rd ed. Chicago: Year Book Medical Publishers, 1974:11–35.

Reinhold JG. Trace elements – a selective survey. *Clin Chem* 1975; 21:476–500.

Sanderson P. Disturbance of electrolyte water and acid-base. *Medicine* 3rd series 1978; 11:565–570.

Taylor WH. *Fluid Therapy and Disorders of Electrolyte Balance.* 2nd ed. Oxford: Blackwell Scientific Publications, 1970.

Wilkinson AW. *Body Fluids in Surgery.* 4th ed. Edinburgh: Churchill-Livingstone, 1973.

CHAPTER 4

ACID-BASE REGULATION

The maintenance of the pH of the blood

The pH of peripheral blood, measured as the pH of plasma in contact with erythrocytes, is normally within the range 7.36 to 7.44: in any individual healthy subject it varies only within narrow limits. Plasma is therefore slightly alkaline in comparison with physicochemically neutral solutions. Arterial blood is slightly more alkaline than venous blood and typical values are: arterial blood pH 7.40; venous blood pH 7.37. The pH is effectively the logarithm of the reciprocal of the hydrogen ion *activity* (a_H), not of the concentration (c_H or [H^+]): in plasma these are not identical and the average arterial plasma pH, 7.40, corresponds to a hydrogen-ion activity of about 40 nmol/l, and to a concentration of about 50 nmol/l. An increase in pH of 0.3 units corresponds roughly to halving the hydrogen ion activity, because log $2 \approx 0.3$.

In the Brønsted-Lowry terminology, an acid is defined as a potential donor of hydrogen-ions (protons), e.g. hydrochloric acid, carbonic acid. A base is defined as a proton acceptor, e.g. (sodium) hydroxide, the bicarbonate ion, namely containing groups that bind hydrogen ions. The terms are restricted here to substances that act as proton donors or acceptors in the aqueous buffers of living systems. The term 'alkali' can be used for a potential donor of hydroxyl ions (OH^-) and is usually confined to compounds of alkali metals. An ion or molecule that is neither an acid nor a base is termed an *aprote*. In practice, in biological solutions, sodium (a cation) or chloride (an anion), may be considered as aprotes: however, in the presence of hydroxyl ions or hydrogen-ions, they can form respectively the strongly ionised base, sodium hydroxide, and the strongly ionised acid, hydrochloric acid. The ammonium ion is an acid, and the bicarbonate ion is a base, because they can form respectively the readily metabolised ammonia with consequent release of hydrogen-ions, and the weakly ionised acid carbonic acid by combining with hydrogen-ions.

Effects of food. On a mixed diet the metabolic processes cause an overall production of acid. To meet this constant tendency to acidify the extracellular fluid (e.c.f.), and to deal with changes in the acid-base balance of the body in disease, the blood contains buffering mechanisms. After intermediate buffering in the cells, final compensation for any change in the hydrogen ion concentration of the e.c.f. is performed by the lungs and the kidneys. The principal acid produced from the solution of the metabolic product carbon dioxide is carbonic acid – this is excreted by the lungs as carbon dioxide. Oxidation of sulphur-containing amino acids, and of organic phosphates (especially phospholipids), produces sulphuric acid and phosphoric acid (formerly called fixed acids): sulphate and phosphate are excreted by the kidneys. Some hydrogen-ions are excreted by the kidneys as ammonium ions, and as organic acids – which are weak acids. A vegetarian diet results in net production of base and a tendency to alkalosis, as oxidation of food then produces salts of organic acids such as sodium lactate, and not lactic acid, whose metabolism then utilises hydrogen-ions.

Buffering. In plasma the carbonic acid-bicarbonate mechanism is the most important buffering mechanism, although plasma proteins (and also phosphates) play a part. In interstitial fluid, protein buffering is absent. In the cells, buffering by proteins is more important. Haemoglobin, within the erythrocytes, plays a major part in the total buffering power of the blood. Buffer base is the sum of all these blood buffer ions.

The pH of erythrocytes is about 7.2 (60 nmol/l of a_H), and of muscle cells is about 6.9 (120 nmol/l of a_H). The diagram (Fig. 4.1) shows the normal distribution of anions and cation in plasma in terms of electro-valency. The buffering power of plasma may, for practical purposes, be considered solely dependent on the carbonic acid-bicarbonate mechanism: $H_2CO_3 \rightleftharpoons H^+ + HCO_3^-$.

The Henderson-Hasselbalch equation

By the laws of Mass Action, at equilibrium

$$\frac{[H^+] \times [HCO_3^-]}{[H_2CO_3]} = K$$

where K is the dissociation constant of carbonic acid.

Therefore, in the Henderson-Hasselbalch equations, as originally expressed without replacement of concentration by activity

$$[H^+] = K \times \frac{[H_2CO_3]}{[HCO_3^-]} \text{ or } pH = pK + \log \frac{[HCO_3^-]}{[H_2CO_3]}$$

The plasma carbonic acid forms a small part (about 1/700) of, and is in equilibrium with, the dissolved carbon dioxide

$$H_2CO_3 \rightleftharpoons CO_2 + H_2O$$

The above equations can now be re-written as

$$[a_H] = K_1 \times \frac{[CO_2]}{[HCO_3^-]} \text{ or } pH = pK_1 + \log \frac{[HCO_3^-]}{[CO_2]}$$

i.e. the hydrogen ion activity of the plasma depends on the ratio of dissolved ('respiratory') carbon dioxide to ('metabolic') bicarbonate. The

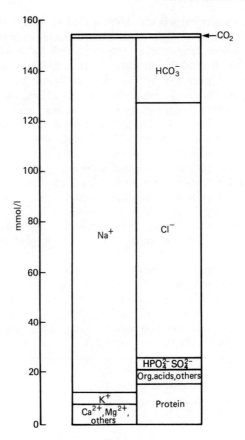

FIG. 4.1. Average electrolyte composition of normal plasma, expressed as millimoles of ion charges per litre of plasma.

plasma carbon dioxide concentration is a function of its partial pressure (P_{CO_2}). The formal chemical name for bicarbonate is hydrogen carbonate.

Methods of measurement

The pH of the plasma (in contact with erythrocytes) is measured with a special glass electrode, and requires anaerobic and iced handling of the blood (arterialised capillary, or arterial) between collection and analysis.

Plasma bicarbonate cannot be found directly: plasma total carbon dioxide (T_{CO_2}) is mainly bicarbonate, but includes dissolved carbon dioxide, carbonic acid and carbamino compounds for which an allowance (1–2 mmol/l) can be made in calculation. It is measured usually by acidifying anaerobically collected plasma, and assaying the carbon dioxide liberated – for greatest accuracy manometrically. Plasma CO_2 content is the same as T_{CO_2}. Plasma CO_2 combining power, or alkali reserve, is a less accurate but more convenient determination which can be done by automated apparatus, and using non-anaerobically collected venous blood: the plasma is resaturated with CO_2 at a hypothetically normal partial pressure of 5.2 kPa (40 mmHg), and its CO_2 content then measured.

Plasma carbonic acid cannot be found directly, and assessment is made by measuring P_{CO_2} on anaerobically collected blood by a special (Severinghaus) electrode – or indirectly by analysis of alveolar air.

Modern automatic blood-gas analysers simultaneously measure P_{O_2}, P_{CO_2}, and pH; and can calculate a value for bicarbonate from the second and third of these results, assuming a constant pK_1. These have largely replaced the Astrup apparatus, which measured the pH of blood after equilibration with gas mixtures of different carbon dioxide tensions and, by application of the Siggaard-Andersen nomogram to the results, calculated the other values. Some workers find other measurements, that are less physiological, useful in patient care. *Standard bicarbonate* is the bicarbonate concentration of fully oxygenated blood equilibrated to a P_{CO_2} of 5.2 kPa at 37°C: this value is presumed to be independent of respiratory changes. *Base excess* is the amount of acid required to titrate (metabolically alkalaemic) whole blood to pH 7.40 at 37°C, P_{CO_2} 5.2 kPa: *base deficit* is the reverse concept, for assessment of metabolically acidaemic changes. At a further remove from the *in vivo* situation are *standard base excess* and *corrected base excess*; these values 'corrected' for P_{CO_2} make the incomplete assumption that *in vitro* and *in vivo* correction are necessarily equal.

Fundamental changes

The diagram (Fig. 4.2) shows the possible ways in which the plasma carbon dioxide and bicarbonate may be altered. Equally valid diagrams are available with pH and P_{CO_2}, or with pH and $[HCO_3^-]$, on the principal axes. The reference range for the partial pressure of plasma carbon dioxide is 4.5–6.0 kPa (35–46 mmHg) corresponding to a concentration in solution of 1.1–1.4 mmol/l: the concentration of bicarbonate (derived from T_{CO_2}) is 24–30 mmol/l, and at pH 7.40 the dissolved carbon dioxide/bicarbonate ratio is approximately 1/20. A primary disturbance which causes (A) an increase in the plasma carbon dioxide or (B) a decrease in plasma bicarbonate leads to a fall in the pH of the plasma. Similarly (C) a decrease in the plasma carbon dioxide or (D) an increase in the plasma bicarbonate leads to a rise in the plasma pH.

The terminology is confusing. Acidosis and alkalosis are here used for conditions which promote an increase or decrease in the hydrogen-ion concentration, hence respectively a fall or rise in the pH, of the blood. If terms are needed to describe the actual changes in blood pH, then

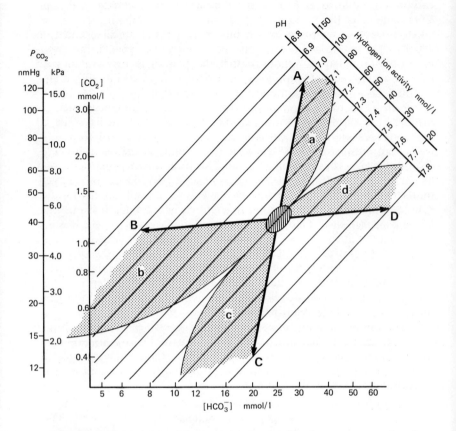

FIG. 4.2. Simplified chart showing the relation between bicarbonate concentration, P_{CO_2}, and pH in normal and abnormal blood plasma. The central shaded area represents the reference range. Direction of changes in primary disturbances are shown by the arrows: A, respiratory acidosis; B, metabolic acidosis; C, respiratory alkalosis; D, metabolic alkalosis. The shaded areas, a, b, c, d, adjacent to these arrows show the range of values found during compensation for the respective primary changes A, B, C, D.

'acidaemia' and 'alkalaemia' have been suggested, though these terms have not become popular. Increase or decrease of plasma CO_2 is sometimes called hypercapnia or hypocapnia.

Compensatory mechanisms for acidosis and alkalosis

Immediate buffering of any disturbance is carried out by the blood and e.c.f. mechanisms, followed by equivalent changes in the general intra-cellular fluid (i.c.f.). The cell membrane (and the cerebrospinal fluid) is readily permeable to H_2CO_3 and CO_2, but much less so to H^+ and HCO_3^-.

Respiratory mechanisms. This compensation for disturbances of the $[HCO_3^-]/[CO_2]$ ratio is rapid, and depends on the sensitivity of the respiratory centre to changes in both the P_{CO_2} and the pH of the blood, and to changes in cerebrospinal fluid pH. When there is an acidosis the respiratory centre responds by causing hyperventilation: this leads to an increased output of carbon dioxide by the lungs, and fall in plasma carbonic acid. When there is an alkalosis the reverse mechanism applies, and the depression of respiration leads to carbon dioxide retention and rise in plasma carbonic acid. However, the respiratory control of carbon dioxide excretion is ineffective when a respiratory disturbance has caused the acidosis or alkalosis, and it is unable to compensate for an acidosis caused by gross additions of acid to the e.c.f. A normal adult excretes each 24 hours about 20 000 mmol of acid as carbon dioxide.

Renal mechanisms. This compensation for the normal tendency to acidification of the e.c.f., and for correction of pathological disturbances of the $[HCO_3^-]/[CO_2]$ ratio, is less rapid, requires a normal glomerular filtration rate, and depends principally on the production of hydrogen-ions by the distal tubular cells, and is helped by a high P_{CO_2}. The hydrogen-ions generated by carbonate dehydratase (carbonic anhydrase) activity are exchanged for sodium ions across the cell membrane, the hydrogen ions passing out into the tubular lumen. Potassium competes with hydrogen for exchange with sodium. For each hydrogen-ion generated, by carbonate dehydratase activity within the tubular cell, there is the simultaneous formation of a bicarbonate ion, which passes back into the peritubular fluid. Thus the kidney, for each hydrogen-ion secreted into the urine, adds to the plasma one bicarbonate ion, so combating acidosis by excreting an acid urine and adding base to the plasma. The hydrogen-ions in the tubular lumen combine with phosphate and sulphate ions forming the titratable acid (fixed acid) of the urine; they also combine with the ammonia secreted into the tubular lumen (produced mainly from glutamine by glutaminase activity) and are excreted as ammonium ions (NH_4^+). The pH and P_{CO_2} of the plasma and the ionic content of the glomerular filtrate affect the rates of excretion of HCO_3^- and the production of hydrogen-ions and ammonia – e.g., acidosis stimulates glutaminase production by adaptive enzyme formation.

A normal adult on a mixed diet excretes daily about 25 mmol of titratable acidity and 40 mmol of ammonia, and less than 5 mmol of bicarbonate. The significant measurement is the net acid excretion: titratable acidity – bicarbonate + ammonia. When there is acidosis, more hydrogen-ions and ammonia are secreted, and the urine contains no bicarbonate, and more ammonia and titratable acidity (ketoacids are also titratable acids): excess ammonia production requires a week to develop fully. When there is alkalosis, less hydrogen-ions and often no ammonia are secreted; the urine contains increased bicarbonate, and titratable acidity may be replaced by titratable alkalinity ($H_2PO_4^-$ is replaced by HPO_4^{2-}). In gross acidosis, to provide still more cations, calcium and sodium may be withdrawn from the bones and potassium from the cells, and these are excreted in the urine; and hydrogen-ions move into cells.

During renal compensation for either acidosis or alkalosis there is usually a diuresis. When there is renal damage the resultant loss of compensatory power will diminish the body's capacity to maintain the constant pH of the e.c.f.

When the disturbance in the acid-base balance of the body is greater than can be reversed by the compensatory mechanisms, a change in blood pH results. In Fig. 4.2 the shaded areas (a, b, c, d) show, in respect of each of the four primary disturbances (A, B, C, D), the range of values for the acid-base variables that are usually found during the normal processes of compensation.

CLINICAL ACIDOSIS AND ALKALOSIS

Uncompensated acidosis itself causes few specific symptoms. In severe acidosis there will be hyperpnoea, and there may be vomiting and drowsiness. The symptoms of uncompensated alkalosis are more specific. There may be confusion nausea and anorexia, there is usually neuromuscular irritability with tetany; and there is often potassium depletion and eventual renal failure. In severe alkalosis respiration is depressed, and both oxygen intake and the release of oxygen from haemoglobin to the tissues are diminished.

Acidosis and alkalosis may be respiratory or non-respiratory (metabolic) in origin (Fig. 4.2). Respiratory disturbances are associated primarily with an increase or decrease of the plasma carbonic acid concentration: in them excretion of carbon dioxide is no longer equal to production of carbon dioxide, and there is a redistribution of hydrogen-ions. Metabolic disturbances are associated primarily with an increase or decrease of the plasma bicarbonate concentration: in them there is either a direct alteration of the e.c.f. bicarbonate, or alteration following changes in other ions – with redistribution of hydrogen-ions.

As with sodium and water, mixed disturbances are common; but the single disorders must first be appreciated.

Primary alteration in carbonic acid

Respiratory alkalosis

This results from hyperventilation, which leads to reduction of plasma carbonic acid. As P_{CO_2} falls, the equilibrium $H_2O + CO_2 \rightleftharpoons H_2CO_3 \rightleftharpoons H^+ + HCO_3^-$ shifts to the left, so $[H^+]$ and $[HCO_3^-]$ also fall. The plasma pH may reach 7.8.

Hyperventilation may occur in fever, at high altitudes (due to compensation for oxygen deficiency), or due to encephalitis, increased intracranial pressure, hepatic coma, anaesthesia and/or automatic ventilation, anxiety, or acute salicylate overdosage. The primary effect of compensation is that the plasma bicarbonate level falls as the kidney excretes excess sodium bicarbonate and an alkaline urine.

Respiratory acidosis

This results from depression of ventilation, which causes retention of carbonic acid. As P_{CO_2} rises, the equilibrium $H_2O + CO_2 \rightleftharpoons H_2CO_3 \rightleftharpoons H^+ + HCO_3^-$ shifts to the right, so $[H^+]$ and $[HCO_3^-]$ also rise. The plasma pH may reach 7.0.

Artificial respiration, by anaesthetist or machine, may produce an acidosis *or* an alkalosis. Diminished respiratory excretion of carbon dioxide results from respiratory obstruction, or may occur in chronic lung disease (either primary such as severe emphysema or secondary to heart failure), may be due to drugs which depress respiration, such as morphine and certain anaesthetics, and can be found in bulbar poliomyelitis and in hypothermia. Coma can develop from a combination of severe CO_2 excess and O_2 lack, as in cardiac arrest with heart failure. Carbon dioxide toxicity, which can accidentally occur in industry, may directly cause retention of carbonic acid.

In acute respiratory acidosis compensation is slight and the bicarbonate may be little raised. The effect of compensation in chronic respiratory acidosis is that the plasma bicarbonate level rises, with a tendency to correct the pH.

Primary alteration in bicarbonate

Metabolic alkalosis

This is associated with an increase in the plasma bicarbonate concentration which is accompanied by either a decrease of the other anions of the plasma (principally chloride) or an increase of cationic sodium. The plasma pH may reach 7.8.

Gain of external base. Patients who treat their indigestion by taking unlimited quantities of sodium bicarbonate (or any other antacids that are alkaline) may become severely alkalotic, with a plasma bicarbonate level higher than 50 mmol/l. Alkalosis may be induced for therapeutic purposes by the use of sodium citrate or sodium lactate, as the catabolism of the anion consumes hydrogen ions.

Loss of hydrogen-ions. This occurs with a secondary rise in plasma bicarbonate following hydrochloric acid loss due to vomiting or nasogastric aspiration. It is commonly seen as a result of the vomiting of pyloric stenosis (including congenital pyloric stenosis of children) and in eclampsia. Patients with a juxta-pyloric ulcer, who are vomiting and are also taking alkali therapeutically, develop a very severe alkalosis. However, if vomiting occurs in a patient who has achlorhydria then alkalosis does not result. If vomiting is prolonged the ketosis of starvation will complicate the clinical and biochemical picture. In chloride diarrhoea (particularly when neonatal) there may be the same disturbance.

Potassium deficiency often produces an alkalosis. This e.c.f. alkalosis is partly due to hydrogen ions entering the cells to replace lost potassium ions (which compete in exchange for sodium ions), or to alterations of renal tubular function – tubular intracellular potassium deficiency enhances bicarbonate resorption, leading to an inappropriately acid urine with an alkalosis.

If a patient who is alkalotic because of vomiting is also very sodium and water deficient, then renal compensation by excretion of sodium bicarbonate will not be effective and the patient will paradoxically excrete an acid urine.

Retention of base. This implies excess reabsorption of bicarbonate (and sodium) by the renal tubules, usually with loss of potassium. It may be due to diuretics such as frusemide and the thiazides.

Combined therapy (diuretics, low dietary NaCl, steroids) of chronic respiratory acidosis often leads to metabolic alkalosis.

Metabolic acidosis

This is associated with a decrease of the plasma bicarbonate level, accompanied by a decrease of the plasma sodium. The plasma pH may reach 6.9.

Gain of external acid. Acidosis can be induced by administration of substances whose metabolism yields hydrogen ions, such as ammonium chloride, hydrochlorides of organic bases, calcium chloride, excess aspirin (acetylsalicylic acid), or resins that release hydrogen ions into the gut. Infusion of sodium chloride to patients with salt depletion tends to cause chloride retention and an acidosis, for isotonic saline (pH 7.0) contains equimolar proportions of sodium and chloride, whereas e.c.f. (pH 7.4) contains appreciably more sodium than chloride.

Loss of bicarbonate (with sodium). Pancreatic juice, is alkaline (the pH of pancreatic juice is about 8 and its bicarbonate concentration may reach 100 mmol/l); bile and high small-intestinal secretions are also mildly alkaline. Such alkaline fluids can be lost through a fistula or ileostomy, or in severe diarrhoea (particularly from cholera) or steatorrhoea, or when there has been excess purgation: the plasma bicarbonate level falls and acidosis is super-imposed on the dominant biochemical picture of water and salt depletion. Sodium and bicarbonate are lost in the urine during treatment with diuretics such as acetazolamide which are carbonate dehydratase inhibitors, or in acquired or inborn renal tubular disorders (renal tubular acidosis, p. 225) where hydrogen-ions cannot be formed for exchange with sodium ions.

Failure to excrete acid. Acidosis due to chloride retention develops after ureteric transplantation into the colon (p. 226).

In renal failure there is diminished production of ammonia and hydrogen-ions in the tubules, and loss of sodium, which with glomerular retention of fixed acids (phosphate and sulphate) and organic acids causes severe acidosis.

Increased internal production of acid. Ketosis lead to an acidosis, whether the ketosis is due to diabetes, to starvation, or to a high fat diet. After the body's oxidative powers for ketone bodies have been fully saturated (p. 79) the keto-acids are retained in the plasma and displace bicarbonate. Sodium is lost in the urine (from the e.c.f.) and potassium (from the i.c.f.) with the excreted keto-acids. In severe diabetic ketosis the plasma bicarbonate level may well be less than 5 mmol/l.

Lactic acid similarly causes an acidosis: this may be due to excess production of lactic acid, or diminished utilisation (p. 71). The acidosis of fetal anoxia due to lactic acid can be monitored by sampling scalp blood at the time of birth.

Methanol poisoning causes a formic acidosis; ethylene glycol produces oxalic acid, and paraldehyde produces acetic acid; in addition all these toxins lead to a lactic acidosis.

The diagnosis of disorders of acid-base balance

Acidosis or alkalosis are often associated with disorders of salt or water balance. The body is less tolerant of osmotic pressure changes, due to total electrolyte loss or gain, then it is of acidosis or alkalosis, due to differential electrolyte loss or gain. In general the osmotic pressure of the e.c.f. is maintained as far as possible, even at the expense of a normal pH.

Acidosis and alkalosis, which cause their symptoms because of changes in the hydrogen-ion activity of the blood, should be evaluated by measuring the pH, P_{CO_2}, and bicarbonate values in the blood: or less rigidly by measuring two and deriving the third. The pK of carbonic acid in plasma, and its solubility coefficient, are not constant in acute conditions of changing blood pH; therefore all three components should be measured separately for the greatest accuracy. It is not possible in practice to measure changes in intracellular pH.

There is a need to distinguish between the primary cause of an acid-base disturbance, changes due to compensation, and changes due to complications. This is especially important in regard to treatment. Fig. 4.2, with knowledge of the history, may be used as a guide. For example, plasma values of pH 7.2, P_{CO_2} 4.0 kPa (30 mm Hg), [HCO_3^-] 12 mmol/l fall within area b, and are therefore likely to represent partially compensated metabolic acidosis. Plasma values of pH 7.0, P_{CO_2} 8.0 kPa (60 mmHg), [HCO_3^-] 15 mmol/l fall between arrows A and B, and are therefore likely to represent combined respiratory and metabolic acidosis as in heart failure (respiratory depression + lactic acidosis). The combination of respiratory alkalosis and metabolic acidosis occurs for example in salicylate poisoning; of respiratory acidosis and metabolic alkalosis in pulmonary oedema treated with diuretics; and of respiratory alkalosis and metabolic alkalosis due to iatrogenic over-ventilation and gastric aspiration.

The plasma bicarbonate level can be used as a measure of the degree of acidosis or alkalosis in all cases when the disturbance is solely metabolic in origin: this is the most commonly performed estimation as it has been automated. Some investigators prefer to use standard bicarbonate or the other 'P_{CO_2}-independent quantities'. In respiratory acidosis or alkalosis the P_{CO_2} ('the plasma creatinine of respiration') is the measure of the primary cause of the change in the plasma pH. In addition P_{O_2} measurements may be useful. Estimation of the plasma sodium, potassium, and chloride levels is also valuable.

Anion gap. In health $[Na^+] = [Cl^-] + [HCO_3^-] + [6-16]$, the last value (in mmol/l) being called the anion gap. An increased anion gap usually indicates an acidosis derived from fixed or undetermined acids, as in renal failure or from lactic or acetoacetic acid.

Some biochemical aspects of treatment

In cases of mild metabolic acidosis, or alkalosis, with water and salt depletion, and in the presence of normal renal function, correction of the water and salt depletion will eventually correct the acidosis or alkalosis – the kidney excretes the unwanted ions. Saline infusion corrects mild alkalosis efficiently, but does not do so for severe acidosis (p. 50). Should intravenous therapy be required for the correction of severe disorders of acid-base balance that do not respond to saline replacement, then a suitable solution, which is approximately isotonic with plasma, is sodium bicarbonate (150 mmol/l; 1.26 per cent w/v), which has now generally replaced sodium lactate (165 mmol/l), for the treatment of *acidosis*. Hypertonic sodium bicarbonate is used for rapid correction, for example when metabolic acidosis is associated with cardiac arrest, and solutions up to 1000 mmol/l (8.4 per cent) are available. If potassium is required when there is acidosis it is usually given as the citrate. Ammonium chloride (165 mmol/l) for the treatment of *alkalosis* is rarely required and must be used with great care, as it is dangerous in liver disease: also it may accentuate sodium or potassium depletion, and in many circumstances potassium chloride, and occasionally dilute hydrochloric acid (150 mmol/l into a deep vein), is necessary. Arginine or lysine, being basic amino acids, may be used as their hydrochlorides.

Primary changes in P_{CO_2}, of respiratory origin, require therapy to that system.

The doses of such replacement fluids, and the duration of treatment and their combination with other therapy, must be judged by the biochemical and clinical degree of alteration of the normal electrolyte balance. It is essential to rely also on the history, on serial estimations of the changes, on a well-kept fluid balance chart, and on experience; and not just to use formulas (e.g. involving base deficit) for correction of disorders of acid-base balance and of salt and water balance.

Unchecked overcorrection of acidosis or alkalosis may lead to the opposite situation.

OXYGEN

Oxygen tension

Measurement of arterial P_{O_2} is being used in conjuction with that of P_{CO_2} in the assessment of respiratory disorders, as the analysis can be done on the same special blood sample with combined electrodes: the reference range on arterial blood is 11–15 kPa (85–105 mmHg) and this corresponds to 95 per cent saturation of haemoglobin with oxygen. A low P_{O_2} is a measure of anoxia, and is found frequently with a high P_{CO_2} whenever there is alveolar hypoventilation due to obstruction or depression of respiration. Less frequently a low P_{O_2} is seen with a low P_{CO_2} when ventilation and perfusion do not change in parallel, particularly when there is pulmonary oedema.

Oxygen availability

Oxygen release to the tissues, at a given P_{O_2}, is diminished by hypothermia, by alkalosis, and by a fall in erythrocyte 2,3-diphosphoglycerate (2,3-DPG), as these affect the dissociation curve of haemoglobin. Measurement of erythrocyte 2,3-DPG, which is not a routine procedure, may become valuable in assessing certain disorders of acid-base balance combined with anoxia. Acidosis causes depletion of 2,3-DPG – accentuated in diabetic ketoacidosis by phosphate deficiency. Restoration of 2,3-DPG is slow when correction of acidosis is rapid, so oxygen availability is then diminished.

Further reading

Campbell EJM. Hydrogen ion (acid-base) regulation. In: Campbell EJM, Dickinson CJ, Slater JDM, eds. *Clinical Physiology*. 4th ed. Oxford: Blackwell Scientific Publications, 1974:232–258.

Clarke S. Respiratory function tests. *Br J Hosp Med* 1976; 15:137–153.

Masoro EJ, Siegel PD. *Acid-Base Regulation: its Physiology and Pathophysiology*. 2nd ed. Philadelphia: W.B. Saunders, 1978.

Robinson JR. *Fundamentals of Acid-Base Regulation*. 5th ed. Oxford: Blackwell Scientific Publications, 1975.

CHAPTER 5

CARBOHYDRATES

A normal adult, living in a temperate climate, has a carbohydrate intake that averages about 400 g/day, and this supplies about a half of the energy requirements – the energy value of carbohydrate is about 17 kilojoules (kJ) (4 kilocalories (kcal)) per gram. Dietary carbohydrate deficiency leads to a deficient energy intake and to starvation: if the protein and fat intake remain normal when the carbohydrate intake is reduced, ketosis develops.

Digestion and absorption of carbohydrate

Most of the carbohydrate of food is the polysaccharide, starch: cellulose cannot be digested by man. Salivary amylase begins the digestion of carbohydrate by converting a little of the starch to α-limit dextrins, maltotriose, and to the disaccharide maltoses. No further chemical digestion of carbohydrate takes place in the stomach. Pancreatic amylase converts unchanged starch and dextrins to maltoses. In the brush border conversion of dextrins to maltoses is completed, and the maltoses are converted by disaccharidases into the monosaccharides, which are absorbed into the portal circulation and pass to the liver. The final digestion of the carbohydrate of the food is performed by maltases, and by isomaltase, which convert maltoses to the monosaccharide glucose. Similarly lactase converts lactose to glucose and galactose, and sucrase converts sucrose to glucose and fructose. Glucose is the principal monosaccharide end-product of carbohydrate digestion; fructose and galactose are also produced when the subject is taking a normal diet. The amount of fructose is increased by a diet which contains excess fruit, or cane sugar (sucrose). The amount of galactose is increased when a high proportion of the carbohydrate intake is lactose, and this happens in infants and in patients on a milk diet.

Any of the disaccharide enzymes may be deficient: this results in an osmotic diarrhoea due to intestinal accumulation of the appropriate disaccharide when it is present in food (p. 73).

Normally more than 99 per cent of the carbohydrate in the diet is digested and absorbed and there is a negligible quantity of carbohydrate in the faeces. When there is an absorption defect of the intestinal mucosa (as in coeliac disease), or when there is intestinal hurry (as in severe diarrhoea), or in the disaccharidase deficiencies, absorption of glucose is reduced – and glucose may be detected in the faeces by the simple tests for urinary glucose. Resection of the small intestine must be considerable to reduce significantly the absorption of glucose.

Absorption of glucose is more rapid in patients with hyperthyroidism, and is delayed in hypothyroidism. The anterior pituitary gland acts on carbohydrate absorption via the thyroid and the adrenal cortex.

Parenteral carbohydrate

The usual intravenous glucose solution is approximately isotonic with plasma (280 mmol/1:5 per cent w/v), but this provides only 800 kJ (200 kcal) per litre. For significant energy input higher concentrations must be used, e.g. 2800 mmol/1:50 per cent w/v (8000 kJ/1) but this is sclerosing and requires the use of central veins. Such hypertonic energy-providers contain less free water than does the same gross volume of an isotonic solution, but produce relatively more water of oxidation. The advantages of related substances whose initial catabolism is not insulin-dependent, as fructose, sorbitol, or ethanol (29 kJ/g) are controversial – they may lead to lactic acidosis.

NORMAL GLUCOSE METABOLISM

Glucose cannot be further metabolised until it has been converted to glucose-6-phosphate by a reaction with ATP: this reaction is catalysed by the non-specific enzyme hexokinase, and also by the specific glucokinase in the liver. The reaction in the reverse direction, a simple hydrolysis of glucose-6-phosphate to glucose, is catalysed by glucose-6-phosphatase. Once glucose has become glucose-6-phosphate it can be converted to glycogen for storage and cannot diffuse out of the cell. The glucose which has not been converted to glycogen passes from the liver via the systemic circulation to the tissues where it can be oxidised, stored as muscle glycogen, or converted to fat and stored in fat depots. The glycogen in the liver acts as a reserve of carbohydrate, and releases glucose into the circulation whenever peripheral glucose utilisation has lowered the concentration of glucose in the blood. Muscle glycogen is converted to lactate by anaerobic glycolysis: it cannot produce glucose as muscle has no glucose-6-phosphatase. For oxidation of glucose, or for conversion of carbohydrate to fat or protein, the glucose-6-phosphate can be converted in stages, via triose phosphates and phosphoenolpyruvate, to pyruvate – the Embden-Meyerhof glycolytic pathway of oxidative phosphorylation. There is an alternative metabolic pathway for the oxidation of glucose, the hexose monophosphate shunt, which leads to the formation of $NADPH_2$ and not of $NADH_2$. Fructose and galactose, after phosphorylation (mainly by fructokinase and galactokinase), enter the common metabolic pathways of carbohydrate. Pyruvate can enter the common metabolic pool or be converted to other compounds. The common metabolic pool represents the series of

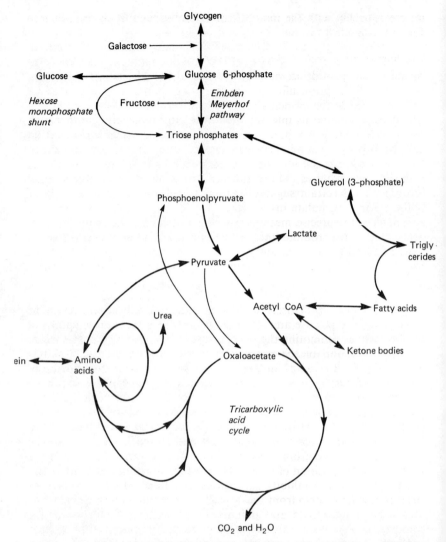

FIG. 5.1. Simplified scheme of the principal pathways of the general metabolism of carbohydrate, protein, and fat (triglycerides). A double-headed arrow indicates that the metabolic process may go in both directions, but not necessarily by the same reaction or series of reactions.

reactions, based on acetyl coenzyme A and the tricarboxylic acid cycle (Krebs' cycle: citrate cycle), within which carbon residues from protein carbohydrate or fat may be oxidised with release of energy, or converted one into another.

The basic biochemistry of the metabolism of glucose, and its interrelationship with the metabolism of protein and lipids, is shown in Fig. 5.1.

The hormonal control of glucose metabolism

Insulin, a polypeptide secreted by the β cells of the Islets of Langerhans, is synthesised as proinsulin, containing two insulin chains connected by C-peptide. It is the principal hormone that controls the metabolism of carbohydrate and its interaction with the metabolism of proteins and lipids. Its structure has been completely elucidated; its modes of action are not fully understood. The secretion of insulin is primarily regulated by the arterial plasma glucose level with secondary influence by stimuli from the vagus nerve. Many other factors, including gastrointestinal hormones, and certain sugars, fatty acids, and amino acids, directly or indirectly may stimulate insulin secretion.

Whatever the precise mechanisms responsible may be, the total effect of insulin is to promote the further metabolism of glucose both to storage and to oxidation, and thus to lower the blood glucose. In the absence of insulin, glucose utilisation is depressed and gluconeogenesis is enhanced.

Insulin acts at the cell membrane to increase the rate of uptake into cells (particularly of muscle and adipose tissue, but not of brain or erythrocytes) of glucose and other sugars. Many of the other actions of insulin, such as promoting the phosphorylation of glucose, are secondary to this promotion of the passage of glucose into cells. The result is acceleration of the entry of glucose into further metabolic processes, either for storage as glycogen in liver and muscle, or for utilisation by conversion or oxidation. (The transport of fructose into cells is independent of insulin control.) Insulin also possibly has a direct stimulant action on the oxidative phosphorylation of carbohydrate at a site further on in the metabolic path. Insulin promotes the conversion of acetyl CoA (derived from pyruvate) to fatty acids, thus promoting the synthesis and deposition of neutral fat: it inhibits lipolysis and the release of free fatty acids. It inhibits gluconeogenesis from protein, and favours the synthesis of protein from amino acids. Insulin also promotes transfer of potassium, phosphate, and amino acids into cells. In liver, the entry of glucose into the cells is only slightly dependent on insulin, and the major action is that glucose output is decreased by insulin.

The hypoglycaemic action of insulin is balanced by the action of hormones from the anterior pituitary and the adrenal cortex. Growth hormone, with the possible involvement of somatomedin, is responsible for the actions of what was formerly thought to be an independent diabetogenic hormone. It increases protein synthesis, and opposes the glucose utilisation actions of insulin – although the secretion of insulin is stimulated. Excess growth hormone causes hyperglycaemia, and the long-term effect of damage to the islet-cells may be due to the hyperglycaemia. Somatostatin (p. 144) inhibits the release of insulin. The glucocorticoids, and indirectly adrenocorticotrophic hormone, stimulate protein catabolism; this releases carbon residues and gluconeogenesis is increased. Glucose utilisation is decreased: the increase of insulin secretion may be an indirect effect.

Hypophysectomy used to be performed for the alleviation of severe diabetic retinopathy in young adults: the rationale is the removal of the source of growth hormone and adrenocorticotrophic hormone.

The pancreatic islets also secrete from the α cells a hyperglycaemic glycogenolytic polypeptide hormone called *glucagon*. As well as having a glycogenolytic action and stimulating the release of insulin and of catecholamines, glucagon promotes protein catabolism, and is lipolytic and ketogenic.

Thyroxine stimulates the rate of intestinal absorption of carbohydrates, and it increases the tissue needs for insulin, perhaps by its general promotion of tissue oxidation.

The adrenal medulla can be stimulated to release adrenaline by vagal impulses when the hypothalamus is stimulated by hypoglycaemia. Adrenaline (and to a lesser extent noradrenaline) raises the blood glucose level in two ways. It has a short-term effect of stimulating hepatic glycogenolysis, and a longer-term effect of promoting the secretion of adrenocorticotrophic hormone: it also inhibits insulin secretion.

Blood sugar/blood glucose

The term 'blood sugar' is loosely used to include glucose and other sugars, and sometimes other reducing substances which may be present in the blood. Originally most methods for sugar analysis depended on glucose being a reducing substance. It is possible to eliminate the non-specific reduction, and to measure only that due to sugars: this is called 'true sugar', and reduction due to sugars other than glucose, e.g. galactose, is normally negligible. Blood for sugar determination is normally taken into fluoride, which inhibits glycolysis.

Methods involving the specific enzyme glucose oxidase (or alternatively using hexokinase) measure only glucose and give results up to 0.3 mmol/l lower than 'true sugar': these are now widely employed, and all figures in this book are blood *glucose*. By using a commercial glucose oxidase stick preparation (p. 274) it is possible to perform a screening blood glucose estimation and to detect hypoglycaemia or hyperglycaemia. Precision is improved by using a reflectance meter to read the colour of the stick and some diabetic patients may thus monitor their own blood glucose levels.

The reference values for fasting venous whole blood glucose at rest are 3.0–5.5 mmol/l in adults, and are lower in infants (p. 269). In capillary blood (which represents arterial blood) the value at rest is about 0.2 mmol/l higher. Because of the widespread use of capillary samples, whole blood glucose is more commonly measured than is plasma glucose, although the latter is preferable. Glucose is freely diffusible between cell water and plasma water, and the different water content of cells and plasma results in the measured concentration of glucose in the plasma being 10–15 per cent higher than in whole blood.

Insulin can be measured in plasma or serum by radioimmunoassay and the assay is mainly used in the investigation of spontaneous hypoglycaemia. The reference range for fasting plasma insulin is 10–30 μu/ml. There is also a variety of difficult biological assays which effectively measure 'insulin-like-activity', and whose results may differ from those found by radioimmunoassay.

The excretion of glucose

Glucose is filtered by the glomeruli, and the average normal tubule reabsorbs more than 99 per cent of the glucose that reaches it in the glomerular filtrate. The proximal renal tubules are responsible for returning glucose to the circulation. If the renal plasma flow is normal, and the kidney is healthy, then at a capillary blood glucose concentration of more than about 10 mmol/l sufficient glucose is filtered into the renal tubules to saturate a significant proportion of their variable reabsorptive capacity, and detectable glycosuria occurs. This concentration of 10 mmol/l is known as the *renal threshold* for glucose. A reduced renal plasma flow (as occurs in heart failure or sodium depletion) or severe glomerular damage will reduce the rate of filtration of glucose through the glomeruli. In such cases a high blood glucose concentration will not cause as high a glomerular filtrate glucose concentration as if the renal plasma flow were normal. If the reabsorptive power of the tubules is unaltered then there is a raised renal threshold for glucose and mild hyperglycaemia will not cause glycosuria. About 2 per cent of diabetic patients, mainly older patients, have a high renal threshold for glucose.

Renal glycosuria. Diminution of tubular reabsorptive capacity for glucose, which may be due to specific or generalised abnormalities of tubular function or to gross tubular disease, can lead to glycosuria when the blood glucose level is normal. Renal glycosuria usually presents in the absence of other evidence of renal damage. The low threshold of pregnancy is attributable to an increase in glomerular filtration.

The effect of carbohydrate on the blood glucose

When a fasting subject ingests glucose, or a meal containing carbohydrate, the blood glucose level rises as glucose is absorbed from the intestine. In a normal person, after a meal, the venous blood glucose level does not exceed 8.5 mmol/l and the capillary level (representing arterial blood glucose) should not rise above 10 mmol/l. The secretion of insulin greatly increases, and that of glucagon (after an initial rise), and of growth hormone, decreases. The mechanisms of tissue oxidation, storage of glucose as glycogen, and diminished gluconeogenesis (all 'anti-hyperglycaemia') are active and counteract the increased blood glucose which results from the absorption of glucose. At about an hour after the ingestion of carbohydrate the rate of removal of glucose from the blood becomes greater than the rate of addition of glucose to the blood, and the blood glucose level begins to fall – these anti-hyperglycaemic actions are not wholly insulin-controlled. The blood glucose may even fall below the fasting level at about 2 hours – the slight hypoglycaemia then mobilises the insulin antagonists and insulin and growth hormone return to normal, glycogenolysis occurs, and the blood glucose level returns to normal at about 3 hours after the meal.

The extent to which the body responds to a carbohydrate load is known as the glucose tolerance and primarily reflects the capacity of the liver to take up glucose. *Impaired glucose tolerance* means that after taking carbohydrate (as glucose) the blood glucose level rises higher, and the rise is more prolonged, than in normal people. *Enhanced glucose tolerance* means that ingestion of carbohydrate causes a diminished rise in the blood glucose level. There is a normal circadian diminution of glucose tolerance in the afternoon.

The detailed response to a carbohydrate load depends both on the previous carbohydrate diet and on the amount of glucose ingested. If a subject is fasting or on a low carbohydrate diet there can be impaired glucose tolerance: fasting increases gluconeogenesis. If a subject is on a very high carbohydrate diet (or has eaten just before the test) there can be enhanced glucose tolerance. The changes in glucose tolerance with alteration of the diet are related to changes in liver glycogen metabolism and also to changes in insulin and growth hormone secretion. The extent of the rise of the blood glucose level after glucose ingestion increases with the dose of glucose, up to a dose of about 1 g/kg body weight. Hence, if measurement of glucose tolerance is required for investigation of disease, standard conditions of diet and of glucose dose must be established.

The effect of insulin on the blood glucose

Insulin has no action orally, even when given in large doses, as it is inactivated by the gastric juice, and then digested. Insulin is given subcutaneously in the normal therapeutic control of diabetes, but for the treatment of diabetic coma or for studying the physiological response it may be injected intravenously. After the intravenous injection, to a fasting subject, of a small dose (0.1 units/kg) of soluble insulin, the blood glucose level falls for about half an hour to about 50 per cent of the resting level – then the hypoglycaemia mobilises the insulin antagonists and the blood glucose returns to normal in about 2 hours.

The response to insulin can be divided into two phases. The rate and degree of fall of the blood glucose concentration after injection of insulin is known as the insulin-sensitivity – insulin-resistance means that the blood glucose does not fall as much as in a normal subject. The rate and degree of return to normal of the blood glucose concentration after the hypoglycaemia is known as the hypoglycaemia-response: hypoglycaemia-unresponsiveness means that the blood glucose fails to return to normal. Both insulin-resistance and hypoglycaemia-unresponsiveness may be present in pathological states.

ABNORMAL GLUCOSE METABOLISM

Hyperglycaemia and impaired glucose tolerance

The level of the blood glucose depends on the balance between intake of carbohydrate and endogenous glucose synthesis and release by the liver on the one hand, and glucose storage utilisation and excretion on the other hand. A carbohydrate meal in a normal person causes only a temporary rise in the blood glucose level: the mechanisms for removal of glucose from the circulation, by storage or utilisation, efficiently restore the normal level.

A temporary hyperglycaemia, due to increased glycogenolysis, may be due to excessive secretion of adrenaline; this occurs in patients who have phaeochromocytoma, and after emotional stress, asphyxia, and anaesthesia. Asphyxia and many anaesthetics also directly stimulate hepatic glycogenolysis. The hyperglycaemia which follows cerebral injury, cerebrovascular accidents, and increased intracranial pressure may be due to increased glycogenolysis. Temporary hyperglycaemia follows over-rapid absorption of glucose from the gut and may occur after gastrectomy, gastroenterostomy, or pyloroplasty. It is also occasionally found, following a meal, in severe liver disease. Peritoneal dialysis with hypertonic glucose solutions can cause severe hyperglycaemia.

An artefactual cause of hyperglycaemia is the blood sample being taken from near the site of an intravenous glucose infusion.

Impairment of glucose tolerance, often with fasting hyperglycaemia, may be seen in patients with cirrhosis, and with severe staphylococcal infections. Glucose tolerance can also be impaired by the chronic action of various toxins, particularly alcohol and barbiturates, on the peripheral utilisation of glucose: 'toxins'' may be responsible for the impaired tolerance of chronic renal failure.

Essential deficiency of effective insulin activity

The β-cell injury in insulin-dependent (juvenile) diabetes mellitus is determined by genetic and immunological mechanisms, and possibly by virus and other factors. Endogenous secretion of insulin is diminished; and plasma insulin is always low at the time of diagnosis.

In noninsulin-dependent (maturity onset) diabetes mellitus the plasma insulin is higher than in juvenile diabetes, and may even be above normal: there is a delayed insulin response to hyperglycaemia. Resistance to insulin is an important mechanism in this disease, as well as genetic and possibly other factors. A high proportion of patients are obese; and insulin-resistance occurs in obesity.

Secondary destruction of insulin secretion

Insulin deficiency results when total pancreatectomy has been performed, and may develop in severe chronic pancreatitis or haemochromatosis.

After total pancreatectomy the patient's insulin requirement is only about 40 units per day, for in such patients there are no primary extrapancreatic metabolic changes, and glucagon secretion is also absent. When there is this type of deficient secretion of insulin, the patient's insulin sensitivity and hypoglycaemia responsiveness are normal, even though glucose tolerance is grossly impaired. Decreased glucose utilisation is more important than increased glucose production.

Excess insulin antagonists

Excessive secretion of the 'anti-insulin' hormones may occur in acromegaly, Cushing's syndrome, phaeochromocytoma, or thyrotoxicosis, and the same effect can develop during treatment with adrenocorticotrophic hormone or corticosteroids; or in pregnancy (gestational diabetes). Impaired glucose tolerance occurs, for the balance of hormonal control of glucose metabolism is disturbed in the same direction as in deficient insulin activity. There may, however, be marked insulin resistance. Increased glucose production is more important than decreased glucose utilisation.

Glucagonoma is rare, and presents with bullous dermatitis. There is hypoaminoacidaemia, and hyperglycaemia is inconstant.

Diabetes mellitus

Diabetes mellitus is a syndrome comprising many disturbances.

Permanent impairment of glucose tolerance is caused by similar deficiencies of insulin activity and alterations of normal glucose metabolism, whatever the initial cause of the disorder. There is impaired liver and tissue utilisation of glucose; and hepatic glycogenolysis, and gluconeogenesis from protein and fatty acid carbon residues, are increased. The blood glucose level rises, and tissue utilisation of glucose increases at a rate proportional to the 'head of pressure' of blood glucose up to a level of about 30 mmol/l. The increased blood glucose level leads to increased glomerular filtration of glucose. The renal threshold is exceeded and glycosuria is present.

Protein metabolism is disturbed as excess protein is broken down in the process of gluconeogenesis. The disturbance of lipid metabolism may lead to ketosis. When there is relative or absolute insulin deficiency excess triglyceride is hydrolysed, which releases excess free fatty acids (FFA): the latter, if not oxidised, are converted to keto-acids if not reconverted to triglycerides. This reconversion, and the capacity of the common metabolic pool, are diminshed because of deficient carbohydrate metabolism (p. 80) and the tissue oxidative power for keto-acids is overloaded. The result is retention of keto-acids in the plasma, and their excretion in the urine.

The clinical features of a patient suffering from untreated diabetes mellitus are results of these metabolic disorders, which result from effective insulin deficiency.

The patient has impaired glucose tolerance, often combined with a high fasting blood glucose level. If the impairment of carbohydrate metabolism is more than minimal, protein and lipid metabolism are also affected. Tissue protein is destroyed during gluconeogenesis, with loss of potassium, nitrogen, and phosphate from the cells to the e.c.f., whence they are excreted. Fat is also drawn on to provide energy requirements as carbon residues for the common metabolic pool. The patient loses weight. The levels of all the lipids in the plasma are raised including FFA, as fat is being transported from depots to liver, and the plasma may appear milky. Excess cholesterol is synthesised from acetyl CoA, and there is an increase in the pre-β lipoproteins. The increased plasma FFA impairs insulin sensitivity and further impairs glucose tolerance. The hyperglycaemia reduces the resistance to bacterial infection, causes itching, and leads to glycosuria. There is often a high value for salivary amylase isoenzyme in plasma, coupled with a decreased pancreatic isoamylase and trypsin due to impaired exocrine function.

Long-standing diabetes mellitus often leads to intercapillary glomerulosclerosis (the Kimmelstiel-Wilson lesion), which is accompanied by proteinuria and renal failure.

The relative parts played by the primary metabolic causes of diabetes mellitus, and by secondary effects such as hyperglycaemia and lipaemia, in the pathogenesis of the vascular and other complications of diabetes, are not decided.

The concentration of glycosylated haemoglobins, particularly HbA_{1c} (p. 127), is increased in diabetes mellitus: a value above 10 per cent indicates, and is a useful investigation for, poor long-term metabolic control.

Diabetic ketosis, acidosis, and coma

When treatment is inadequate, and in the presence of complicating factors such as infection and starvation or anorexia and vomiting, ketosis develops (p. 79); as this becomes severe (the total plasma ketones exceeding about 5 mmol/l), the patient slowly lapses into diabetic coma. The coma is due to the toxic effects of the acidosis and of the acetoacetate on the cerebral cortex. The ketoacids produce a severe metabolic acidosis with a plasma bicarbonate less than 10 mmol/l, and this leads to the characteristic 'air-hunger'. Ketone bodies are excreted in the breath, which has the characteristic odour of acetone, and in the urine, where they can be easily detected (p. 74). The commercial strip or tablet tests for ketonuria can also be used for the detection of excess ketone bodies in plasma: quantitation of plasma ketones is rarely needed. In a few patients there is also a contributory lactic acidosis (p. 71).

The blood glucose is generally above 20 mmol/l and the marked glycosuria (up to 1000 mmol/24 h) causes an osmotic diuresis. This diuresis, vomiting, the ketonuria, and the acidosis, cause severe dehydration with loss of intracellular and extracellular water and electrolytes. The patient shows the symptoms of sodium and water depletion with a slight rise in plasma osmolality, and the loss of extracellular water eventually causes haemoconcentration, oliguria, and a rise in the plasma urea: vomiting causes chloride depletion. From inefficiency of the sodium pump and because of the haemoconcentration, the plasma potassium concentration may be increased, while the plasma sodium is usually slightly lowered. There is increased protein catabolism and a high plasma phosphate, and loss of liver and muscle glycogen. Potassium, nitrogen, and phosphate released from the cells are excreted in the urine.

Diagnosis is made both clinically, and on the demonstration of hyperglycaemia with glycosuria, ketosis with ketonuria, and acidosis – but impaired glomerular filtration may reduce the excretion of glucose and of ketones. Rarely, there is hyperglycaemia without ketoacidosis, or ketoacidosis without severe hyperglycaemia.

Hyperosmolar non-ketotic coma is an unusual complication, mainly in older patients, of unknown cause. The blood glucose usually exceeds 50 mmol/l, which yields a plasma osmolality above 350 mmol/kg and causes cell water deficiency. There is dehydration and often oliguria, and ketosis and acidosis are absent.

Treatment of ketoacidosis is directed to reversing the metabolic disturbances by insulin and by replacing the deficiencies of water and salt with intravenous saline, and base (e.g. as sodium bicarbonate) as necessary. Potassium must be given, orally or intravenously, as soon as the plasma volume is restored and the potassium concentration falls below normal. Close biochemical control of glucose, electrolytes, and acid-base balance is necessary.

A milder diabetic syndrome occurs when glucose tolerance is impaired due to excess insulin antagonists. Ketosis and coma are rare in such conditions.

Hypoglycaemia

In normal adult subjects symptoms of hypoglycaemia occur at or below a capillary blood glucose level of about 2.2 mmol/l. If the brain is accustomed to a lower blood glucose level (as in hyperinsulinaemia or overtreated diabetes mellitus) symptoms occur only when the blood glucose is at a lower level, such as 1.7 mmol/l. If the brain is accustomed to a constantly higher blood glucose level (as in uncontrolled diabetes mellitus), then symptoms can occur at a higher blood glucose level, and the critical concentration may be above 3.3 mmol/l. Hypoglycaemic symptoms may also occur at a blood glucose of 2.8–4.0 mmol/l when the rate of fall of blood glucose is rapid.

Childhood hypoglycaemia. The blood glucose may need to fall below 1.1 mmol/l in infants before there are symptoms, often of convulsions. Chronic hypoglycaemia, particularly in infants, may lead to permanent mental retardation. Although most cases in infants can be diagnosed under one of the general causes of hypoglycaemia described below, there remain a group of 'idiopathic hypoglycaemias of infancy', often with ketosis.

Diminished absorption of glucose

A diet which has been low only in carbohydrate even for a prolonged period does not lead to clinical hypoglycaemia, as the blood glucose level is maintained at a slightly lower level from liver glycogen, which is itself synthesised from non-carbohydrate sources. In kwashiorkor blood glucose is generally low, due largely to deficiency of glucogenic amino acids.

If glucose absorption is diminished, a carbohydrate meal may make little difference to the blood glucose level.

Urinary loss of glucose

A constant drain of glucose, due to a low renal threshold, may result in a persistently low blood glucose level, though this is rarely sufficient to cause symptoms. A patient suffering from renal glycosuria may develop diabetes mellitus as readily as may anyone else.

Treatment of diabetes mellitus

An overdose of insulin is probably the commonest cause of hypoglycaemia: chlorpropamide and other insulin-stimulating anti-diabetic agents may rarely also produce hypoglycaemia.

Insulinoma

Benign or malignant tumours of the islet cells (which can be multiple), or, rarely, hyperplasia of the islet cells, produce excess insulin. This results in a high fasting plasma insulin and a low fasting blood glucose level, and on occasion in attacks of severe hypoglycaemia, with mental or neurological symptoms. The blood glucose is lowest before breakfast, and three to four hours after meals.

As a diagnostic test, it may be necessary to fast the patient for 24–48 hours in hospital under supervision. If hypoglycaemia develops, take blood to look for a diagnostically high insulin (assay of proinsulin may be more sensitive), and treat with intravenous glucose. Alternative tests are to give intravenous *glucagon*, or *leucine*, and to look for the diagnostically high rise in the plasma insulin associated with the fall in blood glucose. The similar, and formerly popular, *tolbutamide test* is too dangerous. To detect autonomous insulin secretion during insulin-induced hypoglycaemia, either C-peptide can be assayed or immunologically-distinct fish insulin can be injected.

A variety of tumours of non-endocrine origin (particularly retroperitoneal fibrosarcoma) may produce hypoglycaemia by secreting an insulin-like hormone.

The hypoglycaemia of childhood which is caused by sensitivity to leucine is associated with high plasma insulin levels, and hyperresponsiveness of insulin secretion to the amino acid.

Neonates of treated diabetic mothers may be hypoglycaemic from insulin excess.

Deficiency of insulin antagonists

In hypopituitarism, adrenal cortical deficiency, and rarely in hypothyroidism, there may be fasting hypoglycaemia because of deficiency of hormones which normally act as insulin antagonists. Patients so affected have enhanced glucose tolerance and are hypoglycaemia-unresponsive.

Hepatic hypoglycaemia

In acute hepatic necrosis and occasionally in viral hepatitis there may be severe hypoglycaemia: renal gluconeogenesis continues on a small scale.

The cause of the hypoglycaemia of galactosaemia (and fructosaemia) is uncertain, but is probably due to diminished gluconeogenesis. The same explanation is offered for the acute alcoholic hypoglycaemia (often with lactic acidosis) which is more often seen in chronic alcoholics who are fasting.

Glycogen storage diseases. These are inborn errors of metabolism: there are many types, some of which are associated with hypoglycaemia. The commonest *von Gierke's disease* (*Cori type I*), is due to deficiency of glucose-6-phosphatase, and resulting inability to complete the breakdown of hepatic and renal glycogen via glucose-6-phosphate to glucose – there is enlargement of liver and kidneys. As well as the episodes of hypoglycaemia with ketosis and lactic acidosis, serum FFA and lipids are increased, there is often hyperuricaemia, and the glycogen deposition in the kidneys may lead to a renal tubular syndrome (p. 225). As a diagnostic test the response to glucagon of the blood glucose is often valuable: normal subjects, after an intravenous injection of 1 mg of glucagon, have at least a 50 per cent rise in the fasting blood glucose within 20 minutes; this fails to occur in von Gierke's disease. The eight other rare types are each due to a deficiency of a different enzyme in the pathway of glycogen synthesis or degradation, and do not all show hypoglycaemia. Diagnosis may require enzyme assay on liver or other tissue biopsy.

Alimentary hypoglycaemia

In patients who have had a gastrectomy or gastroenterostomy a carbohydrate meal rapidly causes a high blood glucose level, often followed by hypoglycaemia between 1 and 2 hours. The high blood glucose level is due to rapid absorption of glucose, as the meal reaches the intestines more quickly than usual. There may be excessive vagal activity. Rapid absorption also occurs in hyperthyroidism. The hypoglycaemia results from rapid acceleration of glucose utilisation with a high plasma insulin at the same time as glucose absorption falls off. This *post-gastrectomy hypoglycaemia* must be distinguished from the *dumping syndrome* (p. 233), which develops in these patients 20–60 minutes after a meal, and whose aetiology is not fully understood.

Functional (reactive) hypoglycaemia

In some otherwise physically healthy subjects hypoglycaemia often occurs about 2 hours after a meal, possibly due to excessive insulin response to glucose. Alcohol may potentiate this effect. This response is also occasionally seen in early diabetes.

Carbohydrate storage diseases

In the glycogen storage diseases (p. 66) the inborn error of metabolism affects carbohydrate metabolism generally. In the several muco-polysaccharidoses, with lysosomal enzyme deficiencies, the disorder is only intracellular, as in the lipidoses (p. 87).

Hurler's syndrome (formerly called *gargoylism*) is typical. There is mucopolysaccharide deposition in brain, liver, reticulum cells and many tissues, and secondarily glycolipid deposition in the nervous system. Detection in the urine of excess sulphated mucopolysaccharides (dermatan sulphate and heparan sulphate), which have not been normally broken down, serves as a biochemical screening test.

INVESTIGATION OF ABNORMALITIES IN CARBOHYDRATE METABOLISM

Investigation of glucose tolerance is of considerable importance in clinical and experimental practice. Conditions should be standardised so that consistent responses may be obtained.

Reliable and reproducible results are obtained only when the patient has been on a normal diet (containing at least 300 g of carbohydrate per day) for at least three days before the test, and is mentally and physically at rest before and during the test. The patient must fast 10–16 hours overnight before all tests (water is allowed), and must not be allowed to smoke.

Consistent results are not found in children who are less than 2 years old. The present customary routine adult dose of glucose is 50 g (280 mmol) and in children 1 g/kg body weight to a maximum of 50 g: recent international recommendations are for an adult dose of 75 g, or of 1.75 g/kg body weight in children to a maximum of 75 g: the larger dose of 100 g is not recommended as this may lead to delay in gastric emptying and even to vomiting. Diagnostic results can usually be obtained without extending the test beyond 120 min.

The test is not needed for diagnosis in cases of clinically overt diabetes mellitus, or if a fasting blood glucose exceeds 7 mmol/l, or a random value exceeds 10 mmol/l.

Standard (oral) glucose tolerance test

Method. Take a fasting blood sample for glucose estimation. Patient empties bladder; collect specimen.

Zero time: the patient drinks a solution of 75 g glucose in a glass of water (250 ml); preferably flavoured, e.g. with lemon.

At 30 min, 60 min, 90 min, 120 min: take blood for glucose estimation.

At 60 min and 120 min: patient empties bladder; collect specimens separately.

Send all blood and urine specimens to the laboratory, clearly labelled with the times of collection.

Interpretation. The figures given here are for venous whole blood. If capillary blood is used, the fasting level is <0.3 mmol/l higher, the level at the peak is 1.1–1.7 mmol/l higher, and the 120 min level is 0.6–1.1 mmol/l higher: for venous plasma the levels are about 1 mmol/l higher. In diabetic patients there may be less difference between the venous and the capillary blood glucose levels.

(a) The normal response.

The fasting blood glucose level is 3.0–5.5 mmol/l. The blood glucose rises by 1.5–4.0 mmol/l to the 30–60 min level which is below 10 mmol/l, then falls to a 120 min level below 7.0 mmol/l. There is no glycosuria.

(b) Impaired glucose tolerance – the diabetic curve.

The curve is raised and prolonged. In diabetes mellitus the fasting blood glucose level is usually above 7.0 mmol/l; if it is not so raised then diabetes may be diagnosed when both an intermediate level and the 120 min level are above 10 mmol/l. Impairment of tolerance not amounting to diabetes is accepted when the fasting level is below 7.0 mmol/l, intermediate levels are below 10 mmol/l, and the 120 min level is between 7.0 and 10 mmol/l; though of course there can be no rigorous boundary between normal and abnormal (p. 4). Glycosuria is normally present, though not always in the fasting specimen.

Special criteria apply in pregnancy.

For the diagnosis of diabetes mellitus, or other causes of impaired glucose tolerance, usually only the 120 min level is *essential*. A normal blood glucose found 120 min after the ingestion of 75 g of glucose under appropriate standardised conditions demonstrates normal glucose tolerance. In many cases of severe diabetes there is no 60 min peak as the blood glucose rises throughout the period of the test. The same type of diabetic curve is seen if there is impairment of tolerance due for example to severe Cushing's disease.

Impairment of tolerance may be found in obesity, late pregnancy (or due to hormonal contraceptives), severe infections (especially staphylococcal), Cushing's syndrome, Conn's syndrome, acromegaly, thyrotoxicosis, gross liver damage, chronic intoxication, chronic renal disease, in old age, and in mild or incipient diabetes mellitus.

The urine results provide a guide to the renal threshold for glucose in that patient, and this is valuable in showing how much reliance can be placed on urine testing in patient management.

Steroid augmented glucose tolerance tests are of some help in the detection of incipient diabetes. If, for example, 100 mg cortisone is given in the early morning before a glucose tolerance test, then the 120 min blood glucose may be raised above 7.7 mmol/l in potential diabetics.

(c) The lag storage curve.

The fasting blood glucose level is normal. There is a steep rise in blood glucose: the maximum level, found at 30 min, is above 10 mmol/l. The curve then falls sharply, and hypoglycaemic levels may be reached before 120 min. There is a *lag* in the initiation of the normal homoeostatic processes, particularly *storage* of glucose as glycogen. Transient glycosuria is usually found. This curve was originally described in certain cases of severe liver disease, and sometimes occurs in thyrotoxicosis, but is more commonly seen due to rapid absorption following gastrectomy, gastroenterostomy, or vagotomy. The lag storage curve is occasionally found in apparently normal subjects.

(d) The flat curve of apparently enhanced glucose tolerance.

The fasting blood glucose is normal or low and throughout the test the level does not vary by more than about ±1.0 mmol/l. This curve may be seen in patients who are suffering from myxoedema (which reduces carbohydrate absorption), or who have deficiency of hormonal insulin antagonists as in Addison's disease and hypopituitarism. There is no glycosuria.

A flat curve is often found in patients who have malabsorption of carbohydrate, as in coeliac disease. In lactase deficiency (p. 54) the blood glucose curve is normal after giving 25 g glucose + 25 g galactose (confirming normal absorption), but is flat (less than 1.0 mmol/l rise) after 50 g lactose because of diminished digestion of lactose to absorbable monosaccharide.

In renal glycosuria the glucose tolerance curve may be flat or normal, depending on the rate of urinary loss of glucose.

(e) The late hypoglycaemia of hyperinsulinism.

In patients with hyperinsulinism the fasting blood glucose is hypoglycaemic or normal, and late blood glucoses estimated 4, 6, and if necessary 24 hours after glucose has been taken may show hypoglycaemic levels.

The diagram (Fig. 5.2) shows typical normal and abnormal oral glucose tolerance test curves.

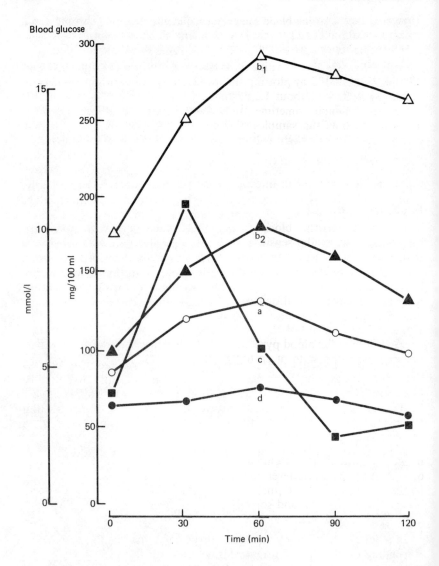

FIG. 5.2. Oral glucose tolerance test curves (75 g glucose: venous blood). (a) Normal, (b₁) Diabetic, (b₂) Mild impairment of tolerance, (c) Lag storage, (d) Flat: enhanced tolerance.

Intravenous glucose tolerance test

Abnormal responses to the oral glucose tolerance test may be masked by defective intestinal absorption. For the investigation of glucose metabolism in such patients the glucose may be given intravenously.

Method. Take a fasting blood sample for blood glucose.

Zero time: 50 ml of 50 per cent glucose is injected intravenously over 2 min.

At 10 min, 20 min, and 30 min: take samples for blood glucose.

Interpretation. The k value (percentage fall in blood glucose per minute) is calculated by plotting the results on semilogarithmic paper. In normal subjects k is about 1.5, in diabetic patients k is less than 1.0.

The test, though sometimes important, is little used because it is necessary to time the samples very accurately: injection of hypertonic glucose also carries a slight risk of thrombophlebitis. Cases for which it is an essential diagnostic measure, such as suspected diabetes in a patient with steatorrhoea, are rare. It is valuable for research on glucose tolerance, as variations in intestinal absorption are eliminated.

Insulin sensitivity test

The response of the blood glucose to insulin has been used for investigation of insulin-sensitivity and of hypoglycaemia-responsiveness in endocrine disease, though because of its dangers this test has now been replaced by appropriate plasma hormone assays. The blood glucose falls further, and remains low for longer, in patients with hypopituitarism or thyroid or adrenocortical deficiency, than in healthy subjects.

Pyruvate metabolism test

The response of the blood pyruvate level to an oral dose of glucose varies not only with the state of carbohydrate metabolism but also with the degree of thiamine (vitamin B_1) saturation of the patient, as thiamine pyrophosphate acts as a coenzyme in the further oxidation of pyruvate to acetyl CoA. Measurement of erythrocyte transketolase, and of its response to thiamine pyrophosphate (p. 122), is more sensitive and specific for the diagnosis of thiamine deficiency.

The reference range for fasting blood pyruvate is 40–80 μmol/l. In a normal subject, after 50 g glucose given fasting, and again at 30 min, the 60 min blood pyruvate level does not exceed 90 μmol/l, and the 90 min level does not exceed 100 μmol/l. Increased values after glucose are seen in thiamine deficiency, and sometimes in polyneuritis of other aetiology. Similar abnormal values occur in chronic barbiturate or alcohol intoxication, due also to disturbance of the peripheral oxidation of glucose.

Lactate

The reference range for venous blood lactate is 0.75–2.0 mmol/l. Accumulation of lactic acid causes a metabolic acidosis, with a reduced anion gap (p. 51).

Lactic acid is produced in excess by anaerobic glycolysis in anoxic tissues, e.g., occasionally during anaesthesia, in severe heart failure especially after cardiac arrest, in muscles after severe exercise, or generally after trauma. Alternatively it may not be normally metabolised, for example in liver failure and von Gierke's disease, or in diabetes mellitus, or due to phenformin therapy. Lactic acidosis is potentiated by alcohol.

Acetate

Acetate metabolism in disease is becoming important because of the use of acetate as base, especially in haemodialysis. Reference values for plasma acetate are <0.4 mmol/l.

GLYCOSURIA

A 24 hour specimen of urine from a normal subject contains a small amount of reducing substances, generally less than 1 g, of which 20–200 mg (0.1–1.1 mmol) is glucose. *Glycosuria* implies that sufficient glucose is present to be detectable by a simple clinical test – the 'correct' term glucosuria is rarely used. The comprehensive tests depend on copper reduction, and these are semiquantitative. The traditional test employed is Benedict's solution, containing alkaline copper(III) citrate [cupric citrate] which is blue because of the presence of copper(III) ions. On reduction of Benedict's solution, by glucose or other substances, the blue colour disappears and an orange-red precipitate of copper(II) oxide [cuprous oxide] is formed. The colour of the reduced mixture varies from green to red, for the more glucose that reduces the reagent the more copper(III) ions are converted to copper(II) oxide. The original, and similar, Fehling's test is no longer employed, as it requires two solutions. In general use Benedict's test has been replaced by Clinitest (p. 271), a commercial modification in which reagents in solid form are added to urine: no external source of heat is required as the heat of solution of the reagents boils the mixture. This is most useful for the ward side-room, for the general practitioner's surgery, and for issuing to diabetic patients to test their urine themselves. Clinitest tablets are less stable, especially in hot damp climates, than is Benedict's solution.

Many substances that reduce copper can occur in urine: reduction due to any sugar is called *melituria*. Glucose is the commonest and most important, and reduction sufficient to form a precipitate must be considered to be due to glucose unless proved otherwise. Quantitative estimation of the 24 hour urinary excretion of glucose is often valuable in the control of treatment of diabetes mellitus if blood glucose estimations cannot be performed.

Many bacterial infections of urine (e.g. due to *E. coli*) lead to absence of urinary glucose. Detection of less than 0.03 mmol (5 mg) glucose per 24 hour urine has been proposed as a screening test for bacteriuria, but gives an unacceptably high proportion of false negative results.

Glucose

The causes of glycosuria may be summarised as:

1 Hyperglycaemia associated with impaired glucose tolerance.

2 Temporary hyperglycaemia.
3 A low renal threshold for glucose.

The causes of these conditions have been discussed above. Hyperglycaemia without glycosuria may be found if there is a raised threshold due to diminished renal plasma flow: this is quite often seen in the elderly diabetic.

A reducing substance found in urine may be identified as glucose by:

Use of the specific enzyme, glucose oxidase. Test strips incorporating glucose oxidase are commercially available for qualitatively testing urine (p. 272): they are simple, sensitive, specific for glucose, and do not react with other reducing substances. Diastix is semi-quantitative, but the reaction is suppressed by ketones. They should not replace copper reduction for the initial testing of urine (especially in children), because diseases such as galactosaemia will be missed.

Chemical tests. Identification of sugars other than glucose is performed in the biochemical laboratory by chromatography. Osazone formation and yeast fermentation are no longer used in clinical biochemistry.

Other sugars

Lactose, galactose, fructose, and pentoses, are other reducing sugars which may be found in urine. Sucrose is not a reducing sugar. Intestinal accumulation of any disaccharide can lead to some absorption and urinary excretion of that sugar as is seen in lactase deficiency (p. 54): a similar alimentary melituria may present when there is flattened intestinal mucosa (p. 240).

Lactose. This is often present in the urine of pregnancy after 20 weeks, and may be found either as the sole reducing sugar, or together with glucose. Lactosuria usually occurs in nursing mothers, and is occasionally found in patients on a milk diet. It is rare for the concentration of lactose in urine to exceed 14 mmol/l (0.5 g/100 ml). Lactosuria is benign.

Galactosaemia (with galactosuria). This occurs as a congenital abnormality. It is due to deficiency of the hepatic enzyme galactose-1-phosphate uridylyltransferase, which is concerned with the conversion of galactose through hexose phosphates to glucose; thus galactose cannot enter into further metabolic processes, and there is hypoglycaemia. Accumulation of galactose-1-phosphate leads to renal tubular damage (p. 225) with aminoaciduria, proteinuria, and acidosis, and to liver damage with jaundice. The high blood galactose leads to cataracts. This disorder should always be considered as a possible cause of failure to thrive in an infant who is on a milk diet. It should be screened for by testing urine for reducing sugars, and the presence of galactose is confirmed by chromatography. The specific enzyme deficiency can be determined in erythrocytes or leucocytes before appropriate dietary therapy.

Fructose intolerance. This is a similar rare disease, due to deficiency of an isoenzyme of (fructose-bisphosphate) aldolase. Fructose-1-phosphate accumulates after ingestion of fructose or sucrose, and this causes hypoglycaemia and liver damage.

Benign congenital abnormalities. Fructosuria due to fructokinase deficiency, and galactosuria (which is associated with cataracts) due to galactokinase deficiency, are rare. Pentosuria (xylulosuria), due to L-xylulose reductase deficiency, is less rare. In addition various pentoses may occasionally be found in the urine after ingestion of large quantities of fruit.

Glucuronides

Glucuronides are conjugates of various compounds with glucuronic acid, and these are urinary reducing substances. Drugs in common use which are partially excreted as ester-glucuronides are the salicylates (including aspirin) and paracetamol.

The glucuronide of any salicylate drug, which is taken in therapeutic dosage, may be excreted in sufficient quantity in the urine to cause a greenish reduction. However the reduction caused by the glucuronide of p-aminosalicylic acid, taken in the usual dosage, may mimic the reduction caused by 1 g glucose/100 ml urine (about 50 mmol/l).

Rare urine components

Amongst other reducing substances are homogentisic acid, phenylpyruvic acid, and melanogen. Homogentisic acid is found in the inborn error of metabolism alkaptonuria (p. 102). Phenylpyruvic acid is found in phenylketonuria (p. 101), and can be further identified by its giving a green colour with iron(III) chloride [ferric chloride] or with the equivalent Phenistix. Melanogen is produced by malignant melanoma: it blackens on oxidation to melanin, and is excreted in widespread disease.

Normal constituents of urine

If urates are present in urine in sufficient quantity to form a sediment, the urine should be filtered before testing it for sugars. A high concentration of urates or of creatinine in urine will cause a slight reduction of copper.

Protein, or a high concentration of phosphates, may precipitate as greyish floccules on boiling the urine with Benedict's solution or Clinitest. This should not be mistaken for reduction.

KETONURIA

The ketone bodies which may be excreted in urine are acetone, aceto-acetic acid, and 3-hydroxybutyric acid. There are two tests available for ketone bodies in the urine. Rothera's test is sensitive to acetoacetic acid and acetone, and is a colour reaction with sodium nitroprusside in alkaline solution. This has now been largely replaced by commercial tablet or stick preparations (p. 272). Gerhardt's test is sensitive to acetoacetic acid and is a colour reaction with the iron(III) [ferric] ion in acid solution (p. 272). The differences in the specificities of the tests to different ketone bodies may be ignored in clinical practice, but there are two important distinctions between them.

(i) Gerhardt's iron(III) chloride test gives a false positive colour with phenolic drugs (particularly salicylates) or their excretion products, and the purplish colour of the iron(III) phenol complex may be indistinguishable from the mauvish colour of the iron(III) keto-acid complex. Phenothiazines usually give a brown to mauve colour with iron (III) chloride; this test is now more commonly used for drugs than for ketones. The nitroprusside tests do not give a false positive with any compound that commonly occurs in urine, and by performing both tests a false positive iron(III) chloride reaction can often be recognised. However, this is not always possible as many patients who have received an overdose of, for example, aspirin, also have a ketosis. Ketone bodies in urine are decomposed by boiling, whereas phenolic drugs remain unchanged.

(ii) Gerhardt's test is much less sensitive than is Rothera's test or even than the more satisfactory and generally used commercial preparations. If these or the iron(III) chloride test is positive, then the plasma ketone level is high and the degree of metabolic acidosis should be controlled by estimation of the plasma bicarbonate level.

Ketonuria occurs when there is ketonaemia. This may be found whenever, in a disorder of carbohydrate metabolism, insufficient carbohydrate is being catabolised to ensure proper oxidation of fat. This incomplete carbohydrate metabolism, combined with excessive fat breakdown, causes the ketosis of diabetes mellitus.

Ketonaemia and ketonuria also develop when the patient is suffering from carbohydrate deficiency. Thus ketonuria is found in starvation (or if the patient is on a badly balanced reducing diet) or after prolonged vomiting. Post-operative ketonuria is commonly seen. It is due to a combination of the starvation that precedes the operation, the vomiting that often follows it, and possibly to the effect of the anaesthetic which depletes liver glycogen.

Just as there may be hyperglycaemia without glycosuria, so ketonaemia without ketonuria may occur if there is a low renal plasma flow. This can be seen, e.g., in the ketosis due to prolonged vomiting associated with starvation and sodium depletion, or sometimes in severe diabetes.

Further reading

Cohen RD, Woods HF. *Lactic Acidosis.* Oxford: Blackwell Scientific Publications, 1976.

Marks V. The investigation of hypoglycaemia. *Br J Hosp Med* 1974; 9:731–763.

Oakley WG, Pyke DA, Taylor KW. *Diabetes and its Management.* 3rd ed. Oxford: Blackwell Scientific Publications, 1978.

LIPIDS

Chemistry and classification

The term 'lipid' is used to include all fats and substances of a fat-like nature. The principal lipids of clinical interest can be classified as:

Triglycerides (neutral fat). These are glycerol esters of long-chain fatty acids – i.e. triacylglycerols. The chief component of olive oil, triolein, is a typical neutral fat. However most triglycerides are mixed, with more than one kind of fatty acid in the molecule.

Phospholipids. These are compounds that contain a nitrogenous base, a phosphoric acid residue, one or more fatty acids, and a complex alcohol, either glycerol or sphingosine. Lecithin (phosphatidyl choline) is a typical phosphoglyceride. Cerebrosides are similar compounds without phosphoric acid.

Steroids. These have a completely different chemical structure, and contain the cyclopentenophenanthrene ring system. Cholesterol is a typical steroid.

Carotenoids. The carotenoids and vitamin A are *not* lipids. They are coloured fat-soluble compounds (lipochromes) and are absorbed with lipids from the small intestine.

The structures of triolein, α-lecithin, cholesterol, and vitamin A, are shown in Fig. 6.1. All these groups of substances are insoluble in water, and are held in solution in plasma by being in combination with specific carrier proteins – the apoproteins A, B, and C.

LIPID METABOLISM

Fat intake and output

Dietary fat

Triglycerides are the main lipid in the diet. They give it palatability and provide a concentrated source of energy: 37 kJ (9 kcal) per gram of fat. The normal daily diet in the United Kingdom at present contains 40–80 g of triglycerides. Fat in the diet carries the fat-soluble vitamins A, D, and K.

The dietary fat contains both unsaturated fatty acids (some of which, particularly linoleic acid, are essential, because they cannot be synthesised in the body) and saturated fatty acids. The proportion of un-

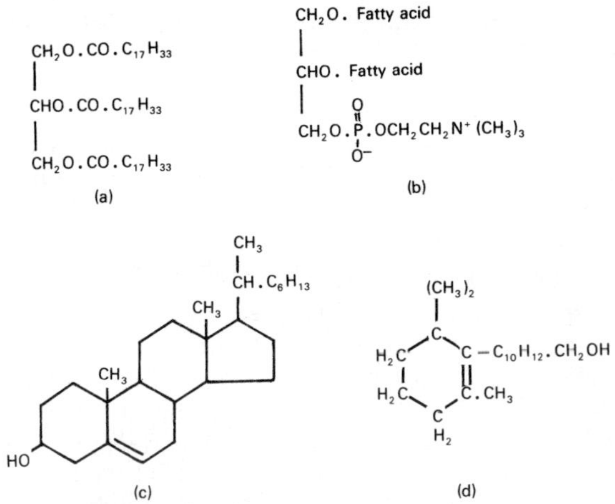
CH2O.CO.C17H33
CHO.CO.C17H33
CH2O.CO.C17H33
(a)
CH2O. Fatty acid
CHO. Fatty acid
CH2O.P.OCH2CH2N+ (CH3)3
O
O−
(b)
CH3
CH.C6H13
CH3
CH3
HO
(c)
(CH3)2
C
H2C
C−C10H12.CH2OH
H2C
C.CH3
C
H2
(d)

FIG. 6.1. Structures of: (a) Triolein, (b) α-Lecithin, (c) Cholesterol, (d) Vitamin A.

saturated to polyunsaturated fatty acids is generally higher in animal fat than in vegetable fat. A high content of fat in the diet, in particular of fat which contains a high proportion of saturated (and a low proportion of unsaturated) fatty acids, is a suggested factor in the aetiology of atheroma.

Fat absorption

Though there is a gastric lipase, negligible digestion of neutral fat takes place in the stomach. In the upper small intestine, under the influence of pancreatic lipase, about a quarter of the neutral fat is completely hydrolysed. There is both partial hydrolysis to monoglycerides, and also complete hydrolysis into glycerol and the constituent fatty acids. The glycerol, which is water-soluble, is readily absorbed into the portal system. Most short-chain fatty acids can be absorbed directly into the blood: the long-chain fatty acids and monoglycerides (normally insoluble in water) in combination with bile salts, form water-soluble micelles. Monoglycerides and fatty acids, with bile salts, promote the emulsification and dispersion of the remaining unhydrolysed fat which is then available for hydrolysis: a little finely dispersed fat can be absorbed directly. The water-soluble fatty acid complex is absorbed into the mucosal cells of the intestine, where the bile salts are released into the portal circulation; the fatty acids and monoglycerides are resynthesised in the intestinal wall to triglycerides. These triglycerides are absorbed into the lacteals as small particles known as chylomicrons, which have an average diameter of 1.0 μm and enter the general circulation via the thoracic duct. Chylomicrons contain about 1 per cent carrier apoprotein.

Bile salts are essential for the adequate absorption of fat. They combine with fatty acids and monoglycerides to form the water-soluble complex described above, and in their absence emulsification of neutral fat is incomplete.

Fat excretion

In a normal subject not more than 10 per cent of the fat that has been taken in the food can be recovered in the faeces. The daily faecal fat excretion of a person on an average diet, which contains about 70 g of fat, is under 5 g (18 mmol), and an increase to a high fat diet (150 g) will not raise this above 7 g (25 mmol): there may be considerable day-to-day variation. Much of the excreted fat is derived from non-dietary sources (bacteria, yeasts, intestinal secretions and excretion, or desquamated epithelium), for up to 2 g of lipid material is found in the faeces even in subjects on a fat-free diet. Fat excretion can be studied by a balance technique, which relates excretion to intake (p. 94). In clinical practice analysis for total fat of three to five days' excretion of faeces, from a patient on an average diet with a fat intake of 60–100 g, gives the same information. Examination of the proportion of fat by weight in dried faeces, or of the proportion of split fat present (as this depends on bacterial action as well as on pancreatic lipase), does not give information of value. Alternatively the effect of an oral dose of vitamin A on its plasma concentration (p. 240) may be used as a measure of total fat absorption.

The investigation, effects, and differential diagnosis of an increase in faecal fat (steatorrhoea) are discussed in chapter 14.

An insignificant quantity of fat is normally lost in the urine and the sebum. Fat is found in the urine in occasional cases of lipid nephrosis or the nephrotic syndrome (lipiduria), or when excess fat enters the blood, often as a fat embolus, after extensive injury to fat depots in bone marrow or subcutaneous tissue. *Chyluria*, the urine having the appearance of milk, is rarely seen. It is usually due to obstruction of the thoracic duct, when chylomicrons reflux through the lymph vessels of the urogenital tract. There can also be *chylothorax* and *chylous ascites* when chylomicrons from the intestinal lacteals leak into the pleural and abdominal cavities.

Intravenous lipid

Various commercial fat emulsions are available, prepared from soyabean oil or cotton-seed oil with phospholipid emulsifiers. They are metabolised as chylomicrons. These preparations provide high energy in low volume (p. 55) for parenteral nutrition: 1 litre of a 20 per cent preparation supplies about 8.4 MJ (2000 kcal).

General lipid metabolism

In the plasma the chylomicrons which have been absorbed are maintained as discrete particles. They are rapidly deposited, mainly in the fat-storage depots (adipose tissue), the remainder in the liver and muscles.

Lipoprotein lipase, which functions on the surface of the capillary endothelium, is responsible for uptake of chylomicrons into extrahepatic tissue; this uptake is accompanied by hydrolysis of triglyceride, and its resynthesis within the cells. There is normally no lipoprotein lipase in plasma except after an injection of heparin – which results in the clearing of lipaemia. There is a rare *lipoprotein lipase deficiency*, in which chylomicrons accumulate in the liver.

Adipose tissue forms about 15 per cent of the body weight in health. This is maintained directly from the gut, from the liver via β-lipoproteins, or by synthesis in situ. Hydrolysis of triglyceride in adipose tissue requires a different lipase, and provides energy with great efficiency.

Free fatty acids

The glycerol which has been released by hydrolysis of fat enters general carbohydrate metabolism via glyceraldehyde and is either converted to glycogen or oxidised. The free fatty acids (FFA; or non-esterified fatty acids, NEFA, as most fatty acids are esterified with glycerol or cholesterol) of the plasma are derived mainly from hydrolysis of chylomicrons or of depot fat; in the fasting state they are a major source of energy. Their plasma concentration (0.3–0.6 mmol/l in the fasting state) is lowered by glucose and insulin which inhibit release of FFA; and is usually raised in diabetes mellitus or after starvation or severe exercise, due to excess lipolysis. The product of oxidation·of fatty acids is the coenzyme-linked 2-carbon atom unit, acetyl CoA, which can be further oxidised in the common metabolic pool (p. 56); or else converted via acetoacetyl CoA to acetoacetate in the liver, normally in small quantities. If FFA are produced at a rate greater than that at which they are oxidised, they are converted by a reaction with glycerol 3-phosphate (from the metabolism of glucose) in the liver and adipose tissue back to triglycerides.

Ketosis

The reference range for plasma total ketones, as acetoacetate, is less than 0.2 mmol/l. Normally acetoacetate is an energy source and is oxidised in skeletal or cardiac muscle via acetyl CoA, by combination with oxaloacetate and entering the tricarboxylic acid (TCA) cycle. Some acetoacetate may be converted to the other 'ketone' bodies, 3-hydroxybutyrate (by reduction: *not* a ketone) and acetone (by decarboxylation) (Fig. 6.2). The state of ketosis exists when acetoacetate and other ketone bodies accumulate in the plasma. The principal causes of ketosis are starvation and diabetes mellitus (p. 63). In starvation, because of lack of carbohydrate, energy requirements are met from depot fat via FFA, and excess ketones are therefore produced in the liver and pass into the plasma – at a rate faster than they can be utilised in the muscles. In diabetes mellitus, glycerol 3-phosphate is not available to take up the excess FFA produced: it is also possible that oxaloacetate

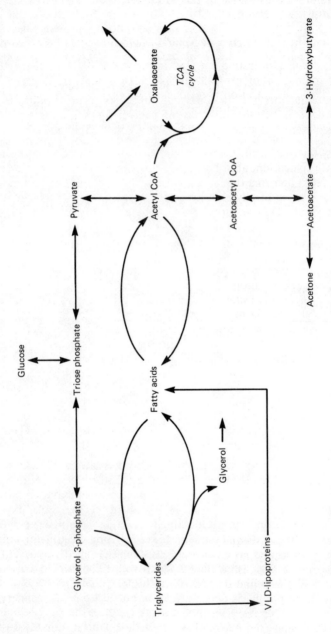

Fig. 6.2. Simplified scheme of the metabolic relations between triglycerides, fatty acids, glucose and the tricarboxylic acid cycle, and acetoacetate and the other ketone bodies.

(from amino acids etc.) has been excessively utilised for gluconeogenesis and is therefore less available to take up acetyl CoA. The excess acetyl CoA is converted to ketones.

Triglycerides and lipaemia

The reference range for fasting plasma triglycerides is 0.3–1.8 mmol/l, this being a combination of exogeneous and endogenous triglycerides in transport. This concentration is insufficient to alter the transparency of the plasma. Pancreatic lipases are present in plasma at too low an activity to have any significant effect on the circulating triglyceride.

Lipaemia means milkiness of the plasma, associated with an increase in its triglyceride content. Generally an increase in the circulating triglyceride concentration above about 5 mmol/l causes an opalescent plasma. In gross lipaemia the fat content may be above about 10 mmol/l, and a creamy layer of chylomicrons appears in the plasma when it is allowed to stand. Diffuse turbidity, without a creamy layer, indicates excess VLDL and not chylomicrons. If there is lipaemia, there is also often an increase in the plasma phospholipid and cholesterol concentrations.

Lipaemia, due to disease or to intravenous lipid, spuriously lowers the total plasma concentration of components such as sodium that are dissolved in the plasma *water*: osmolality (p. 22) however is not affected.

Physiological lipaemia may be seen 1–6 hours after a fatty meal.

Lipaemia may be due to excessive mobilisation of triglyceride (transport lipaemia), and this can occur in diabetes mellitus, liver insufficiency (especially alcoholic cirrhosis and von Gierke's disease), and in alcoholism, severe anaemia and leukaemia. Protein deficiency from any cause often leads to transport lipaemia, and such lipaemia develops in starvation. Hypoproteinaemia and increased production could be a cause of the lipaemia that occurs in the nephrotic syndrome, but there is also impaired utilisation. Lipaemia is seen in chronic pancreatitis, when it may possibly be due to deficiency of a pancreatic lipotropic factor: often recurrent pancreatitis is an outcome of continued lipaemia. Lipaemia is also a feature of some types of primary hyperlipidaemia.

Phospholipids

The most widely distributed phospholipids are the lecithins. They contain glycerol (as the base) and choline (Fig. 6.1): sphingomyelins contain sphingosine as base, and no glycerol. A small quantity of phospholipid is present in food; this is probably hydrolysed before absorption. Phospholipid synthesis and degradation occur within each cell. Most of the lecithin in the plasma is derived from synthesis in the liver, and the reference range for plasma phospholipids (as lecithin) is 1.8–3.0 mmol/l. The estimation of plasma phospholipid is technically difficult and rarely requested.

The plasma phospholipid level is increased in many conditions that cause lipaemia, for example, anaemia, diabetes, nephrotic syndrome, and biliary cirrhosis; and rarely in primary hyperlipoproteinaemias. The phospholipid level is normal in parenchymatous liver disease and in obstructive jaundice without biliary cirrhosis. A low plasma phospholipid level is found in malnutrition and in acute liver insufficiency.

Amniotic fluid. When the fetal pulmonary alveolar lining matures after 35 weeks, it synthesises more dipalmitoyl lecithin which is the major surface-active compound, and this passes into the amniotic fluid: production of sphingomyelin changes little. In suspected abnormal pregnancy, if the amniotic fluid lecithin/sphingomyelin (L/S) ratio is less than 2.0, then the fetal alveoli are immature and the respiratory distress syndrome (RDS) may occur after delivery.

Respiratory secretions. The same analysis may be done on a hypopharyngeal aspirate of a neonate with respiratory distress. An L/S ratio of less than 1.5 is an additional diagnostic aid for RDS.

Cholesterol

Metabolism

Cholesterol is the only steroid that exists in appreciable concentration throughout the body. Dietary cholesterol, which is of animal origin, is absorbed to a limited extent into the lymphatic system in the presence of bile salts and after partial esterification with fatty acids. Plant steroids, except ergosterol (pro-vitamin D), are poorly absorbed by man. Most of the cholesterol requirements of the body are synthesised endogenously from acetyl CoA via β-hydroxy-β-methyl glutamyl CoA. All cells are probably capable of synthesising cholesterol, but most of the cholesterol in the body is produced by the liver. It is carried in the plasma mainly as LDL.

Cholesterol is concerned with the metabolism of lipids, and is a source for synthesis of the steroid hormones. It is excreted into the bile as unchanged cholesterol, or as cholic acid or chenodeoxycholic acid (the bile acids): cholesterol is held in solution in bile by bile salts and phospholipids (p. 205). Cholesterol released from peripheral tissues is esterified in the plasma with fatty acids taken from lecithin by lecithin-cholesterol acyltransferase (LCAT), and transported as HDL to the liver. This ester cholesterol may be transferred to other lipoproteins by exchange with triglycerides. A decrease of plasma ester cholesterol occurs when there is parenchymal liver cell damage, due to deficiency of LCAT which comes from the liver. There is a rare *LCAT deficiency*, in which free cholesterol accumulates in plasma and tissues.

The estimated plasma cholesterol concentration varies with the specificity of the method. Using an enzymatic procedure, acceptable overall reference values for adults are 4.0–6.5 mmol/l, varying with the population sampled, increasing with advancing age, and until age 50 being higher in men. The ester cholesterol is 65–75 per cent of the total plasma cholesterol.

Clinical aspects

In clinical practice the total plasma cholesterol is commonly estimated. It is raised in many of the conditions which are associated with secondary lipaemia, the combination being commonly seen in diabetes mellitus, nephrotic syndrome, primary myxoedema, and biliary cirrhosis. Many types of primary hyperlipidaemia (with or without lipaemia) have a raised plasma cholesterol.

A high value is found in late pregnancy. Retention hypercholesterolaemia, due to failure of cholesterol excretion in the bile, develops in obstructive jaundice and chronic hepatitis of any type. In mild parenchymatous liver damage, e.g. infective hepatitis, the total plasma cholesterol level may be slightly increased, but the percentage of ester cholesterol is diminished. Estimation of plasma cholesterol used to be common practice in following the progress of a case of primary myxoedema, for the level returns to normal as treatment is successful. In atheroma, although cholesterol and other lipids are deposited in the arteries, there is an epidemiological and not an individual relationship (except in the rare familial hypercholesterolaemia) between a raised plasma cholesterol and the existence and extent of atheroma. Even if the plasma cholesterol is not above the reference values, this excludes neither the presence of atheroma nor the risk of a subsequent myocardial infarction.

A lowered plasma cholesterol is found in the presence of severe infection, in severe anaemia, in massive parenchymatous liver damage, and too inconsistently in hyperthyroidism to have any diagnostic value. Findings in malnutrition are variable, but plasma cholesterol is usually low.

Xanthomatosis. In a wide variety of conditions cholesterol and other lipids are deposited in foam cells in the skin with the formation of yellow nodules. This may develop in hypercholesterolaemia associated with lipaemia (as in diabetes), in the hypercholesterolaemia of biliary cirrhosis without lipaemia, or in certain types of familial primary hyperlipidaemia. The xanthomatosis which occurs with lipaemia improves as the lipaemia decreases. Xanthomas can be found with a normal plasma cholesterol and triglyceride levels, as in the Hand-Schüller-Christian syndrome.

Carotenoids

Vitamin A is readily absorbed into the lacteals, whereas β-carotene, which is poorly absorbed from the bowel into the portal system, can be converted to Vitamin A in the intestinal mucosa and in the liver.

The fasting plasma carotenoid level is 1.0–5.5 μmol/l (as β-carotene). Carotenaemia is associated with a yellow pigmentation of the skin and a high icterus index (p. 192) but carotenoids do not react with chemical reagents for bilirubin. Carotenaemia is often present in association with lipaemia (in diabetes mellitus or myxoedema) and as the result of unusual diets such as eating enormous quantities of carrots. There is usually a low plasma carotene level in steatorrhoea; however, a normal level does not exclude malabsorption of fats.

The reference range for fasting plasma vitamin A is 1.0–3.0 μmol/l. Though a low level does not necessarily mean vitamin A deficiency, a consistently high value excludes this.

LIPOPROTEINS IN PLASMA

In the plasma the various lipids (mainly triglycerides, phospholipids, and cholesterol) do not circulate in the free state as they are insoluble, but are combined with carrier apoproteins to form a series of soluble lipoproteins.

Lipoprotein analysis and classification

The reference range for total plasma lipoprotein concentration is 300–800 mg/100 ml, though this measurement is little used. Different analytical procedures divide the plasma lipoproteins into different groupings, though they are a continuous set of decreasing density corresponding to increasing triglyceride concentration. The important methods are electrophoresis and ultracentrifugation, associated with chemical analysis of the separate lipids. Ultracentrifugation is an expensive research technique. Nephelometry, after fractionation of plasma by filtration through pores of different sizes, can be used to express lipoprotein concentrations in terms of Small, Medium, and Large (S; M; L) particles, though the clinical value of this procedure is doubtful. Methods are available for the separate estimation of HDL (cholesterol) and of LDL-β-lipoprotein.

Electrophoresis of normal fasting plasma (on agarose) almost always shows α-lipoprotein, pre-β-lipoprotein, and β-lipoprotein. Chylomicrons are detectable after a fatty meal and remain at the origin (Fig. 6.3).

Ultracentrifugation divides the lipoproteins, by convention, into classes:

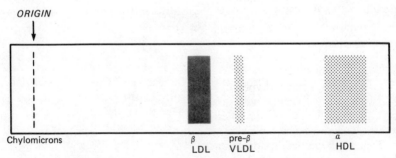

FIG. 6.3. Electrophoresis of normal plasma on agarose for lipoproteins.

(a) high density (HDL) of molecular weight about 200 000 and specific gravity (relative density) >1.063;

(b) low density (LDL) of molecular weight about 2 000 000 and specific gravity 1.006–1.063;

(c) very low density (VLDL) of molecular weight about 6 000 000 and specific gravity <1.006.

When graded in Svedberg flotation units (S_f), LDL are S_f 0–20, VLDL are S_f 20–400, and chylomicrons are S_f >400 (S_f 20 implies the same relative density as protein-free plasma).

There is general correspondence between the classifications. Chylomicrons consist almost entirely of exogenous (dietary) triglycerides, the apoproteins being A, B, and C. β-Lipoproteins are LDL, and contain mainly cholesterol, with carrier protein (apo B) and phospholipid, and little triglyceride. Pre-β-lipoproteins are VLDL, and contain mainly endogenous (hepatic) triglyceride, with some protein (apo B and C), cholesterol, and phospholipid. α-Lipoproteins are HDL, and contain 50 per cent protein (apo A and C), with cholesterol and phospholipid, and little triglyceride. Using nephelometry, S corresponds roughly to LDL, M to VLDL, and L to chylomicrons.

The plasma lipoproteins are derived from the liver, which produces VLDL and HDL. In the plasma LDL is formed from VLDL by the action of lipoprotein lipase.

Hyperlipoproteinaemias

The classification of the hyperlipoproteinaemias and hyperlipidaemias is complex, and no system is ideal. That of Fredrickson, which pays most attention to electrophoretic differentiation, is widely used, and is most satisfactory for consideration of primary genetic abnormalities, whilst less useful for the more common secondary disorders. The main types all represent a variety of conditions, and there are other rarer types.

In the investigation of hyperlipoproteinaemia, it is usual to analyse plasma after 10–14 h fasting (and preferably a normal diet for two weeks), and no alcohol for 24 h. The necessary investigations are visual inspection, and analysis for cholesterol and triglycerides. If any of these are abnormal the electrophoretic pattern is valuable. Plasma should be looked at after being allowed to stand at 4 °C for 18 h. A creamy layer signifies chylomicrons: diffuse turbidity means endogenous hypertriglyceridaemia.

Primary disorders

Fredrickson Type I (hyperchylomicronaemia), which is rare, shows a slightly creamy plasma with a heavy chylomicron band, high triglycerides and slightly raised cholesterol. The clinical presentation includes xanthomas and hepatosplenomegaly with abdominal pain.

Type II (hyperbetalipoproteinaemia) shows (IIa) a clear plasma with a heavy β-band, a high cholesterol and normal triglycerides – this type includes *familial hypercholesterolaemia*, which has a very high incidence of atheroma and of xanthomas. A variant (IIb) also has a slightly increased pre-β-band and triglycerides. Clinically there are xanthomas (and tendon xanthomas), and arterial disease and ischaemic heart disease may develop.

Type III, which is rare, shows a turbid plasma, with an anomalous broad β- to pre-β-band; and a raised cholesterol and triglycerides. Clinically there are xanthomas, and often atheroma and impaired glucose tolerance.

Type IV (endogenous hypertriglyceridaemia) shows a turbid plasma, with an increased pre-β-band, and triglycerides raised more than cholesterol. Clinically there are xanthomas, and often arterial and ischaemic heart disease, and impaired glucose tolerance. The possibly related *Type V* also has increased chylomicrons.

Secondary disorders

In a large number of disease states increase of one or more of the plasma lipid components is usual. An increased plasma cholesterol is usually measured, and increases in triglyceride and phospholipids are often found. The abnormal lipid patterns are variable. In myxoedema, biliary obstruction, and nephrotic syndrome, type IIb is probably the commonest; whilst diabetes mellitus, chronic nephritis, and sometimes alcoholism and myelomatosis, may present as Type IV. Cholestasis often also shows an abnormal group of lipoproteins, known as LP-X (p. 203).

In atheroma and coronary artery disease patients tend to have an increase in pre-β and β-lipoproteins, and in plasma triglycerides and cholesterol. It has been suggested that a high plasma HDL is protective against atheroma, and that HDL should therefore be routinely measured. It appears that a reduction in dietary carbohydrate cholesterol and fat, with a relative increase in polyunsaturated fat, tends to reduce the plasma cholesterol and VLDL concentrations in patients with atheroma. But other factors as diverse as exercise, or exogenous or endogenous oestrogens, and various drugs, may also lower the plasma lipids and may also decrease the liability to coronary artery disease. However, high dose oral contraceptives may increase α-lipoproteins. The causative relationships between diet, plasma lipids, atheroma, and coronary thrombosis are still controversial. In routine individual or epidemiological investigations of atheroma and coronary artery disease, estimation of plasma cholesterol and triglycerides is usually sufficient. Further tests should be done if either of these is abnormal, or if there is reason to suspect a primary hyperlipoproteinaemia.

Hypolipoproteinaemias

There are a number of rare congenital diseases. *Abetalipoproteinaemia* has intestinal malabsorption of lipid, with a very low plasma cholesterol and absent β-lipoproteins and chylomicrons. *Tangier disease* (alphalipo-protein deficiency) has lipid accumulation in the lymphoreticular system, with a low plasma cholesterol and absent α-lipoprotein.

LIPID DEPOSITION

Fatty liver

The liver is important in lipid metabolism, and in many diseases the fat content of the liver may be greatly increased. In starvation and diabetes mellitus, FFA are produced in large amounts, and the excess which is not oxidised is deposited in the liver; liver function is here not seriously impaired. Disturbance of liver metabolism by various poisons results in extensive fatty deposition in the liver without changes in plasma lipids: such toxins may be endogenous (as in toxaemia of pregnancy) or exogenous chemicals (e.g. carbon tetrachloride).

The lipotropic factors are substances responsible for the normal hepatic metabolism of lipids. Choline is an important dietary lipotropic factor, whose essential function may be the synthesis of lecithin. Methionine, which can donate methyl groups for choline synthesis, is also lipotropic; consequently protein-deficiency predisposes to the development of fatty liver.

Chronic alcoholism. Fatty liver is common. Alcohol has a direct hepatotoxic action (causing an early rise in plasma GGT–p. 198), quite apart from the protein- and choline-deficient, vitamins B-deficient, high energy diet of alcoholic patients. There is diversion of fatty acids from oxidation to esterification as triglycerides. These both accumulate in the liver, and are released into the plasma as the characteristic Type IV hyper-lipidaemia.

The lipidoses

Certain rare inborn errors of metabolism are associated with a disturbance of synthesis or disposal of intracellular lipid, whilst the levels of circulating lipids are within the reference range. They are generally due to specific enzyme defects within lysosomes which can be identified in affected organs. The same enzyme defects can often be found in leucocytes, which may be a simpler tissue to obtain for analysis; or in fetal cells to be cultured for prenatal diagnosis (p. 165).

Hand-Schüller-Christian syndrome is a group of disorders in which cholesterol is deposited in the skin (where xanthomas appear), brain, spleen, lymph glands, and bones. *Niemann-Pick's disease* is a group of familial diseases in which the phospholipid sphingomyelin may be deposited throughout the body, particularly in liver and spleen. *Gaucher's disease* is a group of familial diseases in which a glucocerebroside called kerasin is deposited in the reticulo-endothelial system: there is also a high plasma

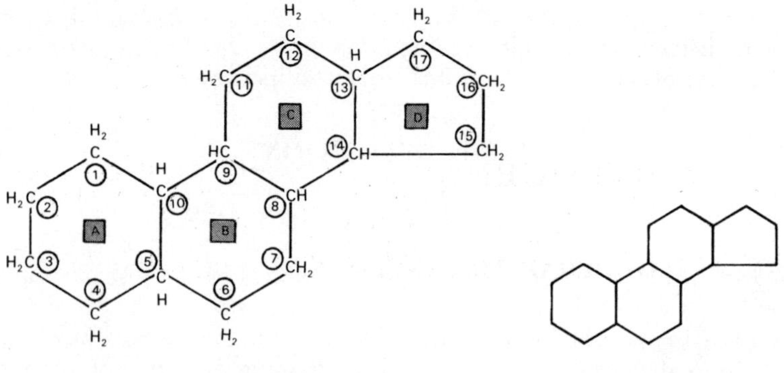

FIG. 6.4. (a) Structure of the saturated unsubstituted cyclopentenophenanthrene ring compound, with the carbon atoms numbered and the rings labelled. (b) Shorthand formula of this compound.

acid phosphatase, derived from the Gaucher's cells. *Tay-Sach's disease* (*infantile amaurotic idiocy*) is a familial disease in which an unusual cerebroside, called ganglioside, is deposited in the central nervous system. *Wolman's disease*, with hepatosplenomegaly, has cholesterol esters and triglycerides as the abnormally stored compounds.

THE STEROIDS

The steroids are a group of substances of great medical and pharmacological importance which contain the cyclopentenophenanthrene ring system (Fig. 6.4). Sterols are steroids which contain a hydroxyl (–OH) group. The steroids differ from one another in the spatial arrangement of their rings and side chains, as well as in the nature of the side chains attached to the rings.

The classes of steroids of interest in clinical biochemistry include cholesterol (p. 82), precursors of vitamin D (p. 176), bile acids (p. 199), adrenocortical hormones (p. 153), oestrogens (p. 161), progestogens (p. 163), androgens (p. 167).

Further reading

Lewis B. Hyperlipidaemia and cardiovascular disease. In: Baron DN, Compston N, Dawson AM, eds. *Recent Advances in Medicine 17*. Edinburgh: Churchill-Livingstone, 1977:245–275.

McGowan GK, Walters, G, eds. Disorders of lipid metabolism. *J Clin Path* 1973; 26:Suppl. 5.

Thompson G. Plasma lipoproteins and their disorders. *Medicine* 3rd series 1978; 11:558–565.

CHAPTER 7

NITROGENOUS COMPOUNDS

GENERAL METABOLISM OF PROTEIN

Dietary protein

A reasonable protein intake for an adult is about 1 g/kg body weight per day, and the actual intake varies according to prosperity and local custom. Protein should provide 10 per cent of the energy requirements – the energy value being about 17 kJ (4 kcal) per gram. The protein allowance for children must be relatively higher to allow for the protein needs of growth: 2–3 g/kg for infants and about 2 g/kg for children have been advocated. In late pregnancy and during lactation the mother's daily diet must contain at least 1 g of protein/kg body weight. These allowances of protein are more than the minimum needed just for equilibrium.

The diet must not only contain sufficient protein, but the protein intake must be qualitatively adequate. Proteins are sometimes classified as first-class and second-class proteins. First-class proteins are capable by themselves of supporting growth, since they contain all the essential amino acids in the right proportions and because these amino acids are readily released by digestion – an amino acid is called 'essential' if it must be provided in the diet because the metabolic requirements cannot be met by synthesis within the body. Second-class proteins do not satisfy these conditions. Most animal proteins are first-class proteins, a notable exception being gelatin. Most second-class proteins are vegetable proteins.

A normal good vegetarian diet, which includes the animal products milk and eggs, contains ample first-class protein. A vegan diet, which is a strictly vegetarian diet omitting all animal products, does not lead to protein deficiency in adults with no extra needs if the diet is otherwise satisfactory.

Effects of dietary protein deficiency

A diet which is moderately inadequate in protein (due to poverty or lack of knowledge) may give rise to fatigue and irritability before symptoms of gross protein deficiency develop. In children protein deficiency retards growth. At all ages prolonged protein deficiency causes anorexia and apathy, muscle wasting, loss of weight (which may be masked by retention of water), poor wound healing, and slow convalescence after illness. There is often a hypochromic anaemia because synthesis of haemoglobin is impaired. Retention of water causes oedema, for which the hypoalbuminaemia is not the only cause. This oedema may develop without detectable change in the levels of the plasma proteins, which are maintained at the expense of the tissue proteins. Eventually, however, there is a marked fall in the level of the plasma albumin and transferrin. Alteration in the plasma globulins is variable, depending on the presence of infections (p. 113). The plasma concentrations of prealbumin and retinol-binding protein are reduced early, and these have also been suggested as markers of protein malnutrition. Liver damage and pulmonary tuberculosis are diseases to which protein-deficient subjects are particularly vulnerable. Damage to the liver occurs because diets which are deficient in protein lack the lipotropic factors (p. 87) that protect the integrity of liver cells. There are also usually associated deficiencies of the vitamin B complex. In kwashiorkor, the protein-deficiency syndrome of children in the tropics who live mainly on carbohydrate, oedema and other symptoms are associated with skin and hair changes. Failure to produce proteolytic digestive enzymes reduces further the small amount of available amino acids. In marasmus, with protein and carbohydrate deficiency, there is less oedema or skin and hair change than in kwashiorkor.

In protein deficiency, 1 kilogram of body weight loss means about 30 grams of nitrogen loss. For biochemical assessment of protein malnutrition, plasma albumin concentration is the most available measure, and due note must be taken of any changes in plasma volume. However, albumin does not respond to rapid changes in nutritional status, and for this the measurement of plasma prealbumin (p. 106) is better.

Protein digestion, absorption, and metabolism

No digestion of protein takes place in the mouth. Gastric juice contains pepsinogen; hydrochloric acid activates pepsinogen to pepsin, and provides the optimum pH for pepsin to digest some protein to polypeptides. Human pepsin also has a rennin-like activity causing coagulation of milk. However, peptic activity is not essential for protein digestion which proceeds satisfactorily when pepsin is deficient, or is inactive due to achlorhydria. Pancreatic juice contains trypsinogen which is activated to trypsin by enterokinase, secreted by the small intestine; chymotrypsin(ogen) and carboxypolypeptidase are other pancreatic proteolytic enzymes. The alkaline pancreatic juice provides the optimum pH for their activity. Trypsin digests protein to short chain peptides and to a limited extent to free amino acids. In chronic pancreatic disease (p. 237) protein digestion may be severely impaired due to trypsin deficiency. A group of intestinal peptidases completes the digestive process by converting peptides to amino acids, though some peptides are not fully digested.

Amino acids from food protein and endogenous protein are readily absorbed by the small intestine. Peptides and possibly even traces of protein can be absorbed undigested: peptides can be hydrolysed by peptidases to amino acids within the brush border. Intestinal disorders associated with malabsorption of fat, such as coeliac disease (p. 240), do not generally cause severe impairment of amino acid absorption. In ulcerative colitis and after massive resection of the gut there is some impaired absorption of the end-products of protein digestion, and also impairment of their digestion (p. 239).

Simple nitrogenous materials, such as ammonium ions, are readily absorbed.

The exogenous and endogenous amino acids pass in the portal system to the liver, and deamination of a proportion of these amino acids takes place there. The amino groups and carbon residues may be used for synthesis of other amino acids, or other nitrogenous compounds. Amino acids as such are not stored: the surplus amino groups are eventually converted to urea, whilst the carbon residues are metabolised in the common metabolic pool and converted to carbohydrate or lipid, or oxidised (p. 56). The remainder are used for protein synthesis in the cells.

Protein stores. There is no absolute distinction between endogenous and exogenous protein metabolism. A few hours after administration of labelled amino acids, isotopic nitrogen can be found in all the protein of the body: and an average adult turns over about 400 g of protein daily. The half-life of plasma albumin is about 15 days, of muscle protein is about 5 months, and of collagen is many years. When a cell dies, its protein is reconverted by lysosomes to amino acids. Although some proteins are more stable than others there is no specialised storage product or deposit protein. There is in the tissues a certain amount of labile protein, which can be utilised when protein intake is insufficient and which serves to stave off the development of the protein-deficiency state. The plasma proteins are maintained at the expense of all the other labile proteins of the body.

Nitrogen excretion

A normal adult ingests 10–15 g of nitrogen per day in dietary protein – on average 1 g nitrogen is derived from about 6 g protein. Faecal excretion of nitrogen is relatively constant, within the limits of 1–1.5 g (70–110 mmol)/24 h, despite changes in the protein intake. It consists partly of nitrogenous material of the diet which has not been digested or absorbed, partly of end-products of nitrogenous metabolism which have been actively excreted into the bowel, and partly of intestinal bacterial and cell nitrogen. In total protein starvation the faecal nitrogen excretion is about 0.5 g (35 mmol)/24 h. Most of the endogenous protein from intestinal secretions (principally enzymes) and desquamated cells, which amounts to about 50 g protein per 24 hours, is digested and reabsorbed. Some urea which diffuses into the gut is hydrolysed (by bacterial ureases) to ammonia which is reabsorbed.

Undigested muscle fibres are not seen in the faeces of healthy persons on a normal diet, but they may be found when faecal nitrogen is increased as a result of impaired protein digestion. Changes in nitrogen excretion in pancreatic disease and in coeliac disease are discussed in chapter 14.

Losses of nitrogen in hair, desquamated skin, and sweat, are about 1 g (70 mmol)/24 h. Nitrogen is also lost in the menstruum. The remainder of the end-products of nitrogen metabolism are excreted in the urine. Only traces of protein (p. 214) are found in the urine in health. Nitrogen is principally excreted in the urine as urea, and with a fall or rise in the protein intake the principal excretory change is in the urine urea; the normal urine urea nitrogen is 80–85 per cent of the total urinary nitrogen. Lesser quantities of nitrogen are lost in the urine as ammonia, as amino acids, as uric acid (the end-product of purine metabolism), as creatinine (the end-product of creatine metabolism in muscles), and as many other identified and unidentified nitrogenous compounds. There is probably no net gain or loss of nitrogen through the lungs as nitrogen or ammonia gas.

Nitrogen balance

A normal adult is in nitrogen equilibrium – the intake of nitrogen in the diet in all its forms is equal to the excretion of nitrogen as metabolic end-products with a measurable daily variation of about ± 10 per cent. A positive nitrogen balance is defined as a state in which the body is retaining nitrogen; and a negative nitrogen balance is a state in which nitrogen is being lost. When the nitrogen intake is reduced (but still remains above the minimum need for equilibrium) a negative nitrogen balance will occur for a few days, then equilibrium will be restored at the lower intake level. When the nitrogen intake is increased the opposite happens: after a short period of positive balance a new steady state is reached.

Effect of hormones. Anabolism and catabolism of protein are to a certain extent under hormonal control. Adrenocorticotrophic hormone and the glucocorticoids, and excess thyroxine, promote protein catabolism and a negative nitrogen balance. Growth hormone, the androgens, to a lesser extent the gonadotrophins and oestrogens, and thyroxine and insulin in physiological amounts, promote protein anabolism and a positive nitrogen balance.

Positive nitrogen balance

This develops during growth and pregnancy, and during recovery from periods of negative nitrogen balance – e.g. in the late post-operative period, if protein intake is adequate. A positive balance develops as a result of the action of excess of the nitrogen anabolic hormones, either due to excess secretion (e.g. in acromegaly) or when given as treatment (e.g. during testosterone therapy). A high protein intake is never harmful in a healthy subject: it is more likely in any person to lead to a positive nitrogen balance and to increase of tissue protein if the diet is adequate in energy with sufficient carbohydrate, fat, and vitamins of the B group.

Negative nitrogen balance

Deficient protein intake. A prolonged negative nitrogen balance leads to protein deficiency. When the protein intake falls below the appropriate minimum, a negative nitrogen balance develops within 48 hours. A negative balance also develops when protein intake is just within the minimum needed for equilibrium and this protein is not qualitatively adequate or the total energy intake is deficient.

Diminished protein digestion. This results from deficiency of proteolytic enzymes due to chronic pancreatic disease (p. 237).

Diminished absorption of amino acids. This develops in severe intestinal disease, or after massive resection of the small intestine (p. 239), or as part of an inherited transport defect (p. 242).

Increased protein catabolism. When there is excess breakdown of body protein the released nitrogen is excreted, and negative balance develops unless nitrogen intake is increased. Certain types of endocrine disturbance directly increase protein catabolism – negative balance develops in thyrotoxicosis or Cushing's syndrome and sometimes at the menopause, and after prolonged treatment with adrenocorticotrophic hormone or cortisone. In wasting processes, including diabetic coma, increased tissue protein breakdown is found. After severe trauma (due to wounds, fracture, or surgical operation), during the course of a severe acute or chronic infection, in malignant disease, or after rest in bed, negative nitrogen balance usually develops, which is partly due to excessive secretion of glucocorticoids. However, patients who have been on a protein-deficient diet do not go into further negative nitrogen balance after injury. Equilibrium may be restored after the protein reserves are exhausted.

Increased protein loss. At each normal menstrual period up to 20 g of protein may be lost, but this is insufficient to cause protein depletion provided an adequate diet is taken. Considerable quantities of protein may be lost from severely burned areas (10–50 g/day), or into the urine in the nephrotic syndrome or in myelomatosis. In exfoliative dermatitis, and similar conditions, skin protein loss may be 20 g/day. Even larger quantities of protein may be lost as pus, for example from a lung abscess or through osteomyelitic sinuses. The *protein-losing enteropathies* are a group of disorders of the gastrointestinal tract, including malignant disease, ulcerative colitis, and sprue, in which there is non-selective excessive leakage of plasma proteins into the gut; although much of the protein is digested and absorbed, the liver cannot resynthesise sufficient extra protein (p. 188). In haemorrhage (to the exterior or into the gut), albumin and globulins, as well as haemoglobin, are lost: 1 litre of blood contains about 200 g of protein, so donation of a 'unit' of blood takes off about 80 g of protein. Formation of ascites causes loss of protein from the circulation into transcellular fluid (p. 21) where exchange is slow, though this loss is not strictly from the body until the ascites is tapped: peritoneal dialysis may remove 25 g of protein per day. In many diseases loss of protein happens at the same time as increased protein catabolism.

Balance tests

Accurate measurement of the state of nitrogen metabolism may be done by means of a *metabolic balance test*. In this the patient's intake and output of nitrogen (or calcium, or other metabolite) are measured over an accurately timed period – usually between three and seven days. A balance test requires skilled ward staff, preferably in a special Metabolic Unit, to ensure that the dietary intake is controlled, and that all the patient's faeces and urine are collected at the correct times.

The results, in the case of a nitrogen balance, will be expressed as:

Average 24-hour intake $\quad\quad\quad\quad\quad$ A g (or A′ mmol) nitrogen
Average 24-hour output in urine $\quad\quad$ B g (or B′ mmol) nitrogen
Average 24-hour output in faeces (or
$\quad$ other source of loss) $\quad\quad\quad\quad$ C g (or C′ mmol) nitrogen
24-hour balance $= A - (B + C)$ grams (or $A' - (B' + C')$ mmol)

The test has a reproducibility of about ± 10 per cent, which is accounted for by slight short-term variations in the patient's nitrogen metabolism, and by errors in collection and analysis. A variation in nitrogen balance during the course of the test may be shown by a change in values for plasma nitrogenous components such as albumin, urea, and creatinine.

Biochemical aspects of treatment

A state of prolonged negative nitrogen balance usually demands treatment; but it may prove impossible to correct the negative nitrogen balance fully by protein replacement, particularly when it is due to toxic destruction of protein or to renal loss. The balance will return to normal when the cause, for example protein loss, is removed, and the lost protein is replaced. In all circumstances the patient must be placed on as high a protein diet as possible, and the diet must also be adequate in its energy and vitamin content – 150 g of protein per day is generally suitable. If the patient is unable to digest ordinary protein food, suitably prepared milk protein or protein hydrolysate (an amino acid mixture) may be given by continuous intragastric drip in a dose of about 150 g daily.

Intravenous therapy. When protein loss cannot be fully replaced by oral feeding, protein substitutes (for general nutrition) or plasma (to replace plasma proteins) can be given intravenously. This method of administration may be used when there are disorders of amino acid absorption.

Commercial amino acid preparations are available for intravenous use that, given adequate carbohydrate and appropriate electrolytes, can maintain a positive nitrogen balance and may be used in connection with major surgery. A 10 per cent solution (casein hydrolysate or a mixture of synthetic L-amino acids) provides about 12 g of nitrogen per litre.

NON-PROTEIN NITROGEN CONSTITUENTS OF THE BLOOD AND URINE

The term 'blood non-protein nitrogen (NPN) comprises urea, urate, creatine and creatinine, amino acids, and minor components; and in health about 50 per cent consists of urea. Total NPN is no longer estimated, for changes in the plasma urea usually reflect adequately total protein catabolism, and the other NPN constituents are estimated individually when required.

Urea

Urea is formed, almost solely in the liver, from the catabolism of amino acids, and is the main excretion product of protein metabolism. The concentration of urea in the blood plasma represents mainly a balance between urea formation from protein catabolism and urea excretion by the kidneys: some urea is further metabolised and a small amount is lost in the sweat and faeces.

The reference range for plasma urea concentration throughout adult life is 3.0–6.5 mmol/l. Urea diffuses freely, at the same concentration, through all the body water. The whole blood urea level is 5–10 per cent lower than the plasma urea level. In the USA results are still often expressed as blood urea nitrogen (BUN), the reference range being 9–20 mg/100 ml – about half of urea is nitrogen.

The classical method for estimating urea requires its conversion to ammonia by the specific enzyme urease, and measurement of the ammonia: a colorimetric method based on a reaction with diacetyl monoxime is now widely used. Analysis of plasma (or often of whole blood) for concentration of urea is perhaps the commonest estimation performed in clinical biochemistry laboratories. There are rapid commercial strip tests (Urastrat: William R. Warner; Azostix: Ames), based on the urease reaction, for approximate estimation of plasma urea.

The plasma urea increases with age even in the absence of detectable renal disease, although the changes are certainly due to alteration of renal function: concentrations are also slightly higher in men. A single protein meal does not significantly increase the plasma urea level. The fasting plasma urea is higher on a high protein diet than on a low protein diet.

High plasma urea

This is one of the commonest abnormal findings in chemical pathology, and its causes are classified as:

Increased tissue protein catabolism associated with a negative nitrogen balance. This occurs for example, in fevers, wasting diseases, thyrotoxicosis, diabetic coma, or after trauma or a major operation. If as is often the case the increase of protein catabolism is small, and there is no primary or secondary renal damage, then urinary excretion will dispose of the excess urea and there will be no significant rise of the plasma urea.

Excess breakdown of blood protein. In leukaemia release of leucocyte protein contributes to the high plasma urea. Erythrocyte haemoglobin and plasma proteins can be released into the gut due to bleeding from gastrointestinal disease, and digested: there is often an associated low blood volume with secondary impairment of renal function.

Diminished excretion of urea. This is the commonest and most important cause and may be pre-renal, renal, or post-renal. A fall in the peripheral blood pressure (as in shock), or venous congestion (as in congestive heart failure), or a low plasma volume and haemoconcentration (as in sodium depletion from any cause, including Addison's disease), diminishes the renal plasma flow. Glomerular filtration of urea falls and there is a rise in the plasma urea. In mild cases, when there is no permanent renal structural damage, the plasma urea will return to normal when the pre-renal condition is restored to normal.

Renal disease that is associated with a fall in the glomerular filtration rate causes a high plasma urea. This is typically seen in acute glomerulonephritis and in chronic renal failure, and is also found in severe destructive renal disease, acute renal failure, and the hepatorenal syndrome. The plasma urea is normal in the uncomplicated nephrotic syndrome.

Obstruction to the outflow of urine, for example by an enlarged prostate gland, leads to a high plasma urea by causing both increased reabsorption of urea through the tubules, and diminished filtration.

Azotaemia is the term used for a high blood/plasma urea concentration. *Uraemia* (as opposed to azotaemia) is the name given to the clinical syndrome that develops when there is marked nitrogen retention due to renal failure (p. 224).

Low plasma urea

This is sometimes seen in late pregnancy; it may be due to increased glomerular filtration, diversion of nitrogen to the fetus, or to water retention. In acute hepatic necrosis the plasma urea is often low, as amino acids are not further metabolised. In cirrhosis of the liver the low plasma urea is due partly to diminished synthesis, and partly to water retention (p. 202): the water retention of inappropriate antidiuretic hormone secretion lowers the plasma urea (p. 169). A low plasma urea, caused by a high rate of protein anabolism, may develop during intensive androgen treatment e.g. for carcinoma of the breast. The plasma urea falls in long-term protein malnutrition. Long-term replacement of blood loss with intravenous dextran, glucose, or saline may lower the plasma urea by dilution.

Urea assays in diagnosis

Because there are so many reasons why a plasma urea may be raised, the estimation has little diagnostic value if performed as a random procedure – but a raised plasma urea is always abnormal. The importance of plasma urea assays in investigating primary or secondary renal disease will be discussed in chapter 13.

The estimation of urine urea is, by itself, of little value. If the nitrogen intake is known a rough indication of nitrogen balance may be obtained. If the plasma urea is known it can serve as a measure of renal function, by calculation of urea clearance (p. 219).

Uric acid/urate

Uric acid is the principal end-product of nucleic acid and purine metabolism in man via a final common pathway of conversion of xanthine, by means of xanthine oxidase, to uric acid. The reference range for plasma urate in men is 0.12–0.42 mmol/l, and in women is 0.09–0.36 mmol/l, increasing slightly with age. There is a urate-binding globulin. The plasma urate level is little affected by variation in the purine content of the diet and represents a steady state between endogenous production and urinary tubular secretion, for filtered urate is normally almost wholly reabsorbed: there is also some intestinal destruction (Fig. 7.1).

Raised plasma urate

Gout. Shortly before, and during, an acute attack of gout the plasma urate rises, to a maximum level of about 0.9 mmol/l, this being usually all that is necessary for diagnosis. In chronic gout, between acute episodes, the plasma urate is usually in the high normal range and moderately raised values may be found in male relatives of patients. The cause of the high plasma urate in gout is not known in all cases, but it is usually due to increased endogenous synthesis of uric acid as an inborn metabolic defect (Fig. 7.1 I) though sometimes there is reduced renal tubular secretion (II). Alcoholism, perhaps by producing lacticacidaemia (II), and an abnormal diet high in purines (III), may be predisposing factors: some patients have hypertriglyceridaemia, associated with obesity. Allopurinol is used in the treatment of gout because, as a xanthine oxidase inhibitor (IV), it blocks the synthesis of uric acid. In gout the urate pool in the body may be over 10 times the normal 6 mmol, and sodium urate is deposited in tissues as tophi (V). Secondary renal damage due to urate deposition, sometimes with calculi, may develop. Clinical gout occurs mainly when the raised urate is due to a metabolic defect and not usually when secondary to other conditions. Urate crystals may be found in synovial fluid of the affected joints, and their identification may be of diagnostic value. In *pseudogout*, which is not a disorder of urate metabolism, the synovial fluid contains crystals of calcium pyrophosphate dihydrate.

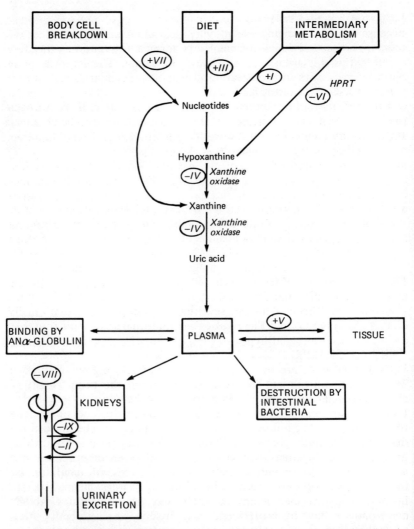

FIG. 7.1. The main pathways of uric acid metabolism and transport. The alterations in gout and other disorders, indicated by roman numerals, are described in the text.

Lesch-Nyhan syndrome. This rare inborn error of metabolism is due to deficient resynthesis of purines to nucleotides (VI), due to deficiency of hypoxanthinephosphoribosyl transferase and consequent excess production and uric acid. There is a high plasma and urine urate with urinary calculi, and sometimes gout; with mental retardation, self-mutilation, and other symptoms.

Breakdown of cell nuclei. A raised plasma urate is found in leukaemia

(especially acute leukaemia during treatment), in myeloproliferative diseases including polycythaemia, often in pernicious anaemia, and sometimes in psoriasis (VII). Treatment with adrenocorticotrophic hormone
or corticosteroids, whose protein catabolic action accelerates nuclear
breakdown, or with cytotoxic drugs, causes a rise in the plasma urate.

Renal causes. In glomerular failure, or when there is obstruction to the
outflow of urine, urate is retained with the other blood NPN constituents
(VIII). The high plasma urate which can develop in eclampsia in the
absence of azotaemia or uraemia may be due to a specific renal lesion or
to altered uric acid metabolism. Both ketotic and lactic acidosis (p. 71)
may increase the plasma urate by diminishing its renal tubular secretion,
as do frusemide and thiazide diuretics (II). The high values (sometimes
causing gout) which occur during therapeutic or other acute starvation
are due to a combination of cell breakdown and ketoacidosis.

Estimation of plasma urate is important principally for the diagnosis
and monitoring of gout and of toxaemia in pregnancy.

Low plasma urate.

This results from urinary loss in a renal tubular syndromes (p. 225), or
from failure of synthesis.

Xanthinuria. This rare inborn error of metabolism is due to deficiency
of xanthine oxidase (IV). The plasma and urine urate are therefore low,
and excess xanthine and hypoxanthine may present as xanthine calculi.

Urine uric acid.

This estimation is of little value; the quantity excreted depends to a large
extent on the purine content of the diet and is normally 1.5–4.5 mmol/24 h.
Uric acid is generally retained before an acute attack of gout, and
the urine uric acid rises during the attack – though these changes are not
diagnostic. Treatment of chronic gout with (e.g.) probenecid (which
diminishes tubular reabsorption of many compounds, including uric
acid) lowers the plasma urate, and improves the patient's condition, by
increasing the urinary excretion of uric acid (IX). Adrenocorticotrophic
hormone or cortisone therapy increases uric acid excretion partly by
diminishing tubular reabsorption, and partly by increasing endogenous
synthesis of uric acid.

Creatine and creatinine

Creatine is principally synthesised in the liver and kidneys from amino
acids. It is taken up from the bloodstream by the muscles, where it is
phosphorylated and enters into muscle metabolism – almost all the
creatine of the body is in the muscles. The end-product of creatine
metabolism in muscles is creatinine, which is metabolically inactive;
creatinine diffuses into the plasma and is excreted in the urine.

Plasma values

The reference range for plasma creatine is 15–60 μmol/l, and for plasma creatinine is 60–120 μmol/l. Creatinine is freely diffusible between cell and plasma water, but the creatine content of erythrocytes is much higher than that of plasma. Urinary excretion of these compounds reflects their plasma levels unless there is renal damage.

In renal failure creatinine is retained with the other NPN constituents of the blood, though creatine is less regularly affected. Plasma creatinine, rather than plasma urea, is widely used to measure chronic failure of renal excretory function, especially in conditions where there is pre-renal alteration of urea metabolism (e.g. a low protein diet). However, the creatinine clearance is a more valuable investigation until it falls below about 10 ml/min (p. 218). In general, if the plasma creatinine is less than about 900 μmol/l then glomerular filtration is normal.

Urine values

The urinary excretion of creatinine in health in an individual varies little from day to day. The magnitude of urinary creatinine excretion is considered to be representative of the total active muscle mass, and estimation of urinary creatinine is used as a very rough check of the accuracy of collection of successive 24 hour urine specimens. In adults urinary creatinine is about 9–18 mmol/24 h, whereas in young children the 24 hour excretion is about 90–160 μmol/kg body weight.

Only trace amounts of creatine (0–400 μmol/24 h) are normally excreted by adults, though creatinuria is regularly present in children of both sexes and in pregnant women.

Creatinuria. This was formerly a useful measurement in patients with muscle disease: estimation of plasma creatine kinase is now a more sensitive way of detecting and measuring acute muscle damage (p. 121). In active primary muscle disease, such as muscular dystrophy, and in secondary muscle disease whether neurological or metabolic (e.g. thyrotoxicosis) conversion of creatine to creatinine is interrupted, and there is creatinuria with a corresponding fall in creatinine excretion.

Amino acids

Changes in amino acid metabolism are only demonstrable to a limited extent by estimation of the total amino acid levels in plasma or in urine. Estimations of all the individual amino acids can be done quantitatively, using expensive automatic apparatus for column chromatography; or semi-quantitatively by simple chromatography.

Plasma values

The reference range for fasting plasma amino acid nitrogen is 2.5–4.0 mmol/l: it rises after a meal. The plasma amino acid level is raised in severe renal failure together with the other NPN constituents of the blood. The most marked rise in the plasma amino acid level, to about 20 mmol/l, is a result of acute hepatic necrosis, because of impaired conversion of amino acids to urea. A slight rise is found in acute hepatitis and cirrhosis, or after severe shock. The plasma amino acid level is lowered by the protein anabolic affects of growth hormone or androgens. A low value may be found in the nephrotic syndrome, due to increased renal tubular loss.

Aminoaciduria

The amino acid excretion in the 24 hour urine of healthy adults is 4–20 mmol of free amino acid nitrogen; and glutamine/glutamic acid, glycine, serine, and alanine are normally detected.

Excess urinary amino acids can be classified as:

Overflow aminoaciduria without primary renal disease. The plasma amino acid levels may be high or normal, depending on their thresholds. The overflow aminoacidurias comprise conditions:

(a) *Acquired secondarily to other diseases.* Generalised aminoaciduria is seen regularly, to a mild extent, in cirrhosis and other chronic liver diseases, and to a marked extent in acute hepatic necrosis. Slight aminoaciduria is seen in wasting diseases, eclampsia, and when there is tissue damage; and also after infusion of amino acids (p. 94).

Hydroxyproline is an amino acid specific to collagen: and is normally excreted in small amounts – 80–250 μmol/24 h. Hydroxyprolinuria is a measure of increased collagen turnover, which includes bone growth, Paget's disease, hyperparathyroidism, and malignant disease of bone. The measurement is more sensitive as the hydroxyproline/creatinine ratio.

(b) *Caused by an inborn error of metabolism.* There are a considerable number of congenital disorders due to enzyme defects, in which one or more amino acids are incompletely degraded, may be present themselves or as metabolites in increased concentration in the plasma, and are excreted in excess in the urine. The examples given are disorders which have specific symptoms and involve different types of amino acid.

Phenylketonuria, a group of related disorders of aromatic amino acids, is in its main variety the commonest aminoaciduria and causes mental retardation: the high phenylalanine also inhibits tyrosinase and lessens melanin formation. Due to deficiency of phenylalanine hydroxylase (phenylalanine 4-monooxygenase), the normal conversion of phenyl- alanine to tyrosine is almost absent and phenylalanine and its deri- vatives, particularly phenylpyruvic acid and phenyllactic acid, are present in excess. Partial deficiency, due to delayed maturation with prematurity, gives the benign hyperphenylalaninaemia. Phenylketonuria should be screened for in all children by detecting a raised blood phenylalanine (from the normal <0.2 mmol/l to >12 mmol/l in homo- zygotes) at 6–14 days after birth, either using the Guthrie test which is a microbiological assay, or by chemical estimation. Screening by detection of the excess phenyl ketones in urine (p. 74), though much simpler, is not satisfactory as there are many false negatives. Further brain damage may then be avoided in affected children by the use of a phenylalanine-free diet. By the use of a modified Guthrie test, or by chromatography, it is possible to screen for many other inborn errors of amino acid metabolism.

Alkaptonuria involves the further metabolism of tyrosine and is relatively benign. Due to deficiency of homogentisate 1,2-dioxygenase, homogentistic acid cannot be further oxidised. It is deposited in cartilage causing arthritis, and excreted in the urine, which turns dark brown on becoming alkaline or oxidised.

Homocystinuria involves sulphur-containing amino acids. In one variety, due to deficiency of cystathionine β-synthase, methionine, homocysteine, and homocystine (excreted in the urine) are present in excess. Diverse clinical features include mental deficiency, skeletal abnormalities, and dislocation of the lens.

Maple syrup urine disease involves branched-chain amino acids. Due to deficiency of 'branched-chain ketoacid decarboxylases', there is a block in the metabolism of valine, leucine, and isoleucine. These and their derivatives accumulate in blood and urine (which smells like maple syrup). Mental damage is severe: its special interest is that treatment by an artificial diet may be possible.

In other (sometimes transient) disorders of which *tyrosinaemia* and *histidinaemia* are examples, symptoms may be absent or not certainly attributable to the metabolic error.

Renal aminoaciduria due to diminished tubular reabsorption. These comprise the renal tubular syndromes, with normal or low plasma amino acids, and can be divided into:

(a) *Aminoaciduria due to specific inborn disorders of the tubular reabsorptive mechanisms, e.g. cystinuria* (p. 225). In some syndromes the same transport defect is present in the small intestine.

Hartnup disease involves intestinal and renal transport of neutral amino acids, especially tryptophan. The patient has nicotinic acid deficiency, with skin and mental effects of pellagra, and cerebellar symptoms. Urinary indoles also are increased, derived from intestinal tryptophan.

(b) *Non-specific aminoaciduria secondary to acquired renal tubular damage.* This can occasionally develop in the nephrotic syndrome, but is commonly due to exogenous toxins (e.g. heavy metal poisoning, p. 136) or to abnormal metabolites (e.g. galactose-1-phosphate, p. 73). In the rare *cystinosis* the primary defect is of cystine metabolism, with deposition of excess cystine intracellularly in various tissues including liver and kidney: the latter causes a secondary Fanconi syndrome and aminoaciduria.

Fanconi syndrome: this includes both congenital and acquired disease of the proximal renal tubules, with generalised aminoaciduria and other reabsorptive defects (p. 225).

Chromatography

In clinical biochemistry chromatographic methods are mainly utilised for the identification and semi-quantitative assay of urinary sugars, amino acids, and barbiturates. The more rapid thin layer chromatography, which employs a thin film of silica gel or cellulose spread on a plate, has mainly replaced the cheaper paper chromatography.

Adsorption or partition chromatography may also be performed using a column of alumina, ion-exchange resin, or other suitable supporting material, as the stationary phase. The differences in principle between adsorption chromatography (separation taking place between a mobile liquid and a stationary solid surface) and partition chromatography (separation taking place between a mobile liquid and a stationary liquid held on a solid, as in paper chromatography) are less important in practice.

Gas-chromatography is used primarily for analysis of steroids, fatty acids, and of drugs – particularly barbiturates and alcohols. High pressure liquid chromatography is, when available, the best procedure for drugs.

Ammonia

A small quantity of ammonia is formed in and absorbed from the gut, and is metabolised in the liver. There is little ammonia in the peripheral blood of normal subjects – but analysis is difficult.

Up to about 350 µmol/l of ammonia nitrogen can be found in the blood in cases of severe parenchymatous liver damage or cirrhosis, particularly when there are neurological complications (p. 204) – analysis is of doubtful clinical value. Excess ammonia is formed because of gastrointestinal bleeding, and this is unable to be converted to urea by the damaged liver. After a porto-caval shunt the blood ammonia rises further; but sterilisation of the gut prevents synthesis of ammonia.

Further reading

Balis ME. Uric acid metabolism in man. *Adv Clin Chem* 1976; 18:213–246.
Scriver DR, Rosenberg, LE. *Aminoacid Metabolism and its Disorders.* Philadelphia: W.B. Saunders, 1973.

CHAPTER 8

PLASMA PROTEINS

The plasma contains very many separate proteins of different chemical constitution – i.e. amino acid composition and sequence. They therefore differ also in such physical properties as relative molecular mass (molecular weight), relative density (specific gravity), solubility, and electrical charge; and also in immunological identity. Most methods which are employed for the routine differential analysis of plasma proteins analyse, apart from albumin, different fractions of the proteins: the number of fractions identified depends on the method of separation.

PLASMA PROTEIN ESTIMATION

Measurement of total protein

The reference range for total protein, estimated in *serum*, is 62–80 g/l; this excludes fibrinogen, which is included in *plasma* proteins. If venous constriction is prolonged, and maintained while blood is being collected, then the concentration of plasma proteins and protein-bound substances (particularly calcium) may be raised by 10–15 per cent because water is lost from the plasma in the veins. Prolonged recumbency may lower the plasma protein concentrations by about 10 per cent, due to redistribution of water in the body.

Nitrogen estimation. The standard procedure is based on the Kjeldahl technique. The protein is digested, and the nitrogen converted to ammonia which can be measured precisely.

Biuret estimation. This is commonly used for clinical work, and depends on a colour reaction between an alkaline copper reagent and the CO-NH peptide linkages. This method relies on there being a constant number of CO-NH linkages per unit mass of protein of whatever nature.

Specific gravity. If serum is dropped into copper sulphate solution of known density, the drop will float or sink according to its density, which largely depends on its protein concentration. This method is useful for field work. If whole blood is used this method becomes a screening test principally for haemoglobin concentration.

Other methods. The refractive index of serum is a measure of its protein concentration: rapid estimation is possible with a suitable instrument. Methods that depend on sensitive procedures for specific amino acids (such as tyrosine and tryptophan) give different results for plasma proteins of different composition.

Differential protein analysis

Colorimetric analysis. Many dyes are bound to albumin. Bromcresol green is commonly used to measure serum albumin: however some α-globulins are included, and some circulating drugs (e.g. salicylates) may also be bound to albumin and the measured value will then be altered.

Fibrinogen is usually estimated after first precipitating it from plasma by the addition of calcium ions and of thrombin.

Total serum globulin is derived as the difference between total protein and albumin.

The reference ranges of plasma proteins by this method are: Albumin 36–50 g/l; total globulins 18–32 g/l; fibrinogen 2–4 g/l.

Precipitation methods. Albumin and the globulins have different solubilities in strong salt solutions: 26 per cent sodium sulphate used to be employed as a precipitant for total globulins.

A number of colloidal solutions are stabilised by albumin and are precipitated by globulins, especially abnormal γ-globulin: many flocculation tests have been devised to detect such qualitative and quantitative abnormalities, and are still used occasionally as 'liver function tests' (p. 196).

Electrophoresis. In a suitable alkaline buffer solution (usually pH 8.6) the plasma proteins become sodium$^+$ proteinate$^-$. The ions of the different plasma proteins have different mobilities in an electric field, and these depend on their net charge, size and shape. This method, devised by Tiselius, can be used to separate plasma proteins within channels in a glass cell into albumin, α_1, α_2, β, and γ-globulins, and fibrinogen, and can detect abnormal proteins, particularly paraproteins.

The Tiselius method of boundary electrophoresis, though very accurate, is time-consuming and the apparatus expensive. When electrophoresis of protein solutions is performed on solid or semi-solid supporting media, almost complete separation of the protein fractions occurs (zone electrophoresis). In routine clinical work cellulose acetate strips, and serum, are employed. The apparatus is simple and inexpensive and the quantity of sample needed is small. After the proteins have migrated they are stained by a basic dye and the stained strip can be scanned.

Quantitative methods of fractional protein analysis yield different results by different techniques. For clinical work an assessment of major changes in the serum protein fractions (excluding fibrinogen) can be obtained by visual examination of the stained strip. This procedure is not sensitive enough to detect changes in proteins that are present in low concentrations, such as IgE. The apparent normal order of magnitude of the different globulin fractions is $\gamma > \beta > \alpha_2 > \alpha_1$ (β_1 and β_2 may be differentiated) and by refined techniques prealbumin and 'fast' post-γ-globulin may be seen (Fig. 8.1, p. 114). Many laboratories, however, use quantitative scanning methods as a routine. Acceptable reference values are:

	Percentage of total protein	Total (g/l)
Albumin	50–70	36.0–52.0
α_1-globulins	2–6	1.0–4.0
α_2-globulins	5–11	4.0–8.0
β-globulins	7–16	5.0–12.0
γ-globulins	11–22	7.0–15.0

By the use of other supporting media (e.g. starch gel, acrylamide gel, or agar gel) many more different proteins can be separated. In electrophoresis, starch or acrylamide gel acts as a molecular sieve, achieving additional separation by molecular size as well as by charge.

Methods are also available for specifically staining lipoproteins (p. 84) or carbohydrate-containing proteins for quantitative analysis.

Ultracentrifugation. When a suitable preparation of serum is centrifuged at 120 000 g the proteins separate into fractions which depend on their sedimentation constants (results given in Svedberg units, S), which are a property of the molecular weight, shape, and density of the protein molecules. This method is used in research work for checking the purity of all types of protein fractions, in molecular weight determination, and in analyses of plasma paraproteins and lipoproteins. Proteins which do not contain lipid and have a molecular weight of about 150 000 have a sedimentation constant of 7S, whilst 19S corresponds to a molecular weight of about 1 000 000. These proteins can also be roughly separated on the basis of their molecular weight by thin layer gel chromatography.

Immunological methods. These procedures, including immunodiffusion, immunoelectrophoresis, and radioimmunoassay are now widely used in specific protein analysis, and are described in detail in immunology texts. They can be employed for the quantitative analysis of most individual proteins including albumin, or for the general qualitative and semiquantitative examination of serum for normal and abnormal proteins. One can automate assay of the immunoglobulin groups IgG, IgA, or IgM by immunoprecipitation and nephelometry.

PROPERTIES OF THE INDIVIDUAL PLASMA PROTEINS

Prealbumin

This has a normal concentration of about 0.3 g/l, and a molecular weight of about 60 000: it transports thyroxine. Its concentration falls early in protein malnutrition, and after infection or injury.

Albumin

The molecular weight of normal plasma albumin is about 70 000 (4 S). Albumin is responsible for 80 per cent of the colloid osmotic pressure of the plasma.

When the plasma albumin level falls below 20–25 g/l oedema is likely to develop. In a patient suffering from severe malnutrition of slow onset the plasma albumin level may be low without there being oedema: conversely, a 'famine oedema' can present with a normal plasma albumin level though there may be excess fluid intake. In hypoalbuminaemia there is increased synthesis, and probably delayed catabolism, of lipids.

Albumin is responsible for the carriage in the plasma of most of the bilirubin and of the protein-bound (non-ionised) calcium. Albumin binds dyes introduced into the circulation (e.g. bromsulphthalein; Evans Blue), and many drugs (e.g. salicylates), metabolites (e.g. FFA), and hormones (e.g. thyroid hormones). It has a stabilising action on colloidal systems (such as those used for the liver function flocculation tests) and on the erythrocyte sedimentation rate (ESR).

Albumin is synthesised in the liver (p. 188) and has a half-life of about 15 days. The albumin which circulates in the plasma probably has no direct tissue nutritive value.

Increase of plasma albumin

An increase in the plasma concentration of albumin is found in disease only when there is loss of plasma water – which may be due to local stasis (p. 257). The concentrations of albumin-bound components such as calcium are then also increased. There is usually an associated haemoconcentration and increase of the plasma viscosity. However, in many of the disorders which cause haemoconcentration, e.g. burns, protein as well as water is lost from the body. In these situations the plasma albumin concentration depends on the relative amounts of water and protein which have been lost or replaced.

Decrease of plasma albumin

Possible causes of a fall in the plasma albumin concentration are: low protein intake, inadequate digestion or absorption of protein, increased protein catabolism, diminished albumin synthesis, increased protein loss, and haemodilution.

Inadequate intake, digestion, or absorption of protein, increased protein catabolism and loss of protein, whilst being causes of albumin deficiency, have been discussed as causes of a negative nitrogen balance (p. 93). A decreased protein intake does not lead to an immediate fall in the plasma albumin: tissue protein is depleted before the plasma protein level falls, and each 10 g/l fall in plasma albumin concentration indicates depletion of about 30 g of tissue protein. Loss of albumin into oedema or ascites from plasma does not of itself change the total body content of albumin.

Analbuminaemia (virtual absence) and bisalbuminaemia (two electrophoretic peaks) are extremely rare familial disorders: the former, rather surprisingly, only shows slight oedema, and the latter is symptomless.

In chronic or severe acute liver disease synthesis of albumin is impaired. The fall in plasma albumin that occurs after trauma, in malignancy and other long continued wasting disease, or in acute or chronic infection and other systemic illnesses, is partly due to liver damage, partly to impaired intake, and partly to an unexplained toxic destruction of protein.

Globulins

The immunoglobulins are synthesised in the reticulo-endothelial system, and the other globulins are synthesised in the parenchymal liver cells.

Increase of total plasma globulins

This is seen in most acute or chronic infections (bacterial or parasitic, but less so in virus infections, except those of the liver) especially in those of long duration. In chronic liver disease and in metastatic carcinoma there is a variable increase in the total plasma globulin. A marked increase is seen in collagen diseases, multiple myeloma, macroglobulinaemia, and sarcoidosis. If there is marked loss of plasma water and haemo-concentration, or severe stasis, the plasma globulins are raised along with the albumin.

Decrease of total plasma globulins

This is seen when there is total plasma protein deficiency, for example from burns or in severe malnutrition or disease of the gastrointestinal tract. When the total plasma globulin is less than 10 g/l agamma-globulinaemia can be suspected.

Additional information of clinical value is obtained by electrophoretic or immunological studies of the separate globulin groups or individual proteins.

α-Globulins

The α-globulins carry metals lipids and carbohydrates. The blue-green copper-binding protein, caeruloplasmin (p. 136), is an α_2-globulin, as are the haptoglobins (p. 127); and there is an α_2-macroglobulin.

Increased α-globulins (principally α_2) are found when there is tissue destruction e.g. malignant disease, in acute inflammatory conditions, and occasionally in chronic infections. In the nephrotic syndrome, the α_2-globulin fraction is increased because of increased lipoproteins and macroglobulin.

The *glycoproteins* are a group of carbohydrate-containing proteins which are electrophoretically mainly α-globulins, and mucoproteins (principally α_1 acid glycoprotein or orosomucoid) are important constituents of the α-glycoproteins – these can be analysed by special methods. Plasma mucoproteins and total glycoproteins are increased in inflammatory conditions and with tissue destruction (including collagen diseases and post-operatively), and are lowered in acute parenchymal liver disease and the nephrotic syndrome. Their estimation is not of diagnostic value except as a non-specific screening test for organic illness.

α_1-*Antitrypsin* is the principal α_1-globulin: its congenital deficiency predisposes to the development of emphysema and of neonatal hepatitis, and may be suspected by electrophoretic absence of α_1-globulin – to be confirmed by immunoassay.

β-Globulins

Much of the β-globulin, as apolipoproteins, is combined with cholesterol and other lipids, and also, as individual binding globulins, carries fat-soluble vitamins and hormones. The iron-binding protein, transferrin (p. 134), is a β-globulin. Clearance of the low molecular weight (12 000) β_2-microglobulin is used as an index of renal tubular function (p. 216).

Increase of the β-globulins is found in conditions where there is increased plasma lipid, for example diabetes mellitus, atheroma, nephrotic syndrome, and biliary cirrhosis, often with characteristic lipoprotein electrophoretic patterns which distinguish between pre-β- and β-lipoproteins (p. 84).

γ-Globulins (immunoglobulins)

Most antibodies are γ-globulins, though α_2-and β-globulins also contain antibodies. Most γ-globulins have antibody activity: the term immunoglobulin includes γ-globulins without antibody activity but formed from immunologically competent cells. All immunoglobulins have the same basic structure. They are composed of two identical polypeptide light chains, each of molecular weight about 20 000, of two possible types called κ or λ; and two identical polypeptide heavy chains, each of molecular weight from 50 000 to 70 000, which are called γ, α, μ, δ, or ε (with some subgroups) and on which depend the class. The main classes of immunoglobulins, and some of their properties, are shown in the table. IgM is a pentamer, and IgA may be present as a dimer in secretions.

The major immunoglobulins IgA, IgG, and IgM may be readily estimated immunologically, though the results are very method-

		Properties of the immunoglobulins		
Class	Heavy chain	Principal sedimentation coefficient	Electrophoretic mobility	Plasma reference values (g/l)
IgG	γ	7 S	γ	8–16
IgA	α	7 S	β–γ	1.5–4.0
IgM	μ	19 S	β–γ	0.5–1.5
IgD	δ	7 S	β–γ	4.0–40 mg/1
IgE	ε	8 S	γ	0.1–1.0 mg/1

dependent. The total immunoglobulin concentration is higher when so measured than when estimated as total γ-globulin by electrophoresis. It has been proposed that the results of immunoglobulin analysis be expressed as international units referred to a standard serum, rather than as g/l (reference ranges: IgG 70–200, IgA 50–280, IgM 50–370 iu/ml).

The different classes of immunoglobulin have different functions. In outline, the usual primary antibody response to a foreign antigen (especially when particulate) is a rise in IgM, and a rise in IgG comes later as the secondary response, especially to soluble antigen. An important function of IgA is protection of the mucosal surfaces of the gut and respiratory tract where it is synthesised. Details of immunoglobulin structure and function may be found in immunology texts. The study of the complement system is also referred to immunologists.

Hypergammaglobulinaemia. Polyclonal increase of γ-globulins is seen in chronic infective states, sarcoidosis, parasitic disease, collagen disease, certain types of liver disease, and autoimmune disorders (particularly systemic lupus erythematosus). Monoclonal increase is paraproteinaemia.

Hypogammaglobulinaemia. There are several types of immune deficiency disease, usually presenting as repeated infections, in which there is primary polyclonal decrease of one or more classes of the immunoglobulins and of their synthetic mechanisms. In transient hypogammaglobulinaemia of the newborn there is normally spontaneous recovery. The congenital anomalies (the commoner type being sex-linked, in premature males) are often called *agammaglobulinaemia*, for simplicity, but immunoglobulins are always present though at a total concentration less than 1 g/l. Adult primary agammaglobulinaemia may occur at any age, the total immunoglobulin concentration being between 1–2 g/l: the cause is unknown (Fig. 8.2).

Secondary decrease of the immunoglobulins is found in the nephrotic syndrome, leukaemia and the malignant paraproteinaemias, and in dietary or intestinal protein malnutrition if infection is absent.

Clotting factors

The study of disturbances of coagulation of blood (including the estimation of fibrin degradation products) is normally the concern of the haematologist, but the chemical pathology laboratory may be responsible for estimation of plasma fibrinogen.

Fibrinogen

Fibrinogen is synthesised in the liver, and has a molecular weight of about 500 000. Excess fibrinogen (with the other acute phase changes in proteins) accelerates the ESR, and increases plasma viscosity.

The plasma fibrinogen concentration is raised in almost all states in which a raised ESR is found, particularly in acute infections and in pregnancy. An increase is also found in patients with carcinoma, as a result of irradiation therapy, and often in the nephrotic syndrome. In some laboratories *plasma viscosity* has replaced the ESR as a measure of disease activity as it is not influenced by abnormalities of erythrocytes.

There may be a marked fall in the plasma fibrinogen in severe liver disease, or in pregnancy as a complication of detachment of the placenta due to release of placental thromboplastin into the maternal circulation. Idiopathic afibrinogenaemia is a rare congenital anomaly. There are syndromes of disseminated intravascular coagulation (DIC) with destruction of fibrinogen by thrombin or plasmin.

Some specific proteins

Bence Jones protein and myeloma globulin

In multiple myeloma specific unusual proteins are formed in the bone marrow by an abnormal clone of neoplastic stem cells, and may be present both in plasma and in urine.

Myeloma globulin can be found in the serum of about 80 per cent of cases. It is usually monoclonal, with a molecular weight of about 160 000 (7 S). There are different types of myeloma globulin, though it is usually IgG or IgA. On electrophoretic analysis of serum it appears as a sharp band (Fig. 8.3) generally intermediate between the β- and γ-globulins (and replacing normal immunoglobulins whose synthesis is suppressed), but it may have other mobility. The myeloma globulin is responsible for the high ESR, and for the significant hyperviscosity, found in multiple myeloma.

Bence Jones protein is one of the κ or λ light chains of the myeloma globulin molecule which has been synthesised in excess: it has a molecular weight of 20 000, or 40 000 as the dimer. Long-standing Bence Jones proteinuria damages the renal tubules. Electrophoresis of concentrated urine is the best test, and this is more sensitive for the diagnosis of multiple myeloma than is electrophoresis of serum for myeloma globulin. The classical heat test for Bence Jones proteinuria (p. 216) detects less than 50 per cent of cases. In *light chain excess* (Bence Jones myeloma) only Bence Jones protein, and no myeloma globulin, is formed.

There is a very rare group of *heavy chain diseases* (α, γ, or μ) which are reticuloses, due to the opposite imbalance of polypeptide chain synthesis, with no excess light chains formed.

Amyloid. The amyloid deposits of multiple myeloma and of primary amyloidosis are composed of fragmented light chains. The deposits of secondary amyloidosis are protein, of unknown nature.

Macroglobulins

A large proportion of the normal α_2-globulins and about 10 per cent of the γ-globulins are of high molecular weight (about 1 000 000: 19 S).

There is a rare Waldenström's primary macroglobulinaemia in which there is excessive synthesis of large quantities of macroglobulin (an abnormal IgM). This is demonstrable in the serum as an irregular dense band in the γ-globulin region, and the normal γ-globulins may be decreased: Bence Jones proteinuria is sometimes present. It presents clinically with high plasma viscosity, consequent vascular disturbances, and immune paresis. Macroglobulinaemia may also be found in myelomatosis, or in reticuloses such as lymphoma.

Paraproteinaemia

This term (much preferred to 'gammopathies') is sometimes used as a general descriptor for diseases of immune globulin synthesis, especially multiple myeloma and macroglobulinaemia, which are associated with proliferation of particular clones of stem cells and an abnormal monoclonal band on electrophoresis. About 10 per cent of cases may be benign, with no suppression of other normal immunoglobulins, and no Bence Jones proteinuria. Differentiation of myeloma globulin from macroglobulin may be difficult on routine electrophoresis, and may require starch gel electrophoresis, immunological studies, or chromatography or ultracentrifugation. The Sia water test is a useful screen: one drop of serum is let fall into a cylinder of water buffered at pH 7.0. Macroglobulins form a heavy precipitate whereas serum containing a high γ-globulin of normal molecular weight, or myeloma globulin, only produces a slight turbidity.

As many paraproteins are cationic, the anion gap is decreased in most cases of IgG multiple myeloma (p. 52). Paraproteinaemia, like lipaemia (p. 81), may spuriously lower the *whole plasma* concentrations of components (electrolytes, glucose, etc.) dissolved in plasma *water*.

Cryoglobulins

These are insoluble proteins which separate as a gel, or even as crystals, from plasma when it is cooled: therefore for diagnosis the blood must be kept at 37 °C between collection and analysis. This rare phenomenon has been observed in polyarteritis nodosa, and occasionally in multiple myeloma, macroglobulinaemia, and leukaemia. Precipitation in small arteries, with a Raynaud's syndrome, may occur *in vivo* in cold weather. The abnormal cryoglobulin is usually but not always a γ-globulin, and may be fibrinogen.

Acute phase proteins

This term includes a number of proteins, such as the glycoproteins, α_1-antitrypsin, the haptoglobins, and fibrinogen, whose plasma concentration is increased when there is acute inflammation or acute cell destruction of any type.

C-reactive protein, so-called because it forms a precipitate with the somatic C-polysaccharide of *Streptococcus pneumoniae*, is a sensitive index of the acute phase reaction.

SUMMARY OF CHANGES IN THE PLASMA PROTEINS IN HEALTH AND DISEASE

Physiological changes

At birth, compared with the values in adults, the plasma albumin is low, and the γ-globulin is increased – it falls below the adult value, however, after about the first month of life as maternal immunoglobulin disappears and infantile synthesis has not fully developed. Hypogammaglobulinaemia may be marked in premature infants. Adult values for all fractions are reached by about two years.

In old age there is a tendency for the albumin level to fall, and the total globulin level rises.

During pregnancy the total plasma protein level falls, principally because of water retention. The albumin level may have fallen by as much as 20 per cent by the eighth month of gestation: however the α- and β-globulin and fibrinogen fractions may rise.

Changes in disease

Malnutrition

In chronic dietary malnutrition the albumin is much lowered, but there may be a secondary increase in γ-globulin due to the generally associated infection, particularly in the tropics: in these states of amino acid deficiency the γ-globulin-producing systems seem to have priority for the available amino acids. In the malabsorption syndrome and protein-losing enteropathies reduction of albumin and decrease of γ-globulins follows the development of protein deficiency; there may be an increase of α_2- and β-globulins.

Infective processes

In the *acute phase* of almost all infections and inflammatory processes, or after acute injury, there is a slight fall in the albumin, and a rise in the α-globulins (principally α_2) which is partly due to extra glycoprotein. C-reactive and other acute phase proteins appear and there may be a slight rise in the γ-globulins, (immunoglobulins, usually IgM) after a week. There is therefore an increase in the ESR and plasma viscosity. The total globulin and fibrinogen levels are slightly increased. As an infection progresses to a chronic state the albumin level continues to fall and the total globulin level continues to rise: with development of the immune response the γ-globulin fraction (usually IgG) progressively increases, whereas changes in α-globulins are variable.

The pattern is non-specific and varies little, whatever the cause of the infection. The more severe and long-lasting the disease, the greater the changes in the plasma proteins. In virus infections the globulin changes are less marked. In parasitic disease, particularly kala-azar, and in lymphogranuloma venereum, a massive increase in γ-globulin

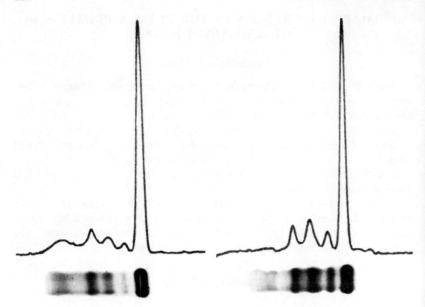

FIG. 8.1. Normal

FIG. 8.2. Agammaglobulinaemia

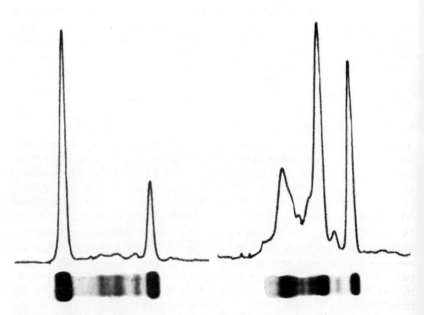

FIG. 8.3. Multiple myeloma

FIG. 8.4. Nephrotic syndrome

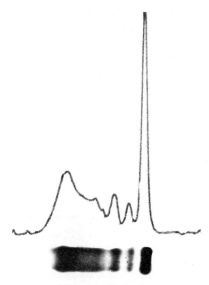

Fig. 8.5. Cirrhosis

Figs. 8.1–8.5. Cellulose acetate electrophoresis of 2 μl serum for proteins. In each case the stained strip is shown below, and a scan is shown above.

(particularly IgM) is often seen. In subacute bacterial endocarditis and in active sarcoidosis the γ-globulin is often particularly increased: in tuberculosis changes are less marked.

The development of amyloidosis, in these conditions or in multiple myeloma, is not in itself associated with any specific changes in the plasma proteins.

Collagen and autoimmune diseases

The tendency in these groups of disorders is for there to be a fall in the albumin, and a rise in the fibrinogen and in total globulin levels due to increase of α_2- and γ-globulins, particularly IgG. In systemic lupus erythematosus a particularly high γ-globulin is seen.

Malignant disease

In advanced malignant disease of any type there tends to be a fall in the albumin, and a rise in total globulin (chiefly the α_2 fraction; with C-reactive protein and acid glycoprotein) and fibrinogen, this being the pattern of non-specific tissue damage: but infection and malnutrition may complicate this picture. In carcinoma of the upper alimentary tract there is usually a marked fall in both albumin and total globulin, due principally to malnutrition. In multiple myeloma the albumin level often falls, and all the normal globulin fractions are reduced. The abnormal myeloma globulin (up to 100 g/l may be present) increases both total globulin and total protein.

Immunological tests: oncofetal antigens. These are a group of proteins, normally produced only by the fetus, that are synthesised by some malignant tumours and can be detected in plasma. Their concentration is proportional to the spread of the tumour and to its response to treatment, and their estimation is more important for follow-up than for diagnosis. Two proteins are commonly measured.

Carcinoembryonic antigen (CEA) is found in most cases of neuroblastoma, and carcinoma of the gastrointestinal tract (especially colon and pancreas) and bronchus, and often in carcinoma of the breast and uterus.

α_1-*Fetoprotein* is found in most cases of primary liver carcinoma and malignant teratoma of the testis. False positives (for either antigen) often occur in non-malignant conditions, particularly hepatitis and colitis. A raised α-fetoprotein is found in amniotic fluid and in maternal serum (p. 165) when there is a fetal neural tube defect, the protein having passed from the fetal central nervous system to the amniotic fluid, and thence been absorbed: exomphalos also gives raised values.

Renal disease

Nephrotic syndrome. Albumin is markedly decreased because of the massive loss of albumin in the urine. α_1-Globulins, γ-globulins, caeruloplasmin and transferrin are also lost in the urine, and are present in decreased concentration in the plasma. Pre β- and β-lipoproteins are increased; both excess lipid and excess protein (α_2- and β-globulins) are present (Fig. 8.4). Fibrinogen is often increased.

Acute and chronic nephritis. In acute glomerulonephritis and chronic renal failure the changes in the plasma protein pattern are slight and of no diagnostic value. Electrophoresis of the urinary protein shows that the excreted protein is principally albumin and this investigation by itself usually has little diagnostic value. However, measurement of the clearance of specific proteins, e.g. transferrin, is valuable in the detailed investigation of renal function (p. 216).

Tubular syndromes. There are no noticeable changes in the plasma proteins in the congenital renal tubular abnormalities. When there is tubular damage the *urinary protein*, however, shows a relatively large amount of low molecular weight globulins (p. 216).

Liver disease

Obstructive jaundice (post-hepatic). There are no particular changes in the plasma proteins except a slight rise in α_2-globulin, unless there is secondary liver damage, complicating infection, or malnutrition.

Acute infective hepatitis. In acute infective hepatitis there is a slight fall in the albumin and α-globulins, β-globulin may be raised, and there is also some increase in γ-globulin. Persistence of a high γ-globulin after the acute phase has passed may indicate progress to chronicity.

Chronic hepatitis and cirrhosis. In cirrhosis and chronic hepatitis there is a decrease in albumin and an increase in globulin which may be considerable, and is principally γ-globulin seen on electrophoresis as a broad band (β-γ fusion, Fig. 8.5). Part of the globulin increase is due to IgA components which run between the β- and γ-globulins, and the pattern (which occurs in cirrhosis but not in active chronic hepatitis) is easily recognised. In biliary cirrhosis, the β-globulins (lipoproteins) are particularly increased in parallel with the rise in plasma cholesterol and other lipids, and there is an increase in IgM. The fibrinogen level rises in cirrhosis, but falls in chronic hepatitis.

Summary of the clinical value of estimation of the plasma proteins

Estimation of *total* plasma or serum protein concentration has value when the patient has lost every type of plasma protein, e.g. as a result of burns or haemorrhage; or when it is necessary to follow the course of haemoconcentration or haemodilution, due to loss or gain of extracellular water. Otherwise changes in albumin and in globulins must be considered separately; the relation between albumin and globulin, expressed as a *ratio*, has no value.

Estimation of plasma albumin is an essential part of the assessment of a patient's nutritional state, and is particularly important as a pre-operative investigation on patients with surgical disease of the gastrointestinal tract. Estimation of differential plasma protein fractions should be done in chronic liver disease, in the nephrotic syndrome, and for the investigation of collagen diseases and of the paraproteinaemias and of chronic diseases of unknown nature. The serum protein pattern of agammaglobulinaemia (Fig. 8.2), multiple myeloma or macroglobulinaemia (Fig. 8.3), nephrotic syndrome (Fig. 8.4), and cirrhosis (Fig. 8.5), may be diagnostic on electrophoretic analysis. Specific analysis of the individual immunoglobulin classes is at present only diagnostically valuable in agammaglobulinaemia and the para-proteinaemias. Estimation of plasma fibrinogen is not usually necessary except in the investigation of haemorrhagic diseases.

PROTEIN ANALYSIS IN OTHER BODY FLUIDS

Changes in the protein composition of urine and cerebrospinal fluid are described in the chapters on renal disease (p. 216) and the nervous system (p. 249). The detection of undigested albumin in meconium is used to investigate cystic fibrosis (p. 237).

Exudates and transudates. In pleural or ascitic fluid a transudate, being a plasma ultrafiltrate modified by circulatory changes, usually has a protein concentration less than 30 g/l (specific gravity <1.015): an exudate, caused by inflammation or malignancy, usually has a protein concentration more than 40 g/l (specific gravity <1.018).

PLASMA ENZYMES

The enzymes found in plasma can be semi-arbitrarily grouped into:

Plasma-active. These act on substrates in plasma: the group includes the coagulation enzymes.

Extracellular fluid-active. These are synthesised in cells close to their site of activity in the extracellular fluid, into which they are secreted: the group includes the digestive enzymes.

Cell-active. These are synthesised in the cells where they act: the group includes the enzymes of intermediary metabolism. Those enzymes found in the plasma mainly originate from the soluble and microsomal fractions of the cell. The cell: plasma gradient of enzyme activity is usually of the order of $10^3:1$, and the plasma half-life of these enzymes is usually about 3 days, though there is wide variation.

The quantity of most enzymes in the blood plasma is low: the *concentration* of prothrombin is about 200 mg/l, and of lactate dehydrogenase is about 100 mg/l. The cell-active enzymes enter the plasma in small amounts as a result of the continuous normal ageing of cells, or due to diffusion through undamaged cell membranes. They leave the plasma through inactivation and catabolism, or rarely by excretion into the bile, small intestine, or urine. This normal steady state of the passage of enzymes from cells to extracellular fluid to disposal maintains the plasma concentration of most enzymes fairly constant. It will be altered:

(i) If there is altered synthesis of enzyme within the cells.

(ii) If there is a change in the amount of enzyme-forming tissue.

(iii) If there is a change in cell permeability. Any damage to a cell which causes an increase in the permeability of the cell membrane, even without actual necrosis, will allow enzymes to escape at a greater rate.

(iv) If there is an alteration in the rate of inactivation or of disposal of enzyme.

(v) If there is an obstruction to a normal pathway of enzyme excretion.

As a result of the operation of one or more of these factors there is generally a rise in the *concentration* of enzyme in the plasma, and this is usually detectable by current methodology (assuming unchanged inhibitors and activators) as an increase in enzyme *activity* – often measured in serum rather than in plasma as some anticoagulants may inhibit some enzymes. Changes in inhibitors or activators may be important: certain poisons act as enzyme inhibitors, and some vitamin deficiencies cause cofactor deficiencies and reduced enzyme activities.

Immunoassays to measure enzyme *concentration* are being developed. They have particular value for assays such as that of trypsin in plasma, where the presence of natural antienzymes renders activity analysis meaningless.

Plasma enzyme changes in disease are related in many ways to cell pathology. Different tissues contain a great number of different enzymes in various concentrations; and following tissue injury plasma enzyme levels do not necessarily change in proportion to those in the damaged tissue. In severe generalised tissue damage, e.g. after heat stroke or cardiac arrest, high values in plasma of almost all cell enzymes may be found. An increase in the plasma activity of any one enzyme is rarely diagnostic of damage to the cells of any one organ or tissue. For example, both myocardium and liver contain the three enzymes, aspartate transaminase, lactate dehydrogenase, and isocitrate dehydrogenase, in high concentration. Yet after a myocardial infarction the plasma aspartate transaminase and lactate dehydrogenase (but not isocitrate dehydrogenase) are increased; whereas after hepatocellular damage the plasma aspartate transaminase and isocitrate dehydrogenase are increased, and less so lactate dehydrogenase. Increased permeability of the damaged cell membrane affects the release of one enzyme more than another; and intracellular location of an enzyme is important, soluble fraction enzymes being released before particulate fraction enzymes when a cell is damaged. Rates of inactivation and of disposal are not the same for all enzymes – 'heart' isocitrate dehydrogenase and 'liver' lactate dehydrogenase are relatively unstable. The different distribution and behaviour of the isoenzymes of the enzymes under consideration can explain many apparent paradoxes.

Isoenzymes

These are different molecular forms of the same enzyme.

In clinical biochemistry two types of isoenzyme are important: when different tissues contain different forms of the enzyme (such as alkaline phosphatase, p. 178), and when different forms of the enzyme are present in all cells but not in the same proportion (such as lactate dehydrogenase, p. 120).

Isoenzymes are generally distinguishable by both biochemical and physical properties. They can usually be separated by electrophoresis, and then visualised by staining. Chromatographic or immunological separations are sometimes used. They may also often be distinguished by their different kinetic properties with related substrates, or by different sensitivities to temperature changes or to inhibitors.

Use of enzyme assays in clinical practice

Because of methodological variations, especially related to temperature of analysis, it is particularly important for enzyme assays that results on patients be referred to the analysing laboratory's own reference values. The values in this book use procedures that are common, but not universal.

The digestive enzymes have been measured for many years, and the value of their assay in plasma or secretions will be considered in the chapter on the gastrointestinal tract (p. 234). The widespread use of plasma enzyme assays as 'liver function tests' will be considered in the chapter on liver (p. 197), and the phosphatases also in the chapter on bone (p. 178). Renal tissue enzymes may be measured in urine to detect local cell damage (p. 217).

Myocardial infarction

Enzyme assays are widely used in the investigation of myocardial infarction: they are not essential in a clinically typical case with an unequivocal electrocardiogram. The enzymes most used are creatine kinase (CK), aspartate transaminase (AST, or aspartate aminotransferase; formerly known as glutamic-oxaloacetic transaminase or GOT) and lactate dehydrogenase (LD). In general, the higher and longer is the rise in plasma enzyme activity, the greater is the extent of myocardial damage: by repeated assay of CK it is possible to calculate the amount of enzyme released from the myocardium, and to quantify the damage.

Creatine kinase. This is present in high activity in cardiac and skeletal muscle and brain, and is absent from liver and erythrocytes – the reference range for plasma CK is 3–70 U/l in women and 5–100 U/l in men at 37 °C.

Two dimeric subunits B and M give rise to three isoenzymes BB, MB, and MM. CK-MB is present almost solely in myocardium and BB in brain (and thyroid): in health only MM (from cardiac and skeletal muscle) is detectable in plasma.

Aspartate transaminase. This is present in high activity in cardiac muscle, skeletal muscle, liver and kidney. The reference range for plasma AST is 5–35 U/l at 37°C in adults. In the first week of life values up to 100 U/l may be found.

Lactate dehydrogenase. This is widely distributed in the tissues, the highest activity being found in kidney, skeletal muscle, liver, cardiac muscle, erythrocytes, and malignant tissue: a slight non-specific rise in total LD occurs in most forms of widespread organic disease. The reference range for plasma LD is 130–500 U/l at 37 °C in adults.

Two tetrameric subunits H and M give rise to five principal isoenzymes, LD–1 to 5 (H_4 to M_4), all normally detectable in plasma. In myocardium the electrophoretically fast-moving LD-1 predominates, and in liver (and also voluntary muscle) LD-5 predominates. Both after myocardial infarction and in hepatitis there is an increase in total LD, but in myocardial infarction this is mainly LD-1 whereas in hepatitis this is mainly LD-5. Separate assay of the 'heart-specific' LD-1 and LD-2 may be useful, and this is usually done by making use of either its heat-stability, or of the preferential reaction of H subunits with the substrate analogue oxobutyrate (as 'hydroxybutyrate dehydrogenase: HBD') – the reference range is 120–260 U/l at 37 °C.

Enzyme pattern. After an infarction the plasma activity of CK is increased from about 6–72 hours with a peak at 24 hours or before: the activity of AST is increased from about 0.5–5 days after the time of infarction with a peak at 24 hours: the activity of LD is increased from 1–10 days after the infarction, with a peak at 2 days. Detection of CK-MB, though often transient, may be possible after 4 hours, and is almost specific for myocardial damage. Heart-specific LD is normally increased between 1 and 12 days after the infarction; many investigators prefer this measurement to that of AST and total LD on account of greater specificity and longer period of application to a patient. The choice of enzyme test, if such investigation is necessary because of clinical doubt, depends on the likely time gap since the onset of the infarction, and also on the possibility of other tissue damage.

Cardiac arrest and congestive heart failure lead to a prolonged rise in enzyme activities, due to secondary damage to liver and skeletal muscle, and probably to delayed disposal of enzyme.

Skeletal muscle disease

The enzymes that are present in cardiac muscle are also present in skeletal muscle, but not in the same relative amounts. In the investigation of muscle disease CK is the enzyme of choice as this gives markedly raised values (mainly of CK-MM) in Duchenne type muscular dystrophy, and abnormal values in female carriers. Raised values are often found in alcoholic and other myopathies, but not in neurogenic disease. It is definitely a more sensitive enzyme assay for disease of voluntary muscle than is aldolase, which is no longer used. However, the plasma CK is raised for 48 hours by severe exercise, or even by large intramuscular injections.

Neuromuscular junction. The succinyl choline derivatives that inhibit the neuronal enzyme acetylcholinesterase [formerly called cholinesterase], and are used in anaesthesia as muscle relaxants, are normally destroyed by the cholinesterase [pseudocholinesterase] present in plasma. Some patients have been found to have prolonged respiratory paralysis (suxamethonium ['scoline'] apnoea) after use of a muscle relaxant such as suxamethonium, and this is usually due to an inborn error of metabolism with the presence of an abnormal cholinesterase in low concentration. Such patients (homozygotes) have a plasma cholinesterase of less than 1 U/l (reference values 2–5 U/l at 37 °C) and in the commonest type of abnormality this is inhibited less than 20 per cent by dibucaine – the normal degree of inhibition being about 80 per cent (or Dibucaine Number 80). Heterozygotes have intermediate values, and are not usually clinically affected.

Acetylcholinesterase and cholinesterase are also inhibited by organophosphorus insecticides, and plasma and erythrocyte cholinesterase assay is therefore used to identify paralytic poisoning by these compounds in agriculture and industry.

Malignant disease

No alteration of plasma or other enzyme activity has been found to be diagnostic of early malignant disease. With the exception of the usually raised plasma acid phosphatase in spreading cancer of the prostate (p. 179) no specific enzyme changes can be found at present even for advanced cancer. However, in advanced malignant disease of many sites a placental-type alkaline phosphatase (the Regan isoenzyme, p. 178) is often produced.

In widespread malignant disease and leukaemia some non-specific elevation of plasma LD, and of other enzymes such as glucosephosphate isomerase, may be found. Leukaemia cells may also leak ALP. A raised plasma (and urinary) lysozyme is found in acute monocytic and myeloid leukaemia.

Other fluids. An LD activity in pleural or ascitic fluid higher than that in plasma suggests local malignancy, provided that there are no excess erythrocytes or leucocytes in the fluid. Similar increased enzyme activity, which is not specific for malignant disease but indicates cell proliferation in local tissues, may be found as a high urine β-D-glucuronidase in bladder cancer, and often a high vaginal fluid phosphogluconate dehydrogenase in carcinoma of the cervix.

Erythrocytes

LD-1 and LD-2, and therefore 'hydroxybutyrate dehydrogenase', are present in high activity in erythrocytes and precursors and have high plasma values in megaloblastic anaemia and haemolytic anaemia. The high plasma LD of pulmonary infarction is partly derived from lung erythrocytes. The transaminases are present in erythrocytes in lesser activity, and CK is absent.

Visible haemolysis of a blood sample significantly raises the plasma LD and acid phosphatase, and to a slight extent the AST.

Malnutrition

Protein malnutrition, through its secondary effects on liver or skeletal muscle, is often associated with raised plasma transaminases and lowered cholinesterase and CK.

Vitamins. Deficiencies of certain vitamins of the B group can be measured by utilising their coenzyme function: erythrocytes are usually analysed as these are easily available cells that reflect the total body stores. In these vitamin deficiencies, although the particular enzyme *concentration* in erythrocytes may be normal, the measured *activity* will be low, but will be raised to normal after *in vitro* addition of the appropriate coenzyme. The most valuable test is of transketolase for thiamine pyrophosphate (p. 71), but aspartate or alanine transaminase can be used for pyridoxal phosphate, and glutathione reductase for riboflavine. There is no such specific test for nicotinic acid.

Further reading

Hobbs JR. Immunoglobulins in clinical chemistry. *Adv. Clin Chem* 1971; 14:219–317.

Putnam FW, ed. *The Plasma Proteins. Structure Function and Genetic Control.* 2nd ed. New York: Academic Press, 1977.

Wilkinson JH, ed. *The Principles and Practice of Diagnostic Enzymology.* London: Edward Arnold, 1976.

CHAPTER 9

THE HAEMOPOIETIC SYSTEM

Chemistry of erythrocytes

The circulating erythrocyte has a life-span of about 120 days. As it is not nucleated, it is a dying cell throughout that period, with a constantly changing composition. The erythrocyte contains about 65 per cent water, and 33 per cent haemoglobin. The average electrolyte composition is Na^+ 8 mmol/l total cell volume, K^+ 90 mmol/l, Cl^- 55 mmol/l, pH 7.2, and the main difference in ionic composition from muscle cells is the high concentration of chloride (p. 24). Because of the relatively low water content of erythrocytes, their total concentration of diffusible substances such as glucose and urea is less than in plasma: hence analyses of whole blood for glucose (p. 58) and urea (p. 95), and for many other substances, do not give the same results as analyses of plasma.

The mature erythrocyte has no mitochondria and therefore maintains its energy flow by anaerobic glycolysis.

When compared to most other cells, cells of the erythroid series have high activity of enzymes of the pentose shunt, of acetylcholinesterase, and (especially in erythroblasts) of LD-1. Excess destruction of erythroid cells may produce an increase in plasma enzymes (p. 122).

HAEMOGLOBIN

Haemoglobin synthesis (Fig. 9.1)

Succinate (as succinyl CoA) and glycine combine in the haemopoietic organs initially to form α-amino β-ketoadipic acid, and δ-aminolaevulinic acid (ALA) is then produced under the influence of ALA-synthase which is the rate-controlling enzyme for the whole synthesis of haemoglobin. Two ALA molecules condense to one molecule of porphobilinogen, a substituted monopyrrole, and four porphobilinogen molecules condense (using uroporphyrinogen I synthase and uroporphyrinogen III cosynthase) to form the cyclic tetrapyrrole (porphyrin) isomeric compounds, uroporphyrinogens of series I and III. Uroporphyrinogen I is the precursor of other porphyrins, but plays no further part in haem synthesis. Uroporphyrinogen III is the precursor of the porphyrin III series, and is converted to coproporphyrinogen III and then via protoporphyrinogen to protoporphyrin IX,

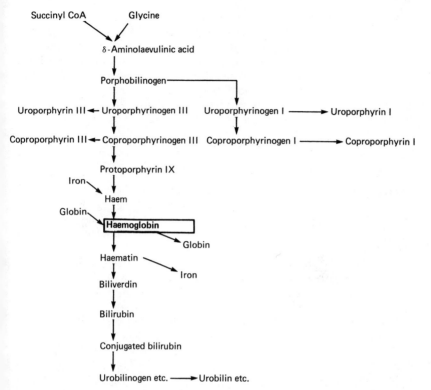

FIG. 9.1. The principal steps in the synthesis and degradation of haemoglobin.

which chelates iron(II) [ferrous iron] to form haem. Haem inhibits ALA-synthase, and this exerts a negative feedback control over the synthesis of porphyrins and haemoglobin.

Each molecule of haem combines with one molecule of globin, and all haemoglobins contain four pairs of haem + globin with a total molecular weight of about 68 000. A number of types of globin polypeptide chains may take part in the haemoglobin molecule: normal adult haemoglobin, Hb A, has two α globin chains and two β globin chains. Erythrocytes also contain a small amount of free protoporphyrin.

Haemoglobin catabolism (Fig. 9.1)

In the reticuloendothelial system erythrocytes are destroyed and the haemoglobin is released. Some haem is released in the marrow during erythroblast maturation or from dead cells of ineffective erythropoiesis. Globin is separated from haem, and haematin is formed in which the iron of the haem is oxidised to [ferric] iron(III). The porphyrin ring is then opened and the iron is removed, with the formation of the straight chain compound biliverdin. This is converted to bilirubin by reduction. A minor pathway first opens the ring to form choleglobin, and then removes the iron and globin to produce biliverdin globin and then biliverdin. The iron, and the amino acids of the globin, are retained; the pyrrole rings are eventually excreted as bilirubin. The normal adult male contains about 800 g of haemoglobin (reference values in blood: 13–18 g/dl), of which about 7 g are produced and destroyed daily. In women the total body haemoglobin is about 600 g (reference values in blood: 11.5–16.5 g/dl).

Haemoglobin derivatives

Oxyhaemoglobin. Haemoglobin without oxygen (reduced haemoglobin) is mauve; fully oxygenated haemoglobin, with each haem + globin pair taking up 2 atoms of oxygen, is yellow-red: 1 g of haemoglobin takes up 1.34 ml of oxygen. The symbol for oxyhaemoglobin should thus be HbO_8, but HbO_2 is conventional.

Carboxyhaemoglobin. Carbon monoxide binds to haemoglobin 200 times more avidly than does oxygen. Therefore in the presence of carbon monoxide (from imperfect combustion of coal or paraffin, or present in exhaust gas or coal gas, or due to heavy cigarette smoking) carboxyhaemoglobin (haem-CO-globin: HbCO) is preferentially formed. Unconsciousness develops when about 50 per cent, and death when about 80 per cent, of the oxyhaemoglobin has been replaced. Carboxyhaemoglobin is cherry-red, especially in dilute solution. Quantitative diagnosis of carboxyhaemoglobinaemia is usually made by differential spectroscopy, which does not detect the traces produced during normal haemoglobin catabolism, nor the slight excess present in haemolytic disease.

Methaemoglobin. This is haematin-globin, containing $Fe^{III}OH$ (symbol: Hi): methaemoglobin cannot carry oxygen for respiration. In normal metabolism haemoglobin is cycled by auto-oxidation and reduction through methaemoglobin, though less than 1 per cent of it is so present at any one time.

Methaemoglobin is brown, and methaemoglobinaemia can be suspected by the colour of the patient and of the diluted blood, and diagnosed by differential spectroscopy. Symptoms of 'cyanosis' develop when about 15 per cent of the haemoglobin (2.5 g/dl), and of anoxia when more than 30 per cent of the haemoglobin, is present as methaemoglobin. Congenital methaemoglobinaemia is rare, being either due to lack of the recycling methaemoglobin reductases, or to an abnormal haemoglobin (Hb M) which easily converts to methaemoglobin. Acquired methaemoglobinaemia may be caused by a number of drugs, particularly phenacetin or sulphonamides; by nitrites which are produced in the intestine from excess nitrates, used as a food preservative or in polluted wellwater (infants being particularly susceptible); by aniline and related compounds via skin absorption, especially in industry. Methylene blue can be used in therapy of methaemoglobinaemia as it activates methaemoglobin reductases.

Sulphaemoglobin. This is of uncertain structure, related to methaemoglobin, and also cannot carry respiratory oxygen. Sulphaemoglobinaemia is produced by the same drugs as cause methaemoglobinaemia, in the presence of *in vivo* (intestinal) hydrogen sulphide which completes the chemical reaction. Conversion of about 5 g/dl of the haemoglobin causes 'cyanosis'. Sulphaemoglobin is also brown: diagnosis of its presence requires spectroscopy and chemical tests.

Glycosylated haemoglobin. Haemoglobin can bind to glucose to form derivatives that are stable for the life of the erythrocyte. The concentration of glycosylated haemoglobin A_1, the major component being Hb A_{1c}, reflects the integrated glucose concentration to which the erythrocyte has been exposed over about the previous two months, and in health does not exceed about 8.5 per cent of the total haemoglobin (p. 63).

Myoglobin. This simplified haemoglobin consists of a single haem + globin (slightly different from that of haemoglobin), containing one Fe^{II} atom, with a molecular weight of about 17 000. It is present in skeletal and cardiac muscle where it can act as a slight oxygen reservoir, and is released after crush injury or ischaemia. Because of its low molecular weight it is rapidly cleared from plasma (cf. Bence Jones protein, p. 111) and presents as myoglobinuria, which is a sensitive index of muscle cell damage, even from violent exercise. The consequent red urine, which does not react with chemical tests for haemoglobin, can be diagnosed spectroscopically. Severe myoglobinuria may lead to acute renal tubular failure.

It is possible to detect myoglobinaemia by immunoassay within a few hours of a myocardial infarction.

Haptoglobins. These are specific α_2-globulins that bind haemoglobin at the globin: there are several haptoglobins with a complex pattern of genetic differences. The reference range for total plasma haptoglobin is 0.3–1.8 g/l. The function of haptoglobins is to conserve iron: after intravascular haemolysis they bind haemoglobin up to about 1.25 g/l of plasma, and only above that concentration is free haemoglobin lost in the urine or bound to haemopexin. Haptoglobins are therefore responsible for the renal threshold for haemoglobin. Haptoglobin bound to haemoglobin is taken up mainly in the liver; the haptoglobin is slowly resynthesised, and the iron recirculates from haemoglobin that is then released. A low plasma haptoglobin concentration is therefore found after repeated or major intravascular haemolysis. A high plasma haptoglobin concentration is non-specific, occurring in malignancy or chronic infections, or as an acute phase reaction (p. 112). Haptoglobins are synthesised in the liver, and (in the absence of haemolysis) are reduced in chronic liver disease in parallel with plasma albumin.

Haemoglobin remaining in the plasma is in part oxidised to methaemoglobin: globin is split off, leaving haem and haematin.

Haemopexin. This is a β_1-glycoprotein that binds remaining haem. The normal plasma concentration is about 0.5 g/l.

Methaemalbumin. This compound is haematin + albumin. It is brown, and its presence in plasma is always abnormal. Methaemalbumin is formed after severe intravascular haemolysis when the haptoglobins and haemopexin are saturated. Other causes of methaemalbuminaemia are bleeding into the abdominal cavity or acute haemorrhagic pancreatitis; pancreatic digestion converts haemoglobin to haematin, which is absorbed and bound to plasma albumin. It is identified spectroscopically, before or after addition of ammonium sulphide (Schumm's test): the haem-haemopexin complex also gives a positive Schumm's test.

Haemoglobinaemia and haemoglobinuria. Intravascular haemolysis from any cause liberates haemoglobin into the circulation, and accounts for about 10 per cent of the breakdown of erythrocytes. If this is at a rate greater than the removal capacity of the binding systems then free haemoglobin can be detected in the plasma. Normally free haemoglobin is less than 50 mg/l in plasma. Haemoglobin is filtered through glomeruli as a dimer, and can be reabsorbed and metabolised in the tubules. When this is saturated haemoglobinuria can be detected, and some haemoglobin is oxidised to methaemoglobin. Haemoglobin in urine accompanied by erythrocytes is usually of renal or post-renal origin: however massive haemoglobin in the glomerular filtrate (as other protein, p. 217) may itself cause renal tubular damage. In some forms of chronic haemoglobinaemia, especially in paroxysmal nocturnal haemoglobinuria, the brown insoluble iron storage compound haemosiderin (an iron(III) hydroxide-protein complex), derived from the tubular metabolism of haemoglobin, is deposited in the renal tubules, and some may be found in a spun urine deposit.

Commercial tests are available (p. 274) for the detection of haemoglobin in urine: they utilise the peroxidase activity of haemoglobin.

Abnormal haemoglobins

The study of different haemoglobins due to changes in the globins has become an important science of its own, with extensions from clinical and laboratory haematology into epidemiology (as the protection against malaria afforded by the haemoglobin of sickle cells), genetics, and molecular biology. For by a knowledge of the small chemical changes in the globin, it has become possible in many cases to predict both the abnormal biochemical properties of the abnormal haemoglobin and the changes in the patient, and to deduce the nature of the primary change in the DNA.

There are also variant myoglobins, not apparently related to muscle disease.

As well as the α and β chains of normal HB A $(\alpha_2\beta_2)$, γ and δ globin chains normally exist. Hb F (fetal haemoglobin) is $\alpha_2\gamma_2$, and constitutes less than 1 per cent of the haemoglobin of an adult, though 75 per cent at birth: Hb A_2 is $\alpha_2\delta_2$, and constitutes about 2.5 per cent of the haemoglobin of an adult.

The haemoglobinopathies

Haemoglobinopathies are conveniently classified into two main groups.

In the first group one or more amino acids are altered in the normal α or β globin chains, giving rise to the formation of an abnormal haemoglobin. More than 100 have been described. With some, such as Hb S (of sickle-cell anaemia) which is the commonest and best-known, presence of the abnormal haemoglobin can give rise to deformation of the cells, anaemia, and other symptoms. In Hb S the α chains are the normal type as in Hb A, but the glutamic acid at position 6 of the β chains is substituted by valine; the symbol for the constitution of this haemoglobin may be written $\alpha_2^A\beta_2^{6\,\text{Val}}$, or $\alpha_2\beta_2^S$.

In the second group there is deficient formation of normal haemoglobin, and these constitute the thalassaemias. In α-thalassaemia, α-chain formation is deficient, with production of the abnormal β_4 (Hb H) or γ_4 (Hb Bart's): the severest homozygous form is incompatible with life but there is a milder homozygous variety, Hb H disease. In β-thalassaemia the deficiency of β-chain formation leads to some compensatory increase in Hb A_2 and Hb F.

One of the principal uses of simple electrophoresis (p. 105) is in the diagnosis of the common haemoglobinopathies.

The haemoglobinopathies are described in detail in haematology texts.

Congenital haemolytic anaemia

Biochemically these are of two main groups – apart from the haemoglobinopathies.

Membrane defects

In these conditions there is a defect of the erythrocyte membrane and an abnormality in the sodium pump: the fundamental causes have not been elucidated. The best-known disorders are hereditary spherocytosis and hereditary elliptocytosis.

Enzyme deficiences (non-spherocytic)

Glucose-6-phosphate dehydrogenase deficiency. This is relatively common, especially in negroes, South Chinese, and Mediterranean people, and may protect against malaria. Glucose-6-phosphate dehydrogenase is the enzyme responsible for the initial deviation of glucose into the pentose phosphate pathway (p. 55) to form 6-phosphogluconate; this pathway provides $NADPH_2$ in the erythrocyte for the conversion of oxidised to reduced glutathione, and for other reactions such as reduction of methaemoglobin. The enzyme deficiency may cause haemolysis per se, but haemolysis chiefly occurs after sensitisation of the erythrocyte by a wide variety of agents, e.g. primaquine, broad beans (favism), or in infections. The cells accumulate methaemoglobin and are deficient in reduced glutathione which is necessary for cell integrity: haemolysis, dark urine, and jaundice are present. Several screening tests are available but definite diagnosis is made by assay of the enzyme in erythrocytes; in homozygotes enzyme activity is reduced to less than 15 per cent of normal. This deficiency may also produce neonatal jaundice.

There are many rarer enzyme deficiencies (the most frequent being of pyruvate kinase) which produce non-spherocytic haemolytic anaemias, but most of these are not related to ingestion of drugs or other sensitisers.

PORPHYRINS

Biochemistry

The porphyrin precursors (ALA, porphobilinogen, uroporphyrinogen, and coproporphyrinogen) are part of the biosynthetic pathway of haem. The classification of the porphyrins into uro-, copro-, and other porphyrins, of series I and III, depends on the nature and spatial distribution of the substituents on the ring system.

Porphobilinogen is a colourless chromogen which can be oxidised to a porphyrin mixture for identification: it also yields a specific reddish pigment with Ehrlich's aldehyde reagent (p. 273). Porphyrins impart a characteristic red-brown colour ('portwine') to urine when they are present in large quantities, and they give a pink fluorescence in ultra-violet light. Identification and quantitative estimation of all the individual porphyrins in urine is a research procedure.

The 24 hour exretion of porphyrins by a normal adult is less than 0.3 μmol in the urine, and less than 0.45 μmol in the faeces: these are mainly coproporphyrins, with protoporphyrins in the faeces. Less than 40 μmol of ALA and 12 μmol of porphobilinogen are excreted daily in the urine, and none in the faeces.

Clinical disorders

Porphyrinurias

In these conditions the excess porphyrin in the urine (usually less than 1.5 μmol/24 h, which does not colour the urine) is almost always coproporphyrin III; the porphyrinuria is secondary to another disease which is not a primary disorder of porphyrin metabolism. Porphyrinuria of about 1.0 μmol/24 h is consistently found in blood disorders associated with excess haemolysis, in liver disease (particularly in cirrhosis, p. 202), and in poisoning from aromatic compounds and heavy metals.

Lead poisoning. Excess lead interferes by multiple enzyme inhibition with haemopoiesis (causing stippled and nucleated erythrocytes) and with haem synthesis. In early lead poisoning, with a blood lead of 4–5 µmol/l erythrocyte ALA dehydratase is decreased, and there is an increase of erythrocyte zinc protoporphyrins (probably the best *screening* test), of urinary coproporphyrins to 0.8–3 µmol/24 h, and of urine ALA to 25–50 µmol/24 h. These analyses need a specialised laboratory.

This is cumulative, from a variety of environmental causes: it may present with anaemia, colic, neuritis, or psychiatric features.

Porphyrias

These conditions are primary inborn metabolic disorders of porphyrin metabolism. There are two general groups, erythropoietic and hepatic, and several varieties.

Erythropoietic ('congenital') porphyria. The metabolic defect in this very rare disorder has not been established, but is probably deficiency of uroporphyrinogen III co-synthase, leading to excessive synthesis in the bone marrow of principally the unphysiological type I uroporphyrin. The urine is coloured red by the porphyrins, as may be the teeth and bones: total urinary porphyrins may be 600 µmol/24 h. The porphyrins in the skin cause severe photosensitivity and blisters. Faecal porphyrin excretion is also high.

Protoporphyria. Deficiency of ferrochelatase leads to protoporphyrin accumulation in erythrocytes, plasma and faeces. There is a rash, and often liver disease.

Hepatic: acute intermittent porphyria. This is associated with increased ALA-synthase activity in the liver, secondary to uroporphyrinogen I synthase deficiency later in the metabolic pathway, with diminished haem synthesis and depression of the normal feedback. This leads to excess synthesis and urinary excretion of ALA and porphobilinogen, and also of some preformed porphyrins. During acute episodes of the disease, which may be precipitated by oral contraceptives, barbiturates, alcohol or many other drugs, or by infection, there may be a fifty-fold increased excretion of the porphyrin precursors: during clinical remissions excretion may return almost to normal. The principal clinical manifestations are related to the gastrointestinal tract, often mimicking an acute abdomen, or to the nervous system with mental, bulbar, peripheral, or autonomic symptoms. It is therefore important, in all clinically suspicious cases, to test the urine for porphobilinogen. A low plasma sodium may be due to alimentary loss or to inappropriate secretion of antidiuretic hormone.

There is a variety with cutaneous and hepatic symptoms, *porphyria cutanea tarda*, in which increased urinary porphyrins are found during attacks.

Porphyria variegata. This has cutaneous and abdominal symptoms, and it is mainly found in South Africa. During the acute phase excess porphyrin precursors are present in urine, whilst during latent phases excess porphyrins are found in the faeces.

THE CONTROL OF ERYTHROCYTE DEVELOPMENT

Erythropoietin

This is a glycoprotein produced by the action of a factor from the kidneys, in response to hypoxia, on a plasma globulin substrate: it acts on and is utilised by the stem cells in the bone marrow. Its bioassay is possible as a research procedure in plasma or urine. It is not detectable in the plasma of normal subjects, but can be found in cases of anaemia.

In polycythaemia vera, erythropoietin production is very low due to negative feedback, whilst in polycythaemia due to carcinoma of the kidney (and occasionally to other tumours and other renal diseases) there is an inappropriate autonomous continuing production of erythropoietin and failure of feedback.

Vitamin B_{12}

The vitamin B_{12} group comprises a set of complex molecules, all of which contain Co^{II} in a porphyrin ring, linked to a nucleotide. Of the two main natural forms, which are interconvertible, deoxyadenosylcobalamin predominates over methylcobalamin. Vitamin B_{12} acts as a coenzyme: its deficiency is thought to cause megaloblastic anaemia by interfering with folate metabolism. The biochemical basis of the neurological lesions of vitamin B_{12} deficiency is not clear.

The normal dietary intake is 10–20 µg daily: vitamin B_{12} is absent from plant foods, so vegans (p. 89) are liable to develop eventual deficiency. All vitamin B_{12} in nature is synthesised by microorganisms, but vitamin B_{12} synthesised in the human colon is not absorbed. The normal requirement is about 2 µg daily, and as body stores are about 3 mg (of which some 50 per cent is in the liver), 3–5 years are required free of dietary B_{12} to develop deficiency.

Vitamin B_{12} in plasma. Vitamin B_{12} circulates bound to specific transport proteins (transcobalamins): the reference range for plasma vitamin B_{12}, measured microbiologically, is 160–900 ng/l (*or* pg/ml): the range by radioassay is 200–1000 ng/l.

The principal causes of a low plasma vitamin B_{12} are dietary deficiency, pernicious anaemia, gastric surgery, small gut disease involving the lower ileum with malabsorption (p. 240), and the blind loop syndrome (p. 239). Intrinsic factor is a mucoprotein, produced by the parietal cells of the stomach, whose synthesis is deficient in pernicious anaemia. It binds vitamin B_{12} (the original 'extrinsic factor'), and the resultant complex is absorbed into the villi of the terminal ileum, where the vitamin B_{12} is slowly split off and enters the circulation. About 1 per cent of a *large* oral dose of vitamin B_{12} can be absorbed in the absence of intrinsic factor.

Investigation of the cause of a low plasma vitamin B_{12}, with the appropriate haematological changes of a megaloblastic anaemia, is best done by measuring radioactive vitamin B_{12} absorption in the absence and presence of added intrinsic factor. There are many procedures, but a urinary excretion (Schilling) test is most popular.

Schilling test. *Method.* After an overnight fast the patient empties his bladder. The patient takes 1 µCi of [^{57}Co *or* ^{58}Co] B_{12} by mouth, and has an intramuscular flushing injection of 1 mg cyanocobalamin (non-radioactive vitamin B_{12}). All urine passed in the next 24 hours is pooled (with a final specimen at 24 hours) and sent to the laboratory.

If pernicious anaemia is suspected the test is repeated after four or five days, with the additional dose of 50 mg intrinsic factor orally taken with the dose of radioactive vitamin B_{12}.

Interpretation. In healthy subjects 10–33 per cent of the dose of radioactive vitamin B_{12} is excreted in the urine in 24 hours. In dietary deficiency, there is normal excretion. In pernicious anaemia less than 5 per cent of the dose is excreted, whilst in malabsorption up to 10 per cent may be found: in pernicious anaemia normal absorption and excretion are restored when the test is repeated with added intrinsic factor. Renal insufficiency depresses excretion of vitamin B_{12}, and invalidates the test.

Other tests. Measuring the ability of the stomach to secrete hydrochloric acid (p. 230) used to be an important part of the investigation of megaloblastic anaemia and is still occasionally useful. It is possible to measure, in serum, antibodies to parietal cells and to intrinsic factor.

The further oxidation of methylmalonyl CoA to succinyl CoA requires vitamin B_{12} as coenzyme. The normal urinary excretion of methylmalonic acid, 30–60 µmol/24 h, is increased up to 4 mmol/24 h in most cases of untreated vitamin B_{12} deficiency: the assay is difficult.

Folate

The parent compound is folic acid, otherwise known as pterylglutamic acid (or folacin), and contains a pteridine double ring, *p*-aminobenzoic acid, and glutamic acid. The various dietary folates are converted to methyl tetrahydrofolate during absorption. This active form enters intracellular metabolism and is converted to the folate coenzymes, which function in amino acid intraconversion and in the synthesis of purines and pyrimidines. Its exact role in erythrocyte maturation is unknown, though its deficiency is thought to cause megaloblastic anaemia through interference with DNA synthesis. Vitamin B_{12} is required for normal folate metabolism.

The normal daily dietary intake of folates from plant and animal food is about 700 µg. The normal requirement is about 200 µg/24 h, being much greater in pregnancy; the body stores are about 20 mg, and 20 weeks free from folate are required to develop deficiency. Folate is absorbed throughout the upper small intestine.

Folate in blood. The reference range for plasma folate is 5–20 μg/l (*or* ng/ml), and for erythrocyte folate is 150–600 μg/l, measured by microbiological assay. Tests for folate deficiency in megaloblastic anaemia, usually nutritional (absolute; or relative as in pregnancy), or due to malabsorption (p. 240) or due to drugs, are less satisfactory than for vitamin B_{12}: the plasma folate falls to less than 2 μg/l, and the erythrocyte folate to less than 100 μg/l. Plasma values fall first, at a subclinical stage of deficiency: erythrocyte values represent body stores – in a full study both should be measured.

Formiminoglutamic acid (FIGLU) requires folate as coenzyme for further metabolism: after an oral loading dose (15 g) of histidine normally less than 15 mg of FIGLU is excreted in 8 hours, whereas in folate deficiency more than 50 mg is excreted. However, this test is non-specific, and gives false positives (e.g. in vitamin B_{12} deficiency and in liver disease) and occasional false negatives.

IRON

Intake and absorption. The normal daily dietary intake of iron is 10–20 mg (200–400 μmol) mainly as complexes containing Fe^{III}. For its absorption the presence of gastric hydrochloric acid, and possibly of ascorbic acid for reduction to Fe^{II}, is desirable. About 10 per cent (1–2 mg) is normally absorbed: as 20–25 mg of iron daily is needed for haemoglobin synthesis, most of this is obtained from recirculated iron. Iron is absorbed, mainly as ferrous ions (Fe^{2+}), into the mucosa of the upper small intestine. There it is absorbed into the portal blood or bound as the soluble storage product ferritin, which is a complex of iron(III) hydroxide, phosphate, and the protein apoferritin, of molecular weight about 400 000. The role of the apoferritin in controlling the rate of iron absorption is uncertain. More iron is absorbed when there is iron deficiency, or when erythropoiesis is increased.

Circulating iron. The iron is then transferred to the plasma where it is bound to the specific β_1-globulin, transferrin (siderophyllin) of molecular weight 80 000. The reference range for plasma transferrin is less than 2 g/l, and plasma has a total iron binding capacity of 45–75 μmol/l. In plasma the concentration of free iron(III), in equilibrium with iron-transferrin, is negligible, and the transferrin is about one-third saturated with iron; the amount of unsaturated transferrin is termed the unsaturated iron-binding capacity. The reference range for plasma iron is 14–34 μmol/l in men, and 11–30 μmol/l in women. There is a marked ciradian rhythm, with a variation of about 7 μmol/l, and highest values at 08:00.

Iron distribution. The main function of iron is acting as the metal component of haemoglobin and myoglobin, and of iron-containing enzymes (cytochromes) of the electron transport system. The total body iron of an adult male is 4–5 g, and of a woman 3–4 g: about 65 per cent is as haemoglobin, 25 per cent as storage iron in the reticuloendothelial system (about equal parts of ferritin and haemosiderin), about 10 per cent as other tissue 'essential' iron (myoglobin, iron-containing enzymes, cytochromes), and only 0.1 per cent as plasma iron. Men lose only about 0.5–1.0 mg of iron daily, mainly in the faeces, with 0.1 mg in urine and 0.2 mg in shed skin. Women lose in addition on average 15 mg at each menstrual period (30 ml blood) and 500 mg at each pregnancy: women therefore are at greater risk of going into negative iron balance. A 'unit' of blood given by a donor contains about 250 mg of iron.

Abnormalities of plasma iron concentration. The concentration is low in iron-deficiency anaemia, whether due to absolute or relative insufficient intake, malabsorption, or blood loss. Low values are also found with the anaemia of most chronic diseases (infection, malignancy, collagen or autoimmune diseases). Plasma iron concentration is high when the marrow cannot utilise iron, in megaloblastic anaemia, in thalassaemia, and in anaemias associated with abnormal haemoglobin and haemolysis: high values are found in severe hepatitis due to release from liver cells, or after oral overdose with iron. In patients with anaemia measurement of plasma iron usually adds little to the information given by full haematological study. Plasma total iron-binding capacity should be measured at the same time as plasma iron: it is high in iron-deficiency anaemia and in pregnancy, whereas it is low in anaemias of chronic infection. The concentration of transferrin (like that of other binding proteins) is decreased in protein malnutrition (p. 113) and by urinary loss in the nephrotic syndrome, and increased by hormonal contraceptives.

Iron stores. Reticuloendothelial accumulation may be determined by histochemistry of bone marrow or liver biopsy for haemosiderin. This is reflected by the plasma ferritin (reference range 15–250 µg/l, males having a higher mean). In iron-deficiency anaemia the concentration is usually less than 10 µg/l, and low values will be found before the haemoglobin falls. In iron overload it may exceed 1000 µg/l, and raised values are also found in liver disease.

Haemochromatosis. It is uncertain whether the primary defect in this inborn error of metabolism is of iron storage or iron transport: iron absorption is excessive. The plasma total iron-binding capacity is low and is fully saturated, with a plasma iron of about 55 µmol/l. Haemosiderin is widely deposited in tissue and can be detected in cells of a urine deposit: the total body iron may be 20–40 g. Iron in the liver may cause cirrhosis, and combined deposition in skin and pancreas cause 'bronze diabetes': there is often hypogonadism.

Secondary haemochromatosis can result from iron overload, particularly due to repeated transfusion but occasionally orally: usually this deposition is mainly in the reticuloendothelial system and is asymptomatic, but hypoparathyroidism may develop.

COPPER

The known biochemical functions of copper are in the electron transport system, and possibly in the synthesis of haemoglobin. The reference range for plasma copper is 13–24 μmol/l, almost all of which is bound to caeruloplasmin, a specific α_2-globulin (molecular weight 150 000) whose plasma concentration is 0.3–0.6 g/l. Less than 1.5 μmol/24 h of copper are lost in the urine.

A low plasma caeruloplasmin results from urinary loss in the nephrotic syndrome, or from malnutrition; and a high value (sometimes with a green plasma) may be due to hormonal contraceptives or is occasionally seen in late pregnancy and primary biliary cirrhosis.

Wilson's disease (hepatolenticular degeneration). In this congenital metabolic disorder the primary defect is probably intrahepatic, with impaired synthesis of caeruloplasmin and impaired hepatobiliary excretion of copper. Plasma copper is low, 6–9 μmol/l; caeruloplasmin (often measured as 'copper oxidase') less than 0.3 g/l; and urinary copper increased to about 8 μmol/24 h. Copper deposition in brain and liver cause the mental and hepatic symptoms, and in the cornea produces the Kayser-Fleischer ring. Deposition in renal tubules may produce a Fanconi syndrome, and the resulting aminoaciduria may be diagnostically useful (p. 102).

Further reading

Elder GH, Gray CH, Nicholson DC. The porphyrias, a review. *J Clin Path* 1972; 25:1013–1033.

Huehns ER. Disease of haemoglobin synthesis. In: Baron DN, Compston, N, Dawson AM, eds. *Recent Advances in Medicine 16*. Edinburgh: Churchill-Livingstone, 1973:365–411.

CHAPTER 10

THE ENDOCRINE GLANDS

Mediation of hormone action by receptors

At a subcellular level many hormones act through a common mechanism. Cell membranes contain receptors for specific polypeptide hormones. When a hormone is bound to a cell of its target organ, the hormone activates adenylate cyclase. This intracellular enzyme converts adenosine triphosphate (ATP) to adenosine $3'5'$ monophosphate (cyclic AMP: 'second messenger'). Cyclic AMP then stimulates enzymes, cell transport systems, and therefore synthetic and metabolic processes, that are specific to the target organ. Other non-polypeptide hormones act via intracellular receptors, and do not use cyclic AMP as an intermediary.

The responsiveness of a target organ may vary in disease.

Hormone assay

Blood analysis gives hormone concentration only at a point in time; whereas urine analysis can represent secretion over a longer period but is influenced by variations in metabolism and excretion. Measurement of actual secretion rate is always difficult and expensive. Carefully selected stimulation and suppression tests are particularly useful in endocrine diagnosis, and may be used to determine the site of a lesion, or to detect loss of organ reserve function in the presence of doubtfully normal resting function. The local laboratory should be consulted for details of tests that are not described here.

The anterior pituitary hormones can be estimated biologically, although the techniques are generally difficult and tedious: new cytochemical procedures measure biological effects of a hormone on target cells, e.g. by microdensitometry. Radioimmunossay and related methods (which may give different results from those of bioassay) for all these hormones in plasma have been developed and they have greatly aided endocrine investigation. If not available locally, the assays can be done (in Britain), if essential for diagnosis, at special centres (p. 255): reference values should be obtained locally.

An increased excretion in urine of the placental hormone chorionic gonadotrophin can also easily be measured semi-quantitatively immunologically as a pregnancy diagnosis test.

In assays of the various peripheral hormones, competitive protein binding and related methods are mainly replacing chemical methods, and gas chromatography is being introduced.

THE HYPOTHALAMUS AND ANTERIOR PITUITARY

Hormones of the anterior pituitary gland.

Six separate hormones, which are probably secreted independently by
different cells, have so far been isolated from the human anterior
pituitary gland and their individual actions are relatively well understood. They are growth hormone (GH: or somatotrophic hormone,
STH); thyrotrophic hormone (TSH, thyroid-stimulating hormone);
adrenocorticotrophic hormone (ACTH); prolactin (PRL); follicle-
stimulating hormone (FSH); luteinising hormone (LH: also in males
sometimes called interstitial cell stimulating hormone, ICSH). The term
'gonadotrophins' combines FSH and LH (from common cells), and also
placental 'human' chorionic gonadotrophin (HCG).

The hormones of the anterior pituitary gland (except GH and prolactin) mainly act on other, target, endocrine glands to stimulate the
production or release of peripheral hormones. An increase in the plasma

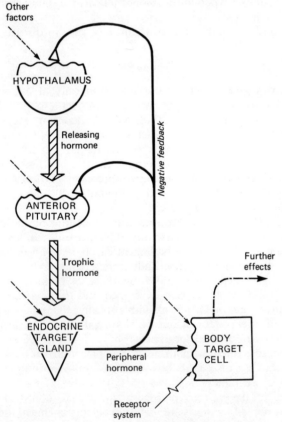

FIG. 10.1. The control of general peripheral hormone secretion by the anterior pituitary
gland and the hypothalamus, and the pathways of negative feedback.

concentration of peripheral hormone, whether secreted by the target gland or administered therapeutically, will depress the secretion by the anterior pituitary of the appropriate trophic hormone, either directly or by acting on the hypothalamus. Removal of the target gland, or cessation of its secretions, withdraws this negative feedback control of the anterior pituitary and an increased secretion of the trophic hormone results. The secretion of the hormones of the anterior pituitary gland is influenced via its hypothalamic regulating hormones directly and indirectly by the central nervous system, by such factors as stress and trauma, by circadian rhythms (p. 18), as well as by the feedback mechanisms of circulating peripheral hormones, and by many drugs (Fig. 10.1).

Hypothalamic regulating hormones

In recent years a number of polypeptide factors or hormones secreted by the hypothalamus have been identified, and their actions on the anterior pituitary are being elucidated. At present these are growth hormone releasing factor (GHRF, specific for GH), growth hormone release inhibitory hormone (GHRIH or somatostatin, with multiple actions including inhibition of glucagon, insulin, and other gastrointestinal hormones and secretions), thyrotrophin releasing hormone (TRH, acts on TSH and prolactin), corticotrophin releasing factor (CRF, specific for ACTH), prolactin inhibitory factor (PIF/dopamine, specific for prolactin), gonadotrophin releasing hormone (LHRH or GnRH, acts on FSH and LH).

The existence in man of a melanocyte stimulating hormone (MSH) independent of ACTH, and of MSH regulating factors, is doubtful: the function of the related lipotrophins is unclarified.

Endocrine disorders due to presumed direct hypothalamic abnormality

Overactivity

Precocious puberty is on rare occasions caused by excessive and premature hypothalamic stimulation of the pituitary, which causes release of gonadotrophins. This may sometimes be due to pressure on the hypothalamus by a pineal tumour, or to its independent effects.

Underactivity

Adiposogenital Dystrophy – Fröhlich's syndrome. This may be associated with a tumour or other lesion of the hypothalamus. At puberty the pituitary fails to produce gonadotrophins. The patient is sexually retarded. Obesity, which may be due to stimulation of an appetite centre, is also present.

General disorders of the anterior pituitary gland

Overactivity of the anterior pituitary need not involve all its hormones; a tumour usually causes excessive secretion of one hormone and may

depress secretion of other hormones. Underactivity of the anterior
pituitary may be complete, or be partial as an isolated hormone
deficiency.

Panhypopituitarism – Simmonds' disease

In this rare disorder there is complete or almost complete destruction of
the anterior of the anterior pituitary gland. It results principally from
post-partum haemorrhage, though local injury or intracranial non-
endocrine lesions may occasionally be responsible. The symptoms result
from deficiency of secondary hormones and measured values for these
and for pituitary hormones will be decreased. Deficiency of TSH lessens
thyroid hormone secretion and results in a low metabolic rate and
bradycardia though the plasma cholesterol is normal; deficiency of
prolactin and gonadotrophins lessens gonadal secretion, prevents lactation, and results in amenorrhoea, loss of libido, loss of sexual hair, and
atrophic skin changes; deficiency of ACTH lessens adrenal glucocorticoid
secretion and results in asthenia, hypoglycaemia (and a flat glucose
tolerance curve), and a very low plasma cortisol and a low corticosteroid
and 17-oxosteroid excretion. As aldosterone activity (independent of
ACTH) is unaltered, plasma electrolytes are normal. The characteristic
pallor is due to the deficiency of the melanocyte stimulating activity from
ACTH. Loss of GH may cause a low plasma phosphate.

Partial hypopituitarism

The above causes of hypopituitarism do not usually destroy all pituitary
activity. When anterior pituitary activity is diminished the secretion of
GH, prolactin, and gonadotrophins is lost first, and the patient presents
with symptoms of failure of lactation, amenorrhoea, and loss of sexual
hair before other symptoms of hypopituitarism develop. Later TSH
secretion, and then ACTH secretion, are impaired. This more common
partial deficiency syndrome, when seen after post-partum haemorrhage,
is often called Sheehan's syndrome. The typical initial biochemical
abnormality is the low gonadotrophins. Due to continuing secretion of
ACTH, plasma and urinary corticosteroids may not be low at first,
through 17-oxosteroid excretion is reduced. Carbohydrate metabolism is
usually unaltered and the patient is relatively well.

   Anorexia nervosa biochemically resembles Sheehan's syndrome. It is a
disorder of psychogenic origin, and the patient is suffering from malnutrition. Hormone production in general is slightly depressed, there is
usually a low to normal thyroid function, and a low or normal corticosteroid and 17-oxosteroid output. Secretion of gonadotrophins is
decreased early, leading to amenorrhoea. The glucose tolerance test is
normal in the early stages of the disease, and later flat, and hypersensitivity to insulin may develop: there is hypoglycaemia which leads to
increased GH secretion. The malnutrition, and vomiting, commonly
cause hypokalaemic alkalosis. The condition can respond to psycho-

therapy and to feeding. Rarely, prolonged anorexia nervosa may cause a permanent hypopituitarism.

Single hormone deficiencies. Pituitary myxoedema, pituitary Addison's disease, or pituitary amenorrhoea/eunuchoidism, may occur. These terms imply that there is defective pituitary secretion specifically of TSH, or of ACTH, or of gonadotrophins, but that there is no general pituitary deficiency nor primary disease of the thyroid, adrenal cortex, or gonads. These diseases are rare, and must be distinguished from mild general hypopituitarism in which perhaps the particular target organ (thyroid, adrenal cortex, or gonads) responds less readily to stimulation by its trophic hormone.

Investigation of central versus target gland deficiency

Primary deficiency of target glands (Fig. 10.2; such as myxoedema), typically show low resting plasma (and urinary) values of the appropriate peripheral hormone (Fig. 10.2, I) (such as thyroxine), and these values are not raised by stimulation with the specific pituitary trophic (II) or hypothalamic releasing hormone (III) (such as TSH, or TRH). The plasma concentration of the trophic hormone (TSH) will be high due to withdrawal of negative feedback.

When primary pituitary deficiency is causing deficiency of target gland function. (Fig. 10.3), the low resting values for peripheral hormone (Fig. 10.3 I) will respond to stimulation by the appropriate trophic hormone (II). The plasma (and urine) values for the pituitary trophic hormone will be low, and these (and the peripheral hormone values) will not respond to stimulation by the hypothalamic releasing hormone (III).

To test hypothalamic function it is possible to modify feedback controls (e.g. insulin-hypoglycaemia p. 161, metyrapone p. 160, clomiphene p. 163) and then to measure changes in trophic hormones or in peripheral hormones. Releasing hormones cannot be measured in plasma.

Investigation of central versus target gland overactivity

Determination of the level of the primary lesion is usually less of a problem here than for deficiency.

Autonomous primary overactivity of target glands (Fig. 10.4; such as Cushing's syndrome due to adrenal tumour) typically shows high resting plasma or urinary values for peripheral hormones (Fig. 10.4, I; such as cortisol): these are not lowered by suppressing the stimulant system (II) (e.g. by dexamethasone). The plasma value for the trophic hormone (ACTH) will be low due to excess negative feedback.

When primary hypothalamic-pituitary excess is causing target gland overaction (Fig. 10.5), the resting plasma values for the trophic hormone will be high as feedback is ineffective (Fig. 10.5, I); the high values for peripheral hormone will respond to appropriate suppression (II) – except for pituitary tumours which do not so respond, being autonomous.

142

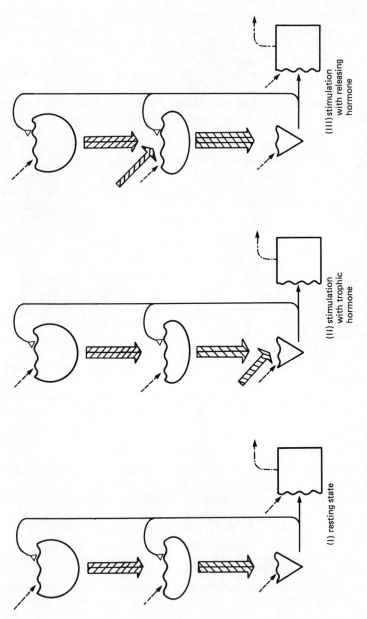

FIG. 10.2. Effect of stimulant tests on hormone secretion in primary deficiency of target glands (for use of symbols, see Fig. 10.1).

(I) resting state

(II) stimulation with trophic hormone

(III) stimulation with releasing hormone

143

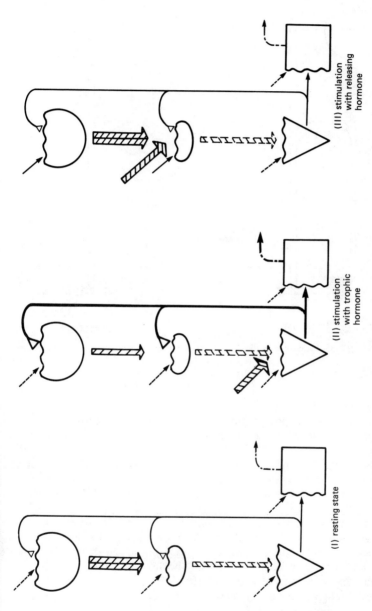

FIG. 10.3. Effect of stimulant tests on hormone secretion in primary pituitary deficiency.

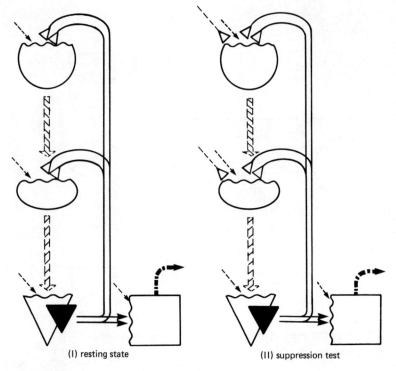

(I) resting state   (II) suppression test

FIG. 10.4. Effect of suppression tests on hormone secretion in autonomous overactivity of target glands.

Growth hormone

Secretion of GH, a polypeptide, is controlled by a releasing factor, and by a non-specific inhibiting hormone, somatostatin. GH acts mainly via a circulating polypeptide from the liver, somatomedin, which affects tissues to promote nitrogen retention and growth. It has diabetogenic and anti-insulin actions. Normally the fasting plasma GH level (reference values <10 µg/l) falls after glucose, and rises (due to hypoglycaemia) after insulin.

Pituitary dwarfism. This rare condition is due to decreased activity of its acidophil cells. There is usually a destructive lesion, and other manifestations of hypopituitarism are present; though there may be pure GH deficiency. The plasma GH may be low, and does not rise after insulin. The biochemical effects of the deficiency of GH are increased tolerance to glucose and increased sensitivity to insulin: there is a low urinary corticosteroid and 17-oxosteroid excretion.

Acromegaly. This results from excessive secretion of GH, caused by a tumour of acidophil or chromophobe cells, or less usually by hyper-

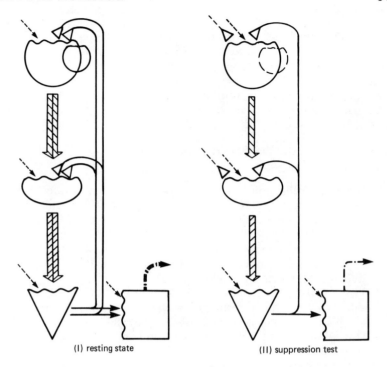

FIG. 10.5. Effect of suppression tests on hormone secretion in hypothalamic-pituitary overactivity.

plasia. In children, before the epiphyses have closed, it leads to gigantism. The fasting plasma GH level is usually raised, and there is no suppresion by a 75 g oral glucose load. The most marked effect is a stimulation of growth of bone and cartilage: in acromegaly hands, feet, nose, chin and ears are typically affected but internal organs may also be enlarged. There is demineralisation of the skeleton; the plasma calcium is normal with a high urinary calcium, but the plasma phosphate is usually raised. During the active phase there may be a goitre but not necessarily hyperthyroidism. Occasionally lactation is present. Patients with acromegaly may develop diabetes. Late destruction of basophil cells by the tumour diminishes gonadotrophin secretion and causes loss of sexual functions: if the disease stabilises there is generalised hypopituitarism but GH remains high.

THYROTROPHIC HORMONE AND THYROID FUNCTION

Secretion of TSH, a glycoprotein, is controlled by a tripeptide releasing hormone (TRH). TSH acts on the thyroid gland to promote the production and release of thyroxine and triiodothyronine. There are thyroid-stimulating immunoglobulins (thyroid receptor antibodies), whose production and relation to thyrotoxicosis, exophthalmos, and the mucopolysaccharide deposition of pretibial myxoedema are not fully elucidated.

Free thyroxine and triiodothyronine, by acting on the anterior pituitary, partly control the secretion of TSH as a negative feedback control by opposing the action of TRH.

Hormone synthesis in the thyroid gland

This may be summarised as follows (Fig. 10.6).

1 The acinar cells remove iodide from the plasma at a rate which is controlled by the plasma/gland iodide gradient (normally about 1:20), and by TSH activity.
2 Iodide is oxidised to iodine.
3 The iodine is immediately taken up by a tyrosine component of an intrathyroid globulin to produce mono- and di-iodotyrosine globulin – this forms the colloid.
4 Two of these molecules condense to form thyroxine and triiodothyronine, which are coupled to globulin as thyroglobulin: those which are not condensed are dehalogenated and recycled.
5 Thyroglobulin is hydrolysed and thyroid hormones are released into the circulation.

The actions of TSH on the thyroid gland are both anatomical and physiological. It causes hypertrophy and hyperplasia of the thyroid cells. It acts to promote iodide uptake into the thyroid gland and release of thyroid hormones. It stimulates most aspects of the intrathyroid synthesis of thyroxine.

Iodine

The minimum daily requirement of iodine in adults is about 20 μg, the normal intake being 70–200 μg. Iodine is concentrated in certain secretions (e.g. saliva, milk) as well as in the thyroid. A deficiency of iodine in the diet or drinking water, which occurs in certain inland mountainous areas, causes a simple goitre, and cretinism develops when there is gross iodine deficiency in infancy. Iodine-deficiency goitre can be prevented by the addition of sodium iodide to table salt (sodium chloride) in the proportion of 1/10 000.

When iodine is given for the treatment of thyrotoxicosis it acts principally by inhibiting the action of TSH, possibly by reducing the sensitivity of the thyroid cells to the hormone. Reduced secretion of thyroxine results, and this inhibition reaches its maximum in 10–14 days.

Goitrogenic agents

The thioamides (e.g. carbimazole) act principally by restricting the utilisation of iodide in the thyroid gland; and diminish the synthesis of

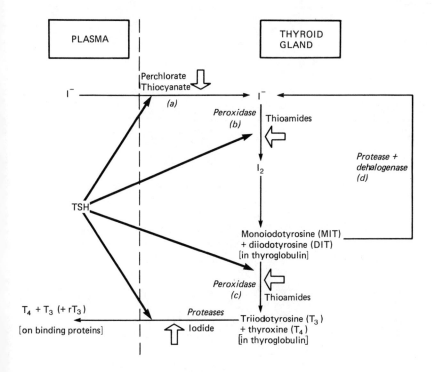

FIG. 10.6. Scheme of main pathways of thyroid hormone biosynthesis and control. The probable sites of action of antithyroid drugs are indicated, and the locations of the commoner genetic enzyme defects shown as (a), (b), (c), (d). See p. 152.

thyroxine. The activity of TSH is unhindered. There may be hypersensitivity of the thyroid cells to TSH, and secretion of TSH increases because of diminution of circulating thyroxine. The result is hypertrophy and hyperplasia of the thyroid. Thiocyanates and perchlorates, on the other hand, act competitively to diminish iodide uptake by the thyroid.

Thyroid hormones

3, 5, 3'-Triiodothyronine (T_3) is more potent than thyroxine, and has a shorter half-life. The relative importance of these two hormones in affecting cell metabolism, and to what extent T_4 is a prohormone, are uncertain. About 0.02 per cent of the thyroxine in plasma is active and in the free state; the remainder being bound to a T_4-binding α-globulin (TBG), to prealbumin, and to albumin, and triiodothyronine is about 0.3 % free. Reverse-T_3 (rT_3) is an *inactive* alternative to T_3 from deiodination of thyroxine; in malnutrition and in severe disease generally its production increases, so its concentration rises and that of T_3 falls, and general catabolism is thus reduced. Fig. 10.7 shows the structures of the compounds that are important in thyroid metabolism.

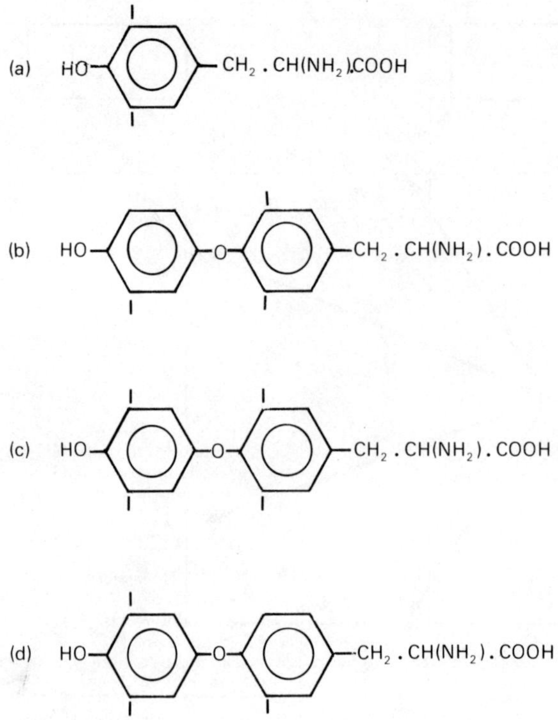

FIG. 10.7. Structures of the thyroid compounds: (a) Diiodotyrosine, (b) 3,5,3'-Triiodothyronine (T_3), (c) Thyroxine (T_4), (d) Reverse-T_3.

Calcitonin, from the parafollicular (C) cells, is unrelated to the other thyroid activities (p. 175).

The principal biochemical action of the thyroid hormones is acceleration of tissue oxidation. In physiological concentrations they are protein anabolisers, but in excess they are protein-catabolic, causing a negative nitrogen balance, and stimulating breakdown of muscle creatinine. Specific actions on carbohydrate and lipid metabolism, apart from secondary effects by the general stimulation of all metabolic processes, are uncertain. T_4 and T_3 are to a certain extent diabetogenic and anti-insulin for they stimulate gluconeogenesis, but the abnormally high glucose tolerance test curve (lag storage or diabetic) found in thyrotoxicosis is principally due to rapid absorption of carbohydrate from the intestine. The thyroid hormones lower the plasma concentration of cholesterol and the lipoproteins; they also directly stimulate the breakdown of bone.

About 10 per cent of the synthesised T_4 and T_3 is excreted in the bile, and the remainder is deiodinated.

The assessment of thyroid function

There are three complementary approaches: measurement of circulating thyroid or pituitary hormones, of thyroidal metabolism of iodine, and of secondary effects of thyroid hormones.

Thyroid hormones. Protein bound iodine (PBI) includes thyroxine and triiodothyronine (and rT_3 and mono- and di-iodothyronines), and also contaminating organic iodine such as X-ray contrast media.

Specific methods for plasma thyroxine have almost universally replaced measurement of PBI, and these avoid interference from iodine-containing drugs: reference values 60–130 nmol/l. In thyrotoxicosis the value is usually > 160 nmol/l, and in myxoedema is < 50 nmol/l. It is possible to measure T_3 (though less precisely): reference values 2–3 nmol/l.

Free thyroid hormones. Assay of *free* thyroxine is possible; of *free* T_3 (perhaps the ideal), is difficult and still a research procedure.

Resin uptake. A widely used but indirect procedure for determining the unsaturated binding capacity for thyroid hormones involves mixing serum (or plasma), a resin, and $[^{125}I]$ T_3. If plasma thyroxine is high (with a normal thyroxine-binding globulin, as in thyrotoxicosis), then the $[^{125}I]$ T_3 cannot be taken up by the plasma because the binding sites on TBG are saturated. It therefore is absorbed on to the *resin* where the high uptake can be measured. Conversely, the resin uptake is low in hypothyroidism because binding sites are unoccupied.

Changes in thyroxine-binding. With normal thyroid function, the nephrotic syndrome lowers thyroxine-binding globulin by urinary loss and produces a low plasma thyroxine and a high result on the resin test, whilst excess oestrogens and pregnancy increase thyroxine-binding globulin and produce a high plasma thyroxine and a low resin test result. Salicylates displace thyroxine from binding-globulin, usually leading to increased resin uptake and to increased free hormone concentrations. Protein malnutrition may also reduce thyroxine-binding globulin.

A few laboratories, instead of measuring resin uptake, measure *supernatant* activity which is low in thyrotoxicosis, and high in myxoedema.

Complex tests. It is possible to combine the above tests and express plasma thyroxine corrected for changes in protein-binding – i.e. 'free'. The usual measure is *free thyroxine index* (reference values 52 per cent to 142 per cent), calculated as plasma thyroxine × resin uptake. *Normalised thyroid ratio* and *effective thyroxine ratio* are similar investigations. The free thyroxine index is a useful derived measurement in pregnancy, or in patients receiving oestrogens including oral contraceptives: or conversely in thyroxine-binding globulin deficiency.

Pituitary hormone. The assay of TSH can distinguish between pituitary hypothyroidism, in which plasma TSH is low, and primary myxoedema, in which it is high at an early stage. In thyrotoxicosis, plasma TSH is low or normal (difficult to distinguish with current methods), and there is no discrimination from euthyroid patients.

TRH stimulation test

A valuable test for depression of pituitary thyrotrophic function is to measure the response of plasma TSH to intravenous TRH: the procedure, and reference values for the responses, vary locally but the following is acceptable

Method. 09:00; Collect 10 ml blood for TSH assay. Inject i.v. 200 μg TRH.
09:20, 10:00; Collect further blood samples for TSH assay.

Interpretation. In a normal subject the basal value is less than 5 mU/l, the 20 minute value 5–20 mU/l, and the 60 minute value 2–10 mU/l.

An impaired response is found even in early hyperthyroidism due to the excess circulating thyroxine causing pituitary suppression. A low response is also found in pituitary (but not hypothalamic) hypothyroidism: primary hypothyroidism may give an enhanced response.

Tests based on iodine metabolism

All tests of thyroid function which are based on investigation of iodine metabolism are disturbed by the presence of circulating exogenous iodine. Organic iodine received within the year before the test, or large doses of inorganic iodine taken within the previous three months, will depress the uptake of iodine by the thyroid gland and invalidate the results of the tests. In states of iodine deficiency, radioactive iodine uptake is increased.

Tests using radioactive iodine generally employ ^{131}I: however isotopes with a shorter half-life have great advantages in safety. Technetium is widely used as [^{99}Tc^{m}] pertechnetate.

These dynamic tests of thyroid function include thyroid iodine uptake, plasma ^{131}I concentration, plasma iodine clearance, and urinary iodine excretion. They are less sensitive than the hormone assays described above, even when combined with stimulation by TSH or suppression by T_3. The use of *in vivo* uptake studies and scanning for the localisation of disease in the thyroid, such as tumour nodules, is usually not the responsibility of chemical pathology.

Indirect tests – basal metabolic rate

The basal metabolic rate (BMR) of a patient is the basal (fasting and at rest) energy output, measured as oxygen uptake (assuming a constant respiratory quotient, 0.82) compared with the mean average energy output of normal subjects of the same age, sex, and size (conveniently measured by the surface area). Accurate measurement of the BMR is difficult; and the test, which is non-specific, is now obsolete. The reference values are -13% to $+13\%$.

A raised BMR is typically found in hyperthyroidism, when it is usually above $+20$ per cent and is proportional to the degree of toxicity. However fever, anxiety states, and other hormonal over-secretory states (e.g. acromegaly) also raise the BMR. A low BMR is typically found in hypothyroidism, when it is usually below -20 per cent. However, other endocrine deficiencies (e.g. Addison's disease) also lower the BMR.

Unlike the hormone assays and *in vivo* iodine tests, the BMR takes account of possible altered tissue sensitivity to thyroxine.

Other indirect biochemical tests

The plasma cholesterol concentration is occasionally lowered in thyrotoxicosis, but this is of no value in diagnosis. A raised plasma cholesterol is usually found in myxoedema, and the value is proportional to the severity of the disease in an individual patient: this has been used in following the effects of therapy. Phospholipids are similarly altered, and in myxoedema there is also carotinaemia. Effects of thyroxine on muscle can be shown by an increase of urinary creatine: plasma creatine kinase does not increase. In thyrotoxicosis, by an effect on the sodium pump, the erythrocyte sodium is increased.

Choice of tests

A proposed order of biochemical investigations to combine efficiency with economy, later tests being unnecessary if earlier tests answer the question, is

1 Plasma thyroxine
2 Resin uptake
3 Free thyroxine index
4 Plasma TSH
5 TRH test
6 Plasma T_3 (for T_3-toxicosis)

Summary of biochemical changes in thyroid disease

Hyperthyroidism

Most of the symptoms are due to increased metabolic oxidation and in severe thyrotoxicosis this may lead to hyperpyrexia and thyrotoxic crises. The principal laboratory finding of diagnostic value at present is an increased plasma thyroxine, supported if necessary by a raised free thyroxine index. Doubtful cases may be detected by an impaired TSH response to TRH. In the rare T_3-*toxicosis*, plasma T_3 is raised, but not thyroxine. As T_3 is also raised in 'standard' thyrotoxicosis, it has been suggested that estimation of plasma T_3 should replace that of plasma thyroxine in *all* cases.

A lag storage or diabetic type of glucose tolerance curve, and a low plasma cholesterol may be present, but these findings are insufficiently consistent to be of more than secondary interest. Demineralisation of the skeleton, with increased urinary calcium, is found in severe cases. If there is secondary renal damage, hypercalcaemia may be present.

Other procedures, such as a radioiodine scan for thyroid nodules, may be necessary to determine the pathological cause of the hyperthyroidism.

Thyrotoxicosis may be brought about by excessive intake of thyroxine – thyrotoxicosis factitia – and this occurs typically during self-medication for obesity. Dynamic iodine tests may be diagnostically confusing as a high plasma thyroxine is associated with depressed thyroidal iodine uptake.

Hypothyroidism

In cretins (congenital hypothyroidism is the commonest inborn error of metabolism) thyroid function is deficient from birth. In neonates measurement of serum TSH on the blood sample taken for the Guthrie test for phenylketonuria (p. 101) is probably the best screening test, and a value >80 mU/l is diagnostic: perhaps thyroxine should also be measured.

Most of the symptoms of hypothyroidism can be generally explained as being due to deficient tissue oxidation throughout the body. In severe myxoedema the reduced metabolism may lead to hypothermia and coma. The retention in the interstitial tissues of mucopolysaccharide (myxoedema tissue) is not satisfactorily explained. The laboratory finding of diagnostic value at present is a low plasma thyroxine, supported if necessary by a low free thyroxine index. Doubtful cases may be detected by a raised plasma TSH.

Other abnormal findings of secondary interest are a high plasma cholesterol and β-lipoproteins. A flat glucose tolerance curve is sometimes found. The urinary corticosteroid (and oxosteroid) excretion is often low.

Other procedures, such as measurement of thyroidal antibodies for Hashimoto's disease, may be necessary to determine the pathological cause of the hypothyroidism.

There are various rare *genetic defects* causing goitre and hypothyroidism which are thought to be due to the enzyme deficiencies shown at *a, b, c,* or *d,* in Fig. 10.6. More detailed hormone studies are needed for their elucidation, and biochemical analysis of a biopsy may be required.

In *endemic goitre,* due to dietary iodine deficiency, compensatory hypersecretion of TSH often maintains the euthyroid state by enlarging the gland.

ADRENOCORTICOTROPHIC HORMONE AND ADRENAL CORTICAL FUNCTION

ACTH is a polypeptide whose secretion is controlled by CRF from the hypothalamus, with feedback from the level of circulating plasma cortisol. ACTH acts on the adrenal cortex to produce hyperplasia, and to

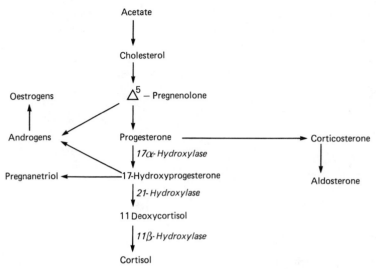

FIG. 10.8. The principal steps in the synthesis of the hormones of the adrenal cortex.

promote the conversion of cholesterol to pregnenolone and progesterone, and thus stimulates the formation of the glucocorticoids and
adrenal androgens. There is a marked circadian rhythm of ACTH
secretion. It also has a slight direct melanophore expanding activity
because the ACTH polypeptide contains the active amino acid sequence
of melanophore stimulating hormone activity.

As a result of various stimuli, such as cold, injury, mental stress,
attacks of depression, operations, or infections, the secretion of ACTH by
the anterior pituitary gland is increased due to excess production of CRF
which overrides the negative feedback control. This ACTH secretion
promotes an increased output of adrenal glucocorticoids: if the external
stimulus is long continued, exhaustion of the adrenal cortex occurs and
resistance to further noxious stimuli is lowered.

Hormones of the adrenal cortex

Two main types of hormone, corticosteroids and androgens, are synthesised in and secreted by the adrenal cortex (Fig. 10.8); it also probably
normally secretes a small quantity of oestrogens and progestogens.

Corticosteroids

The principal corticosteroids secreted by the human adrenal cortex are
aldosterone (from the zona glomerulosa), cortisol (in pharmacy called
hydrocortisone, from the zona fasciculata), and corticosterone (from both
layers). Cortisol is synthesised from progesterone by the action of successive
hydroxylases (steroid monooxygenases), and aldosterone by a different

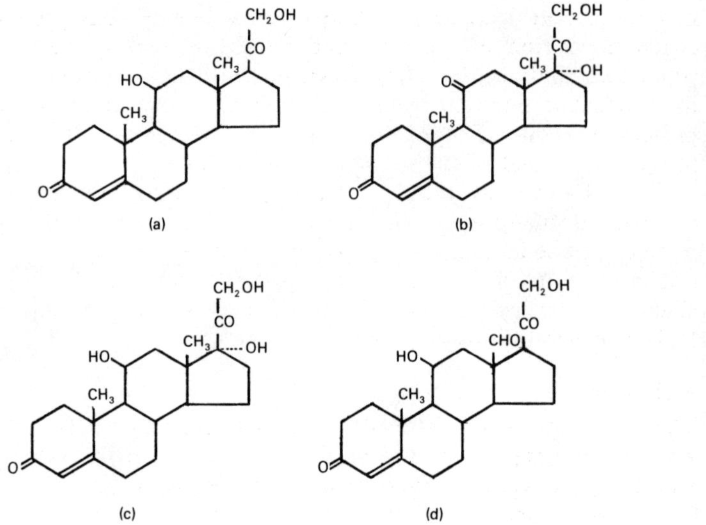

Fig. 10.9. Structures of the corticosteroids: (a) Corticosterone, (b) Cortisone, (c) Cortisol (hydrocortisone), (d) Aldosterone.

pathway via corticosterone. Cortisone is a synthetic steroid, not a normal secretion. Their structures are shown in Fig. 10.9. Aldosterone is very potent, and is secreted in small amounts, about 0.5 μmol/24 h: the normal secretion of cortisol is about 70 μmol/24 h.

Mineralocorticoid activity

Aldosterone is called a mineralocorticoid. By a cell membrane effect, particularly by an action on the renal tubules (and to a lesser extent on the small intestine, and salivary and sweat glands) it promotes sodium reabsorption and potassium exchange. The result is retention of sodium, chloride, and water, and loss of potassium.

The final stages of the secretion of aldosterone are not under primary ACTH control. Renin is produced in the juxtaglomerular cells of the kidney (p. 210) by a feedback mechanism involving volume changes of the extracellular fluid that affect renal perfusion pressure. Renin produces the decapeptide angiotensin I from a circulating α-glycoprotein angiotensinogen, and converting enzyme in the lung transforms it to the active octapeptide angiotensin II, which stimulates release of aldosterone. Sodium or water depletion promotes aldosterone secretion, and vice versa, by affecting the production of renin.

Cortisol and corticosterone have some mineralocorticoid activity.

Glucocorticoid activity

Corticosterone and cortisol are called glucocorticoids. They act on carbohydrate metabolism in opposition to insulin, stimulating gluconeogenesis and decreasing carbohydrate utilisation, but promoting glycogen deposition in the liver and fat deposition. In excess they are protein catabolisers, breaking down protein to carbohydrate, and causing a negative nitrogen balance; though physiological amounts may be protein anabolic. They help in the maintenance of the glomerular filtration rate and of the normal blood pressure.

Cortisol and its synthetic derivatives, but not corticosterone, suppress antibody formation and the inflammatory response, and depress the number of circulating eosinophils and lymphocytes.

The secretion of the glucocorticoids is stimulated by ACTH. The very slight glucocorticoid activity of aldosterone has no significance at physiological concentrations.

Androgens

Their secretion in the adrenal glands is stimulated by ACTH, possibly with gonadotrophin synergism. They include dehydro*epi*androsterone and 11-hydroxylated compounds, but not testosterone. They are only feebly androgenic and protein anabolic, and are excreted as 17-oxosteroids.

The adrenal androgens and oestrogens act as promoters of growth of hormone-dependent carcinoma of the prostate and breast respectively. The rationale of adrenalectomy, when performed (in combination with gonadectomy) as palliative treatment of these tumours, is the removal of the 'controlling' hormonal background. Hypophysectomy is performed for the same purpose. The rationale here is the removal of ACTH, the gonadotrophins, and GH. It has been claimed that a high ratio of urinary aetiocholanolone to total 17-hydroxycorticosteroids in patients with carcinoma of the breast is a positive discriminant in favour of a response to such endocrine ablative therapy.

Adrenocortical hormones in plasma and urine

Cortisol is the principal glucocorticoid in the plasma. About 5 per cent of it is active and circulates in the free state, the remainder being bound to a relatively specific β-globulin (CBG, transcortin); and a little to albumin. The plasma concentration of binding-globulin, therefore of transcortin-bound and of total cortisol, is increased by endogenous and exogenous oestrogens – particularly pregnancy and hormonal contraceptives. Plasma cortisol is usually estimated either fluorimetrically as 'corticosteroids' (which includes corticosterone and non-steroid components; and spironolactone) or specifically by competitive protein binding. There is a marked circadian variation – the reference values for plasma cortisol at midnight are 50–280 nmol/l, and at 09:00 are 200–700 nmol/l. The glucocorticoids are excreted in the urine principally in reduced forms, conjugated with glucuronic acid. Methods for urinary cortisol and its metabolites ('corticosteroids') as 17-oxogenic steroids give reference values of 20–75 µmol/24 h in adult males and 15–60 µmol/24 h in adult females: the alternative measurement of 17-hydroxycorticosteroids gives similar results except in cases of biochemical disorders of adrenal hormone synthesis. More specific methods for urinary free cortisol, whose excretion follows the plasma free cortisol, are available.

Estimation of plasma aldosterone is a specialised radioimmunoassay, the reference values being 100–500 pmol/l: urinary assay is equally difficult, and the normal excretion is 15–20 nmol/24 h.

The plasma corticosteroid level reflects adrenocortical secretion of cortisol (and corticosterone) at that time, or exogenous cortisol administration. The urinary corticosteroid excretion reflects these blood levels (p. 137) unless there is renal excretory impairment, or sometimes in metabolic disorders of the adrenal cortex when unusual derivatives are excreted. These values are therefore in general increased when there is increased ACTH secretion, or hyperplasia or tumour of the adrenal cortex; and decreased when there is decreased ACTH secretion, or damage to the adrenal cortex.

Plasma ACTH may be measured by radioimmunoassay, and a cytochemical method of bioassay has been developed as a research procedure. This is a direct measure of pituitary or ectopic hormone production in diagnostically difficult cases, and may distinguish between primary and secondary adrenocortical deficiency.

Adrenocortical hyperactivity

Oversecretion of adrenal cortical hormones may arise from hyperplasia or tumour of the adrenal cortex, and may be secondary to increased ACTH secretion. The symptomatology depends on the nature of the cortical hormones which are secreted in excess.

Cushing's syndrome

This is characterised by an increased circulating free cortisol concentration.

It is often associated with excess secretion of ACTH by an overactive anterior pituitary with abolition of the circadian rhythm: the negative feedback cycle is impaired and sensitivity to the high plasma cortisol level from the hyperplastic adrenals has been lost. The syndrome may be caused by an ACTH-secreting pituitary tumour; or by an adrenal tumour that autonomously secretes excess cortisol, with suppression of ACTH secretion. There may also be extrapituitary ectopic secretion of an adrenocorticotrophic hormone by a 'non-endocrine' tumour, such as carcinoma of the bronchus. Excessive treatment with ACTH or corticosteroids can cause a similar syndrome, and this may also be seen in chronic alcoholics due to 'stress' stimulation.

Insulin-resistant diabetes and glycosuria result from effects on carbohydrate metabolism; cessation of growth, muscular wasting, osteoporosis, and atrophy of collagen leading to the characteristic striae, from effects

on protein metabolism; the moon-face and buffalo-hump from effects on
fat metabolism. A moderate hypokalaemic alkalosis, and sodium and
water retention, from effects on electrolyte metabolism, are found.
Hypertension, polycythaemia, lymphopenia, and eosinopenia, generally
occur. Adrenal androgen secretion is usually little altered (except in
adrenocortical carcinoma), hence in women virilism is rare though
hirsutism may be seen.

The plasma cortisol level is high, with characteristic abolition of the
circadian rhythm and high midnight levels. The plasma ACTH value
depends on the aetiology of the syndrome. The response to dexamethasone (p. 160) may help in diagnosis. Specific measurement of the
increased cortisol secretion rate is a research procedure. Urinary corticosteroids are typically more than 90 μmol/24 h, with a high 'free' cortisol;
the urinary 17-oxosteroid excretion may be normal or only slightly
raised.

Adrenogenital syndrome (congenital adrenal hyperplasia)

These common inborn errors of metabolism, in contrast to Cushing's
syndrome, are due to excess secretion of androgens and present as
virilism without glucocorticoid metabolic effects. They are caused by a
metabolic block, usually at the stage of 21-hydroxylation (Fig. 10.8) in
the synthesis of cortisol from progesterone, and the deficiency of
circulating cortisol (generally low-normal) results in excess ACTH secretion by removal of feedback inhibition. There may be pseudo-
Addison's disease with sodium deficiency, because of deficient cortisol
and aldosterone secretion, when the enzyme deficiency is more complete.
The excess ACTH stimulates the production of androgens along other
pathways and these are excreted in excess in the urine as 17-oxosteroids:
excess pregnanetriol is also produced and excreted in the urine. These
two findings (which require a 24 hour collection of urine) are valuable in
diagnosis, and the significant levels depend on the age of the patient. A
high plasma 17-hydroxyprogesterone is also found. The 11-oxygenation
index is useful in that it can be measured in infants on a random urine
sample: the ratio of 11-deoxy to 11-oxy metabolites of 17-oxogenic
steroids, normally <0.5, diagnostically exceeds 1.0. A recent development may lead to prenatal diagnosis by analysis of steroids in amniotic
fluid.

One rare variety of the syndrome, with a block at 11-hydroxylation,
also shows hypertension, possibly due to excess 11-deoxycortisol (and
aldosterone) that is produced (Fig.10.8). This compound is measured as a
urinary 17-oxogenic steroid, so this value may be normal even though
cortisol secretion is deficient, and urinary steroid fractionation may be
needed for diagnosis.

Treatment with cortisone depresses the excessive ACTH secretion, and
reverses the syndrome.

Tumours

Benign or malignant tumours of the adrenal cortex usually give rise to a syndrome with mixed metabolic and virilising aspects, either of which may predominate: ACTH secretion is depressed. In general, benign tumours produce one hormone (but are often non-endocrine), and malignant tumours can produce multiple hormones. Urinary excretion of corticosteroids and of 17-oxosteroids are often both increased to more than 150 μmol/24 h, and may be more than 2 mmol/24 h. Adrenal tumours give rise to excess 3β-compounds such as dehydro-epiandrosterone.

Primary aldosteronism (Conn's syndrome)

There are rare tumours of the adrenal cortex, or occasionally hyperplasia, which produce only excess aldosterone and cause primary aldosteronism – inappropriate secretion. This is characterised by hypokalaemia (due to urinary and intestinal potassium loss) and muscular weakness, alkalosis, polyuria, hypertension, and generally sodium retention. There is often a diabetic glucose tolerance curve. Renin secretion is suppressed. The diagnosis can be confirmed biochemically, when the patient is on a standard Na/K intake, by showing a high plasma and urinary aldosterone, or aldosterone secretion rate, with a low plasma renin.

Secondary aldosteronism. This common condition may be found in conditions where there is loss of sodium from the extracellular fluid, such as nephrotic syndrome, cirrhosis and ascites, congestive heart failure, and due to many diuretics. In these conditions hypokalaemia is rarer, and plasma renin and aldosterone are increased – appropriate secretion.

Adrenocortical hypoactivity

Chronic secondary hyposecretion of adrenal cortical hormones may result from hypopituitarism; other features of hypopituitarism are then usually present, but aldosterone secretion is retained so sodium and potassium balance are then little altered. Specific ACTH deficiency can follow excessive treatment with corticosteroids.

Addison's disease

This is a primary lesion of the adrenal glands due to destructive or atrophic disease, usually autoimmune or tuberculous. The symptoms that develop are due to defiency of all adrenocortical hormones. There is salt depletion due to excess urinary sodium and chloride loss, and potassium retention. Plasma electrolyte changes are a sign of loss of adrenal functional reserve. A low renal plasma flow is caused by the sodium deficiency and hypotension; and this leads to prerenal azotaemia. Asthenia, loss of weight, hypotension, and gastrointestinal disturbances,

regularly occur. Increased glucose utilisation and decreased gluconeogenesis lead to hypoglycaemia (p. 66) in severe cases: there is a flat
glucose tolerance curve, and hypersensitivity to insulin. There is secretion
of excess ACTH: this stimulates the adrenal remnant, and causes the
characteristic pigmentation because of its melanocyte stimulating action.

Whilst adrenal reserve is still present plasma and urinary corticosteroids may only be low-normal, and a stimulation test may be needed:
in severe cases these hormones will be undetectable. Urinary
17-oxosteroids are similarly low.

Acute adrenal insufficiency

This may develop in Addison's disease or in the Friderichsen-
Waterhouse syndrome (adrenal haemorrhage in meningococcal or similar septicaemia). In an Addisonian crisis the metabolic features of
Addison's disease are severe, in particular hyponatraemia and hypotension with a high plasma urea, and hypoglycaemia.

It is not uncommon for long-term corticosteroid therapy markedly to
suppress the secretion of ACTH. These patients, who show mild adrenocortical deficiency on cessation of treatment, may develop acute adrenal
insufficiency when 'stressed' – e.g. by severe infection or surgery.

Stimulation and suppression tests for adrenocorticoid function

Although measurement of base-line plasma or urinary corticosteroids,
and if available plasma ACTH, will often be diagnostic in cases of overt
disease of the anterior pituitary-adrenocortical axis, further information
can be obtained from appropriate stimulation or suppression tests in
doubtful cases (Figs. 10.2–10.5).

Short tetracosactrin test

The standard rapid procedure is to measure the plasma cortisol response
to synthetic corticotrophin polypeptide, tetracosactrin (Synacthen, Ciba).

Method. A midnight sample may be collected for studies of the circadian
rhythm.
09:00. Collect 10 ml heparinised blood for cortisol assay (baseline).
Inject intramuscularly 250 μg tetracosactrin.
09:30. Collect blood for cortisol assay.

Interpretation. In a normal subject, the base-line value is more than
200 nmol/l, and there is an increase of at least 300 nmol/l over the base-
line at 30 minutes. In Addison's disease there is a low base-line and less
than 150 nmol/l response to tetracosactrin, and in hypopituitarism there
may be a subnormal rise at 30 minutes. In Cushing's syndrome (hyperplasia) there may be an exaggerated response; an autonomous adrenal
tumour gives no response.

Prolonged tetracosactrin test

This gives a greater stimulus than does the short test, and is useful in doubtful cases and especially in checking function after long-term steroid therapy. All hormonal treatment must be discontinued from at least three days before the control period until the end of the test.

Method. First test day; 09:00. Collect 10 ml heparinised blood for cortisol assay (base-line).
Inject intramuscularly 1 mg depot tetracosactrin.
17:00. Collect blood for cortisol assay.
Second and third test days. Repeat the blood collections and the stimulant injections.

Interpretation. In a normal adult there is a rise in plasma cortisol on the first day to above 1400 nmol/l. In Addison's disease there is no rise even after three days, whereas in adrenocortical hypofunction secondary to pituitary deficiency the value may exceed 700 nmol/l after the third injection.

Dexamethasone suppression tests

Dexamethasone is a synthetic steroid that inhibits ACTH secretion, and suppresses the plasma and urinary corticosteroids in normal subjects. The test is used to differentiate adrenal hyperplasia from tumour.

Method.
(i) Collect 24 hour urine samples for base-line corticosteroid estimation for 2 days (Days 1 and 2).
(ii) Collect blood samples for base-line cortisol estimation at 09:00 on Days 1 and 2.
(iii) Dexamethasone is given 6 hourly in 0.5 mg oral doses for 8 doses (low dose test: Days 3 and 4) followed by 2.0 mg oral doses 6 hourly for 8 doses (high dose test: Days 5 and 6).
(iv) 24 hour urine samples are collected for corticosteroid estimation while on dexamethasone (Days 3, 4, 5, and 6).
(v) Blood samples for cortisol are collected preceding the dexamethasone dose on Days 4, 5, 6, and 7.

Interpretation. In a normal subject the urine and plasma corticosteroids are suppressed on the lower dosage below 50 per cent of the base-line values. On the lower doses of dexamethasone patients with Cushing's syndrome will show no suppression irrespective of cause. On the higher dose, those with hyperplasia have a 50 per cent or more suppression, while those with either adenoma or carcinoma, or ectopic ACTH production, are unaffected.

Metyrapone test

Metyrapone (Metapirone) inhibits the action of the enzyme 11β-hydroxylase in the adrenal cortex (Fig. 10.8), thus reducing cortisol synthesis. This triggers the feedback mechanism, causing CRF and

ACTH secretion. The result is excess adrenocortical secretion of 11-deoxycortisol, which is measured as a urinary corticosteroid. The test is used for investigating hypothalamic or anterior pituitary deficiency if plasma ACTH assays are not available.

Method.
(i) Collect 24 hour urine samples for base-line corticosteroid estimation for 2 days (Days 1 and 2).
(ii) Metyrapone is given 4 hourly in 750 mg oral doses for 6 doses (Day 3).
(iii) Collect 24 hour urine samples for corticosteroid estimation on day of, and after Metyrapone administration (Days 3 and 4).

Interpretation. A normal subject shows an increase in urine corticosteroid values of at least 35 μmol/24 h, or a twofold increase above the resting level. A subnormal response, in the presence of known normal adrenocortical function, shows deficiency at the level of the hypothalamus or anterior pituitary. In addition, patients with autonomous tumours of the adrenal cortex fail to show a response.

Alternatively, but less usually, an increase in plasma 11-deoxycortisol is measured as the normal response.

Other tests

These are used mainly in special circumstances, and local procedures should be followed. They involve the use of either *insulin*-induced hypoglycaemia or *pyrogen* as stress agents to the hypothalamus via higher centres, or of *lysine-vasopressin* as a synthetic corticotrophin releasing factor to stimulate the anterior pituitary.

GONADOTROPHIC HORMONES AND GONADAL FUNCTION

Hypothalamic control of pituitary gonadotrophin secretion by the specific releasing hormone is influenced both by higher centres and by feedback from circulating oestrogens and androgens.

The somatic effects of FSH and LH are due to the actions of the sex hormones whose production they stimulate from the gonads. It is doubtful whether these pituitary hormones have any independent metabolic activity.

Female sex hormones

Oestrogens

The three principal human oestrogens are oestradiol, oestrone, and oestriol: a steroid ring is not necessary for oestrogenic activity, as shown by the original synthetic oestrogen, stilboestrol. Their structures are shown in Fig. 10.10. Apart from their actions on the sexual organs and activities, the oestrogens are protein anabolisers, and are occasionally given therapeutically, but with little success, to promote a positive

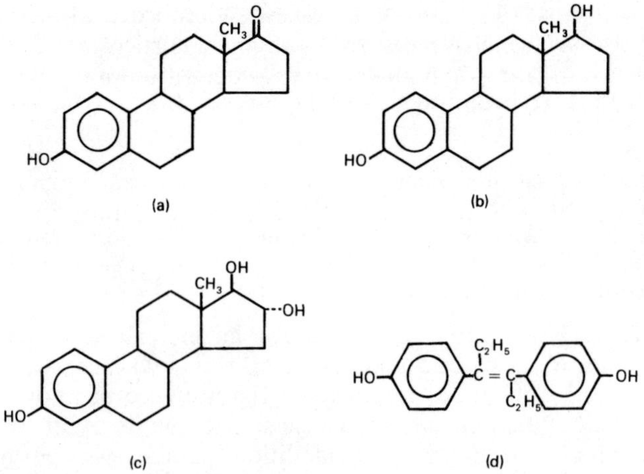

FIG. 10.10. Structures of the oestrogens: (a) Oestrone, (b) Oestradiol, (c) Oestriol, (d) Stilboestrol.

nitrogen balance especially for post-menopausal osteoporosis (p. 183). They also have a slight sodium and water-retaining activity.

There is a plasma sex hormone binding globulin (SHBG), with limited affinity for oestradiol, and greater affinity for testosterone.

Oestrogens are used for the treatment of carcinoma of the prostate: prostatic growth is maintained by androgens, and oestrogens depress the pituitary production of gonadotrophins, thus reducing in males the secretion of androgens. Oestrogens in large doses have a limited value in the treatment of post-menopausal carcinoma of the breast with meta-stases; but about 50 per cent of cases of pre-menopausal carcinoma of the breast are hormone-dependent, namely their growth is stimulated by oestrogens. The continued presence in malignant breast tissue of oestrogen-receptors, and also of progesterone-receptors (as are present in normal breast tissue) is a valuable indication of likely response to endocrine therapy. This may also indicate general freedom from re-currence, and response to chemotherapy. Their assay is still a research procedure.

An increase in the production of oestrogens in relation to androgens, from any cause, causes gynaecomastia. Excess oestrogen production, and consequent excretion, takes place in occasional tumours of the ovary, testis, or adrenal cortex.

Oestrogen assays. Oestrogens are excreted in the urine principally after conjugation with glucuronic acid in the liver; and in cirrhosis there is increased excretion of free oestrogens, with diminished conjugation. Total urinary oestrogen excretion is a common assay, but separate estimation of the individual oestrogens is technically complex. The main use of oestrogen assay is in a possibly abnormal pregnancy to monitor the fetoplacental unit. Low values are found in primary and secondary amenorrhoea, and assay of gonadotrophins is used for differential diagnosis. In the successful treatment of amenorrhoea, generally for infertility, by human chorionic gonadotrophin or by clomiphene, there is a rise in the urinary oestrogen excretion and this must be monitored for the control of therapy.

Plasma oestriol assay is becoming available, and this may replace analysis of urine.

Progesterone

The estimation of progesterone in plasma is a recent introduction, and studies of progesterone metabolism are generally made on the inactive urinary excretion product, pregnanediol. Their structures are shown in Fig. 10.11. The normal excretion of pregnanediol is: males, and females (follicular phase of menstrual cycle) 0.6–3 μmol/24 h: females (luteal phase of menstrual cycle) 5–20 μmol/24 h.

An increased excretion of pregnanediol occurs in pregnancy because there is an increase in the secretion of progesterone. The excretion steadily increases to a maximum of about 150 μmol/24 h at about 30 weeks, and falls to normal about a week after delivery, though the rise is too inconstant to be used as a test for pregnancy. An increase is often also found in patients with adrenocortical tumours.

The detection of an increase in plasma progesterone in the second half of the menstrual cycle may be used to check that ovulation has occurred.

Hormonal contraceptives

The most frequently administered sex hormones are the oral hormonal contraceptives (the Pill), which are usually a mixture of an oestrogen and a progestogen and have a complex mode of action. These may have marked effects in healthy women on normal biochemical patterns, principally due to the oestrogen component. By increasing the specific binding proteins, the hormones cause raised plasma levels of thyroxine (p. 149), corticosteroids (p. 155), iron (p. 135), and copper (p. 136): the free fractions are unaltered. In some subjects there is diminished glucose

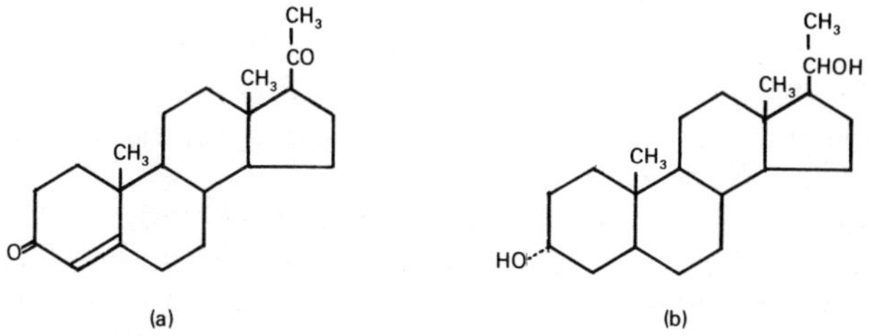

(a) (b)

Fig. 10.11. Structures of the progestogens: (a) Progesterone, (b) Pregnanediol.

tolerance ('steroid diabetes') and also an increased plasma free fatty acids. An increase in plasma triglycerides, and to a lesser extent, in cholesterol, is significant where there is preexisting hyperlipoprotein-aemia (p. 86). Abnormal liver function tests from cholestasis may develop. An effect on tryptophan metabolism may be the cause of the occasional deficiency of folate and of vitamin B_6.

Menstrual cycle

At the beginning of the menstrual cycle hypothalamic stimulation of the anterior pituitary causes release of FSH, and the ovum matures. Before midcycle there is a peak of ovarian oestrogen secretion which depresses FSH secretion, and stimulates the midcycle peak of LH. There is a second, sharper, FSH peak and ovulation occurs, and the follicle ripens to form the corpus luteum. This, under the influence of LH, secretes progesterone, and more oestrogen with another peak 10 days after ovulation. The progesterone secretion depresses LH production, the corpus luteum ceases to function, the oestrogen and progesterone then fall, and there is menstrual bleeding. The final fall in oestrogen is responsible for triggering the hypothalamus to restart the cycle by initiating the release of FSH.

Pregnancy

If fertilisation occurs the regular alternation of hormone secretion is altered. Progesterone secretion by the corpus luteum increases, and after the third month of gestation progesterone production is taken over by the placenta. This is converted in the fetal adrenal to dehydro*epi*-androsterone, which back in the placenta becomes oestrogens: many steroids are produced by such two-organ metabolic processes. In the last month urinary oestrogen excretion, mainly oestriol, rises to 30–150 μmol/24 h.

The placenta also secretes, with a plateau at 36 weeks, a lactogen (HPL) with similar properties to prolactin and GH; and a 'human' chorionic gonadotrophin (HCG), which has similar properties to LH and can both increase ovarian weight and cause ripening of the follicles; and other hormones.

Changes in plasma proteins and metal-binding, due to the increased oestrogens, are as for hormonal contraceptives.

Pregnancy diagnosis tests

All reliable methods for the laboratory diagnosis of pregnancy depend on detection of the increased urinary excretion of HCG which occurs in early pregnancy. The classical biological tests depended on the HCG stimulat-ing the sex glands of a test animal and have now been almost completely replaced by immunological tests. Commercial preparations have variable sensitivity, but most give a positive reaction with about 2000 iu of HCG/litre of urine. Serum may also be used.

Excretion of HCG in pregnancy begins to be detectable by sensitive techniques at about the 10th day of gestation, rises to a peak from the 50th to 70th day of gestation, has fallen off by the 120th day, and stays constant thereafter till delivery. A fall may be due to fetal death or incipient miscarriage. If the urine of a patient who is thought to be in early pregnancy gives a negative result the test should be repeated two weeks later. The test usually become negative in the first week after delivery.

Hydatidiform mole, chorion carcinoma, or testicular teratoma contain chorionic tissue, produce HCG, and give strongly positive results with 'pregnancy diagnosis tests', the two former tumours with a rising titre after delivery. Progress and response to treatment should be followed by quantitative immunoassay. There is a cross reaction between this reaction and LH: for the investigation of tumours a specific β-HCG assay is available.

At the peak of HCG excretion in pregnancy a positive reaction is usually given by urine diluted 1/20, whilst in late pregnancy the test may be positive only on undiluted urine. Urine from a patient suffering from a hydatidiform mole may give a positive reaction at a dilution of 1/100 or more.

Assessment of fetal and placental integrity

Failure of urinary oestriol or total oestrogens to rise in late pregnancy reflects the integrity of the fetoplacental unit, and may indicate imminent fetal death or placental insufficiency, e.g. pre-eclamptic toxaemia. Urinary pregnanediol (or plasma progesterone) reflects placental function only, as does plasma HPL (measured by radioimmunoassay). The results of isolated assays are of little value because of the wide range of normal; a falling titre of urinary oestrogen or plasma placental lactogen is serious. There is a placental alkaline phosphatase which increases in plasma during normal pregnancy, but the changes are too variable to be an index of placental damage.

Prenatal diagnosis. Further biochemical tests that may be useful in prenatal diagnosis of neonatal disease are the measurement in amniotic fluid of bilirubin for the assessment of erythroblastosis (p. 190), of the lecithin/sphingomyelin ratio for the assessment of the respiratory distress syndrome (p. 82), and of (maternal) plasma and amniotic fluid α-fetoprotein (and amniotic fluid acetylcholinesterase: p. 121) for the diagnosis of spina bifida and other neural tube defects (p. 247). Specialist laboratories can assay enzymes in cultured fibroblasts from amniotic fluid taken at 14–16 weeks, and thereby diagnose a number of inborn errors of metabolism, mainly of lysosomal enzymes.

Ovarian hyperactivity

Various tumours of the ovary of mixed histological and endocrine pattern may be seen; the vast majority are not endocrinologically active and are often destructive. The arrhenoblastoma is a virilising tumour, and there is a raised urinary 17-oxosteroid excretion.

Hirsutism (excess hair in women) may be associated with a slightly raised plasma testosterone, possibly of ovarian or adrenal origin; with a decreased plasma sex hormone binding globulin as a secondary and exacerbating effect. However in many cases of hirsutism no abnormality of androgen metabolism can be demonstrated.

Virilism implies other evidence of masculinisation, and is associated with androgen-producing ovarian or adrenal tumours, or with the adrenogenital syndrome.

Ovarian hypoactivity

Menopausal symptoms occur when oestrogen secretion falls off, and excessive secretion of gonadotrophins develops. Osteoporosis may appear after the menopause partly due to lack of the protein anabolising action of the oestrogens; though replacement therapy has variable success.

Turner's syndrome (gonadal dysgenesis) is a combination of primary ovarian agenesis and other congenital abnormalities. Oestrogen excretion is absent, 17-oxosteroid excretion is variable, and gonadotrophin excretion is increased. Investigations which detect the genetic sex of a patient by examination of somatic cell nuclei for the presence of the female XX chromosome structure have shown that many cases of so-called ovarian agenesis are in fact cases of chromosome abnormality, usually XO.

Polycystic ovarian disease (Stein-Leventhal syndrome), of amenorrhoea hirsutism and enlarged cystic ovaries, may be due to a metabolic block in oestrogen synthesis from androgens, or to a hypothalamic disorder: androgen production is sometimes increased.

Investigation of pituitary-ovarian failure

An increase in plasma FSH results from primary ovarian failure. If FSH is low, or normal, then failure of plasma LH to respond to injected LH-RH is evidence of failure of pituitary function, which may be secondary to a hypothalamic deficiency. Amenorrhoea may be due to an alteration of feedback; here both oestrogen and gonadotrophin values may be normal.

Male sex hormones

FSH promotes spermatogenesis.

LH stimulates the secretion of the androgens from the interstitial cells of the testis; the principal androgen is testosterone, which is converted to the more active dihydrotestosterone, and both circulate bound to sex hormone binding globulin and other proteins. The androgens have a feedback action on the secretion of LH from the anterior pituitary gland.

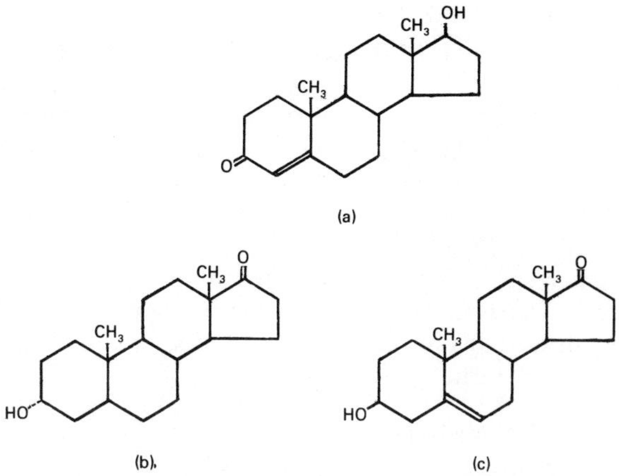

FIG. 10.12. Structures of the androgens: (a) Testosterone, (b) Androsterone, (e) Dehydro*epi*androsterone.

The actions of the male sex hormones on the sexual organs and activities will not be further described here. Testosterone is a protein anaboliser, and when given therapeutically in large doses raises the plasma calcium level. The protein anabolic action of less virilising analogues may be utilised therapeutically to promote a positive nitrogen balance.

Testosterone and its analogues are sometimes used for the treatment of carcinoma of the breast with bony metastases. Recession of the metastases with diminution of pain often occurs, but the treatment may have to be stopped because of masculinisation or because of hypercalcaemia and consequent renal damage.

Testosterone is almost fully metabolised in the body. The urinary excretion products are 17-oxosteroids, the most important of which is the weakly androgenic androsterone. The structures of the principal androgens are shown in Fig. 10.12.

Plasma testosterone estimation is becoming available. The low values found in hypogonadism are diagnostically more useful than the inconsistently high values found in hirsutism.

Testicular hyperactivity

Tumours of the testis vary in their histological and endocrine pattern. Teratoma and chorionepithelioma of the testis usually produce HCG, (and often α-fetoprotein) and the urine of patients suffering from these tumours gives a positive 'pregnancy diagnosis test' at a dilution which may be more than 1/100. In these conditions the urinary 17-oxosteroid excretion is generally normal, but interstitial cell tumours give an increased excretion. Seminoma of the testis may produce HCG or FSH. There are also rare oestrogen-producing tumours.

Testicular hypoactivity

The eunuchoid syndrome of impotence, obesity, and muscular wasting (due to loss of the protein anabolising power of testosterone), may be primary, i.e. due to absence or disease of the testes, or be secondary to pituitary or hypothalamic disease. There is delayed epiphyseal closure if the disorder was present before puberty. There is a low plasma testosterone, and 17-oxosteroid excretion. Measurement of plasma FSH and LH, if necessary with stimulation tests, may be used to distinguish between primary and secondary eunuchism.

Klinefelter's syndrome (small testes and other abnormalities) corresponds to Turner's syndrome in that an endocrine disorder is due to a chromosome defect (usually XXY).

17-Oxosteroids (17-Ketosteroids)

These are excretion products of testicular androgens (one-third; in males) and adrenal androgens (two-thirds), and a small amount originates from ovarian androgens and from corticosteroids. Reference values are: adult females 15–60 μmol/24 h, adult males 25–80 μmol/24 h.

The estimation of total 17-oxosteroids is a measure of overall androgen production. Differential analysis is complex, but is valuable in the differential diagnosis of adrenal virilism.

PROLACTIN

Prolactin, in combination with oestrogens and progesterone, initiates and maintains lactation. Its inhibitory factor (PIF) is much more important than its releasing factor. Its secretion, stimulated by suckling, also inhibits ovulation.

Galactorrhoea in both men and women may be due to a pituitary tumour causing hyperprolactinaemia, often with low gonadotrophin secretion. Some drugs (e.g. chlorpromazine) cause lactation by blocking secretion of PIF.

Many symptomless chromophobe adenomas are prolactinomas.

OTHER ENDOCRINE ORGANS

Neurohypophysis

The hypothalamus, mainly under neural control, secretes two independent peptide hormones.

Oxytocin

This causes contraction of uterine muscle when it is under the influence of oestrogens, and promotes ejection of milk during suckling. Oxytocin abnormalities are not measurable.

Antidiuretic hormone (ADH; vasopressin)

This acts on the kidneys to promote distal tubular reabsorption of water: in pharmacological doses it causes peripheral vasoconstriction. The posterior lobe of the pituitary acts as a store for ADH, whence it is released in response to water deprivation, due to the effect on plasma osmolality and/or blood volume.

Diabetes insipidus. This results from deficient secretion of ADH, of many pathological causes, and the patient suffers from polyuria of low osmolality, and polydipsia. The polyuria of diabetes insipidus causes slightly increased plasma osmolality, responds to ADH or an analogue, and is not improved by temporary reduction of the fluid intake or by infusion of hypertonic saline (p. 34): plasma ADH is low.

In differential diagnosis, the polyuria of severe renal disease, or of the rare specific nephrogenic diabetes insipidus with receptor defect, does not respond to ADH. The polyuria of psychogenic polydipsia (usually with a decreased plasma osmolality) responds to water deprivation.

Inappropriate secretion. 'Non-endocrine' tumours, particularly those of the bronchus, may occasionally 'ectopically' synthesise, and produce a syndrome of inappropriate secretion of ADH, and such SIADH may also be seen after brain damage and in lung disease (p. 33). There is water retention with a low plasma osmolality and low concentrations of all plasma components (sodium, protein, etc.) with slowly developing hyponatraemia symptoms (p. 34); and a concentrated urine.

Adrenal medulla

This secretes adrenaline and also some noradrenaline: the manifold pharmacological properties of these hormones will not be discussed further here.

A rare endocrine tumour of the adrenal medulla (phaeochromo-cytoma), or of chromaffin tissue elsewhere, produces noradrenaline and adrenaline in excess; this leads to progressive paroxysmal hypertension, and often to increased glycogenolysis with impairment of glucose tolerance with hyperglycaemia and glycosuria. Similar tumours arising mainly in the sympathetic nervous system (neuroblastoma) produce primarily excess noradrenaline, and dopamine.

Estimation of the plasma concentration or urinary excretion of the actual hormones (catecholamines, pressor amines) is difficult but may be necessary for differential diagnosis of tumours. A major end-product of catecholamine metabolism is vanilmandelic acid (VMA: preferably called HMMA, 4-hydroxy-3-methoxymandelic acid) which is excreted in the urine, and this is estimated in the investigation of paroxysmal hypertension. Urinary HMMA is normally less than 35 mmol/24 h, whereas in phaeochromocytoma values above 50 mmol/24 h are found in at least one specimen on repeated testing. The patient must be off treatment with monoamine oxidase inhibitors (and vanilla, e.g. in bananas and coffee) for 48 hours beforehand. Measurement of total urinary metadrenalines (i.e. metanephrine and normetanephrine, normally less than 5 µmol/24 h) may be of diagnostic value in doubtful cases.

In essential hypertension all these hormonal values are normal.

Other hormones

The principal independent endocrine organs, the parathyroid glands and the pancreatic islets, are discussed respectively in the chapters on calcium (p. 175) and on carbohydrates (p. 57). The gastrointestinal hormones are discussed in the chapter on the alimentary tract (p. 242).

At present no certain chemical pathology is attributable to abnormalities of the prostaglandins and the related thromboxanes and prostacyclin.

ECTOPIC HORMONE PRODUCTION

Tumours of tissues of other than endocrine organs may occasionally produce a hormone 'inappropriately', and this is most often seen with bronchial carcinoma. The commonest ectopic hormones are ACTH, ADH, and parathyroid hormone, but many others have been described. The cause is uncertain, and may be due to derepression; or in some cases to production of hormone from pluripotent APUD cells (p. 242). The ectopic hormone is not always identical with the natural hormone, either biologically or immunologically.

Further reading

Anderson DC. Endocrine function of the testis. In: O'Riordan JLH, ed. *Recent Advances in Endocrinology and Metabolism 1*. Edinburgh: Churchill-Livingstone, 1978:111–136.

Besser M. The adrenal cortex, *Medicine* 3rd series 1978; 9:418–429.

Hall R, Gomez-Pan A. The hypothalamic regulatory hormones and their clinical applications. *Adv Clin Chem* 1976; 18:173–212.

Hoffenberg R. The thyroid. *Medicine* 3rd series 1978; 8:392–404.

Holton JB. Diagnostic tests on amniotic fluid. In: Marks V, Hales CN, eds. *Essays in Medical Biochemistry*. London: Biochemical Society, 1977; 3:75–107.

London DR, Shaw RW. Gynaecological endocrinology. In: O'Riordan JLH, ed. *Recent Advances in Endocrinology and Metabolism 1*. Edinburgh: Churchill-Livingstone, 1978:91–110.

Rees L. Endocrine manifestations of cancer. *Medicine* 3rd series 1978; 10:485–490.

Tepperman J. *Metabolic and Endocrine Physiology*. 3rd ed. Chicago: Year Book Medical Publishers, 1973.

CHAPTER 11

CALCIUM, PHOSPHORUS, AND THE BONES

GENERAL METABOLISM

Calcium and phosphorus intake and absorption

The usual daily dietary intake of calcium in adults is about 25 mmol (1.0 g), with a wide variation; and calcium balance can be maintained on a minimum intake of about 10 mmol (0.4 g). During late pregnancy and lactation a higher intake is required to provide calcium for the fetus and for the milk – which contains about 7.5 mmol (0.3 g) of calcium per litre; and 30 mmol (1.2 g) per day has been recommended. A higher intake is also necessary during periods of active growth.

The absorption of calcium ions, which takes place principally in the upper small intestine, is promoted by 1,25-dihydroxycholecalciferol (and other active metabolites of vitamin D) with a synergistic action of parathyroid hormone. To stimulate calcium absorption, by promoting the synthesis of calcium-binding protein in the enterocyte, the active metabolites must be present in the general circulation, not within the lumen of the intestine. Calcium absorption can be reduced by giving oral phytate, or by excess phosphates or fatty acids (p. 240).

The normal daily intake of phosphorus in adults in 1.5–3.0 g, and 1.0–1.5 g is the minimum recommended. A diet which is otherwise satisfactory is never deficient in phosphorus. Inorganic phosphate is absorbed as the phosphate ion, whereas phospholipid or nucleic acid phosphate has to be liberated by hydrolysis before it can be absorbed. When there is defective absorption of calcium then defective absorption of phosphorus usually results, as the excess calcium in the gut causes precipitation of calcium phosphate. Vitamin D has a stimulatory action on the net absorption of phosphate, but this is probably only secondary to its effects on the absorption of calcium. Phosphate absorption can be reduced by giving aluminium hydroxide because this forms a insoluble aluminium phosphate.

Calcium and phosphorus in the blood

The reference range of plasma/serum calcium in adults is 2.1–2.6 mmol/l. Approximately 50 per cent of the plasma calcium is ultrafiltrable calcium, and most of this is present as free calcium ions (Ca^{2+}), reference range 1.0–1.2 mmol/1; the remainder being non-ionised and bound to citrate and other small ions. The other 50 per cent of the plasma calcium is bound to proteins, particularly albumin. It is the free calcium ions that are physiologically active and are responsible for the effects of calcium on the parathyroid glands, bones, and neuromuscular tissue. The tetany of citrate poisoning, due to massive rapid transfusion of citrated blood, is caused by the complexing of the free calcium ions. The concentration of the non-ultrafiltrable or protein-bound fractions in plasma varies with the plasma protein concentration, and blood for calcium estimation must therefore be collected without stasis because venous constriction raises the plasma protein concentration (p. 257): some laboratories correct all plasma calcium values for plasma albumin or total protein concentration, but the ideal correction formula has not been agreed. Measurement of the ionised calcium requires a special electrode (p. 22), and this is not universally available.

The reference range of plasma inorganic phosphate in adults is 0.8–1.4 mmol/l. Plasma also contains organic phosphorus, most of which is as phospholipids (p. 82). The phosphorus content of erythrocytes is high, and phosphate estimations should always be performed fasting (there is a circadian variation of 0.3 mmol/l), and on unhaemolysed plasma or serum, either freshly separated or preserved with fluoride because erythrocyte organic phosphates are easily hydrolysed.

In infants the normal plasma calcium and plasma phosphate levels are higher than in adults (p. 269).

Calcium-phosphate product. There is in general a reciprocal relation between the plasma calcium and phosphate, maintained homeostatically by solution of bone salt. This can be expressed that the product of the concentrations in the plasma of 'ionised calcium' and of 'phosphate' is about 1.2 (15 in traditional mass units), and of 'total calcium' × 'phosphate' is about 2.8 (35 in mass units). Plasma is not quite saturated with calcium and phosphate: metastatic calcification becomes a hazard when the total calcium-phosphate product exceeds about 5.5.

The excretion of calcium and phosphorus

The calcium and phosphorus in the faeces consists both of unabsorbed calcium and phosphorus from the diet, and also of calcium and phosphorus which have passed from the plasma into the intestine. Of a daily intake of 25 mmol (1 g) of calcium, 2.5–7.5 mmol (0.1–0.3 g) is excreted in the urine, and the remainder is recovered in the faeces. A large increase in the faecal calcium excretion is found when calcium absorption is diminished, particularly in steatorrhoea. Normally about one-third of the intake of phosphorus is excreted in the faeces and two-thirds in the urine.

Normally almost all of the filtered calcium is reabsorbed: calcium behaves as a threshold substance, and when the plasma calcium level falls below about 1.8 mmol/l its excretion in the urine normally ceases. When renal function is normal, the amount of calcium excreted in the urine increases as the plasma calcium level increases: however in 'idiopathic' hypercalciuria (p. 186) the plasma calcium is normal. A high excretion of calcium is also found in chronic acidosis.

The urinary phosphate excretion of a healthy subject on a normal diet is 15–50 mmol (0.5–1.5 g) per 24 h. The clearance of phosphate is altered both by disorders of the glomeruli and of the tubules, phosphate excretion falling when there is glomerular damage (p. 211) and increasing in renal tubular syndromes (p. 225). Excess parathyroid hormone decreases phosphate reabsorption, thereby increasing its clearance.

About 2.5 mmol (0.1 g) of calcium is lost daily in the skin and sweat.

Bone

In biochemical studies a bone may be considered principally as a metabolic pool of calcium and phosphate: its mineral fraction (65 per cent) consists largely of a hydroxyapatite type of crystal, $3Ca_3(PO_4)_2.Ca(OH)_2$. More than 99 per cent of the body calcium (about 30 mol: 1200 g) and more than 75 per cent of the phosphate is in the bones, and about 150 mmol (6 g) of calcium is readily exchangeable. Bone contains a considerable store of sodium (amounting to at least one-third of the total body sodium), of magnesium and potassium, and of carbonate, fluoride, and citrate. These ions are absorbed on the hydroxyapatite crystals. The hypothetical metabolic pool has two very large 'surfaces' because the actual crystals are small. At one of these surfaces bone salt is deposited, at the other bone salt is withdrawn. Bones are not static structures, for calcium, phosphate, and other ions are continuously being laid down and reabsorbed, and there is a state of dynamic equilibrium.

The diagram (Fig. 11.1) shows an idealised bone, and the general processes of calcium transport.

The different bone cells are interconvertible. The deposition surface of the bone is lined by osteoblasts. These have two functions:

(i) They manufacture the protein of the bone matrix (osteoid) which is composed of collagen, mucopolysaccharide, and osteocytes. The manufacture of matrix requires supply of suitable precursors, and there must be a proper balance between the protein anabolic and the protein catabolic hormones. Hence matrix formation may be deficient when there is protein malnutrition, or when there is deficiency of oestrogens, or excess glucocorticoids.

(ii) They secrete alkaline phosphatase. This enzyme is released from the osteoblasts spontaneously, and in response to local strain. The mechanism by which alkaline phosphatase secretion leads to deposition of bone is uncertain but hydrolysis of pyrophosphate, which is an inhibitor of hydroxyapatite formation, plays a part. Phosphatase is also concerned with matrix production. The normal process of development and mineralisation of bone depends on adequate active vitamin D metabolites being available, and also requires vitamins A and C. The function of citrate is uncertain.

The withdrawal surface of the bone is lined by osteoclasts. Reabsorp-

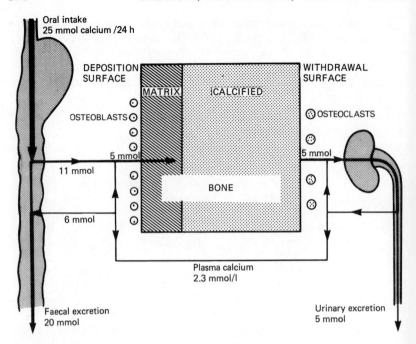

FIG. 11.1. The general processes of calcium transport (excluding recirculation of gastro-intestinal secretions), and an idealised structure of bone, in a normal adult.

tion of bone occurs by demolition of matrix and release of mineral by the osteoclasts and osteocytes. This process is encouraged by a low plasma concentration of calcium, phosphate, or bicarbonate. Parathyroid hormone, by stimulating osteoclast activity, acts at the withdrawal surface to cause release of calcium and phosphate ions from bone salt – and hydroxyproline (p. 101) is released from bone matrix.

Other sites of metabolism

Although the largest part of the calcium and much of the phosphorus of the body is concerned with the metabolism of bone, these elements have many other important functions. Calcium ions are essential for the conversion of prothrombin to thrombin, and for the normal action of heart muscle and for neuromuscular conduction generally. Phosphate is involved in very many ways in cell metabolism as a constituent of nucleic acids, and of ATP, metabolic intermediates, and phospholipids. The normal metabolism of glucose under the influence of insulin lowers the plasma phosphate: cell breakdown from any cause raises the plasma phosphate. Phosphate plays an important part in the buffering mechanisms of plasma and of urine.

SPECIAL FACTORS

Hormones and vitamins

Parathyroid hormone

Only a single active polypeptide is produced by the parathyroid glands. The secretion of parathyroid hormone (PTH) is not governed by a trophic hormone of the anterior pituitary gland, but is stimulated by a low plasma calcium ion concentration. The effects of PTH are to raise the plasma calcium and lower the plasma phosphate: chemical solubility of bone salt would alone maintain the plasma calcium at about 1.7 mmol/l, and it is raised above that level by the influence of PTH. The accepted actions of PTH are:

(i) On the bone, via the osteoclasts and osteocytes, to promote dissolution of matrix, breakdown of bone salt, and liberation of calcium, phosphate, and some hydroxyl ions. Bone citrate production is stimulated. Adequate vitamin D must be present.

(ii) On the kidney, (a) to promote the 1α-hydroxylation of 25-hydroxycholecalciferol, (b) to diminish tubular reabsorption of phosphate and thus promote phosphate excretion. The increased excretion of phosphate lowers the plasma phosphate concentration, and this probably causes a rise in the plasma calcium by a mass action effect in promoting further dissolution of bone salt. To a limited extent, PTH increases tubular reabsorption of calcium, and also of hydrogen ions promoting an acidaemia. These actions are independent of vitamin D.

Urinary cyclic AMP increases, derived from both bone and kidney.

(iii) Some promotion of calcium absorption from the gut is also likely.

Measurement of plasma PTH (by radioimmunoassay) may be valuable in the investigation of problems of hypercalcaemia or hypocalcaemia.

Calcitonin

This polypeptide hormone was originally thought to arise from the parathyroid glands but it is primarily of thyroidal origin (p. 147), embryologically from the ultimobranchial bodies. It plays an important but unclarified role in the maintenance of a steady plasma calcium level, and its secretion is modified by the plasma calcium ion concentration. It diminishes bone resorption by inhibition of osteoclast activity, increases the renal excretion of calcium and phosphate, and lowers the plasma calcium and phosphate.

The rare medullary cell carcinoma of the thyroid secretes excess calcitonin, but the plasma calcium is usually normal.

Other hormones

Thyroxine stimulates the activity of osteoclasts. In hyperthyroidism there may be decalcification with an increase in urinary calcium excretion, and sometimes hypercalcaemia.

The oestrogens and androgens influence bone metabolism by their effects on the production of the bone matrix. When there is oestrogen or androgen deficiency matrix production is diminished, and this can sometimes be reversed by appropriate replacement therapy.

The glucocorticoids also influence bone metabolism by their actions on protein catabolism affecting the production of bone matrix. When excess glucocorticoids are present, in iatrogenic or idiopathic Cushing's syndrome (p. 156), matrix production is diminished. They stimulate bone breakdown, causing an increased urinary calcium, and have an anti-calciferol effect. Growth hormone raises the plasma phosphate, as seen in acromegaly.

Vitamin D – the calciferols

There are a number of related substances that have vitamin D activity (Fig. 11.2). The most important are ergocaliferol (vitamin D_2) which is produced by artificial irradiation of ergosterol (from plants) with ultra-violet light; and cholecalciferol (vitamin D_3) which is produced by irradiation of 7-dehydrocholesterol in human skin by the ultraviolet component of sunlight (which opens the B ring, p. 88), and also occurs naturally in some animal food sources. Cholecalciferol is converted in the liver (and probably the gut) to 25-hydroxycholecalciferol, then in the kidney, under the influence of PTH and with stimulation by a low plasma phosphate, to 1,25-dihydroxycholecalciferol (the most active form), and 24,25-dihydroxycholecalciferol: there are other active metabolites. Ergocalciferol is metabolised similarly. The increased synthesis of vitamin D in the skin during the summer in Britain causes a seasonal variation in the reference values for all related substances.

Because cholecalciferol is produced naturally in the skin, and the body's requirements are only supplemented from the diet, 'vitamin D' can be considered to be a hormone.

The actions of vitamin D (via the active forms) raise the levels of both the plasma calcium and the plasma phosphate. The principal site of action is on the intestine, where the net absorption of both calcium and phosphate is promoted. It raises the blood and bone citrate. Vitamin D acts directly on bone to promote normal growth and development, and utilisation of calcium. It may have a PTH-like activity on the kidneys, especially in states of parathyroid deficiency.

Measurement of serum 25-hydroxycholecalciferol is now possible, and may be useful in the investigation of some cases of hypocalcaemia or hypercalcaemia.

Hypervitaminosis D. The primary effect of therapeutic overdosage with vitamin D is excessive absorption of calcium, and possibly some excessive absorption of phosphate. There is progressive hypercalcaemia with a normal or raised plasma phosphate, and secondary depression of

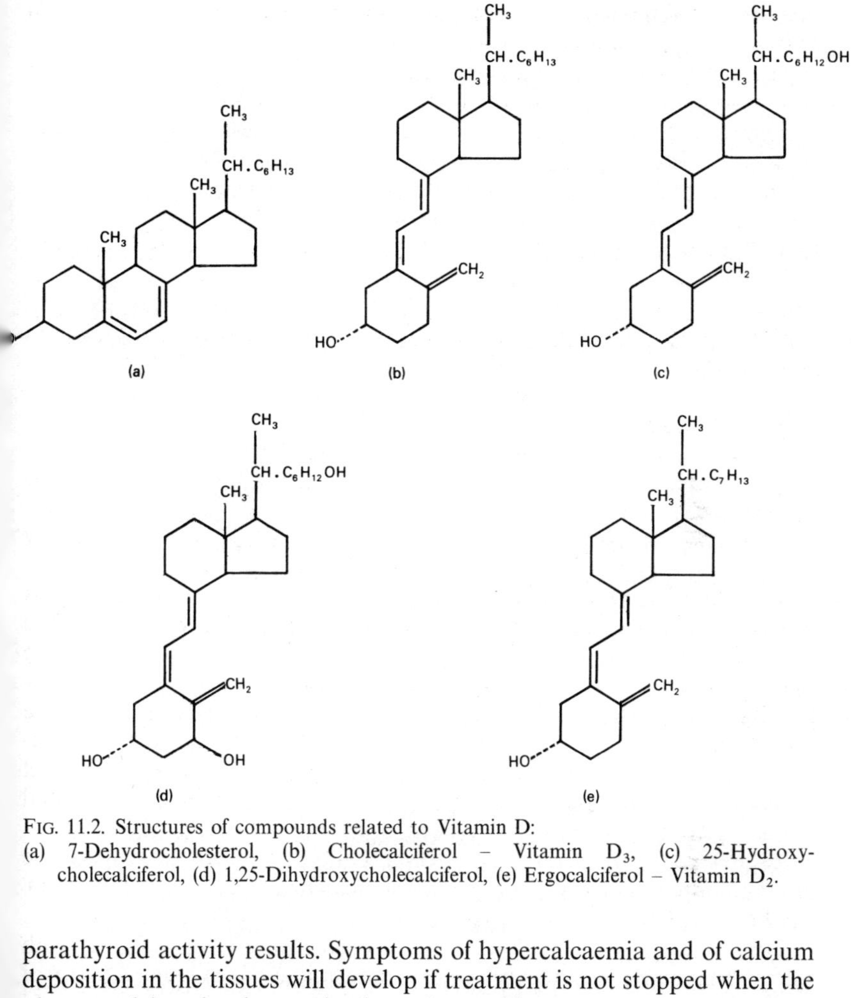

FIG. 11.2. Structures of compounds related to Vitamin D:
(a) 7-Dehydrocholesterol, (b) Cholecalciferol – Vitamin D_3, (c) 25-Hydroxy-cholecalciferol, (d) 1,25-Dihydroxycholecalciferol, (e) Ergocalciferol – Vitamin D_2.

parathyroid activity results. Symptoms of hypercalcaemia and of calcium deposition in the tissues will develop if treatment is not stopped when the plasma calcium level exceeds about 3 mmol/l.

Enzymes – the phosphatases

The phosphatases are a group of enzymes which promote the hydrolysis of organic phosphates with liberation of phosphate ions. They can be divided into two main groups, the classification depending on whether the enzyme has maximum activity in an alkaline or an acid medium. Alkaline phosphatase has a major concern with bone metabolism: acid phosphatase is involved with lysosomal activity and is for convenience included in this section although it is not concerned with bone metabolism.

Alkaline phosphatases

These enzymes are produced in many cells of the body, and one important site of secretion is the osteoblasts: the main other alkaline phosphatase isoenzymes in plasma of diagnostic importance come from the liver, and sometimes from intestinal mucosa and placenta. Alkaline phosphatase is found both in urine and in bile, in both cases arising from local cells. The reference range in adult plasma is 25–95 U/l in men; 20–80 U/l in women (3–13 King-Armstrong units/dl): this is derived from the liver and bone – other methods, with different reference values, are in use. The plasma activity varies with age (p. 269), tends to be higher in males, and is higher (up to 200 U/l) during late pregnancy and periods of active bone growth, from excess placental and osteoblastic isoenzyme respectively.

A raised plasma alkaline phosphatase is found either when there is excess production or release of the enzyme, or perhaps when elimination of the enzyme is reduced. When there is increased osteoblastic activity excess alkaline phosphatase is secreted. In hyperparathyroidism with bone disease, malignant disease with an osteoblastic response (osteosarcoma or certain secondary carcinomas), rickets and the other forms of osteomalacia, and the healing phase of fractures, the plasma activity is usually 150–350 U/l, and in Paget's disease the value may be over 500 U/l. Normal plasma values are almost always found in osteolytic bone disease, for example in multiple myeloma and some types of malignant deposits in bone.

Isoenzymes. Liver alkaline phosphatase is increased in various types of hepatobiliary disease (p. 197). In cases where both osteoblastic and liver isoenzymes may be present it is necessary either to perform electrophoresis to identify the isoenzymes, or to measure an enzyme which has similar hepatobiliary behaviour to alkaline phosphatase but which is absent from osteoblasts, e.g. 5′-nucleotidase, γ-glutamyltransferase (p. 198). Placental alkaline phosphatase is measured in plasma as a test for placental insufficiency (p. 165). Other abnormal alkaline phosphatases, usually of placental type, may be produced by malignant tissue (p. 122). Intestinal alkaline phosphatase has the interesting feature of being absent from the plasma of subjects of blood group A, or who are non-secretors of ABH.

Hypophosphatasia. This is a rare hereditary disorder, which presents as a skeletal condition resembling rickets. There is deficient tissue synthesis of alkaline phosphatase, a very low plasma alkaline phosphatase, and high urinary excretion of phosphorylethanolamine, a natural substrate for the enzyme.

Acid phosphatases

Acid phosphatases are produced in many organs. The acid phosphatase that is clinically important for diagnosis is derived from mature prostatic epithelium and secreted into prostatic fluid. Other acid phosphatases are present in erythrocytes and in platelets, and escape into the plasma only if the blood is haemolysed or during clotting: most 'normal' plasma acid phosphatase originates *in vitro* from platelets. The reference range for total acid phosphatase in adult plasma is 0.5–5.5 U/l (0.3–3.0 King-Armstrong units/dl). A raised plasma acid phosphatase value is usually due to an increase in the prostatic phosphatase. However, a slightly raised acid phosphatase is occasionally found in severe osteoblastic bone disease (including Paget's disease) or cholestatic liver disease, in Gaucher's disease, and when there is excessive destruction of platelets. Such abnormalities can be identified by special biochemical techniques: in particular prostatic phosphatase is L(+) tartrate-labile. The normal tartrate-labile phosphatase is < 1.0 U/l. A recent development is specific immunological estimation of plasma prostatic acid phosphatase *concentration* – reference values < 4.0 µg/l.

Prostatic disease. A high plasma (prostatic) acid phosphatase is generally found in malignant disease of the prostate when malignant tissue has spread outside the gland capsule, and particularly when there are metastatic deposits in bone: when, as is usual, these metastases are osteoblastic the plasma alkaline phosphatase is also raised. A plasma total acid phosphatase > 9 U/l or a 'prostatic' acid phosphatase > 2 U/l is strongly suggestive of metastasising prostatic carcinoma, and with widespread dissemination of the disease a value above 200 U/l may sometimes be found. Estimation of the plasma acid phosphatase is of use both in diagnosis, and in monitoring hormonal treatment of patients suffering from carcinoma of the prostate. Normal values are found in benign prostatic hyperplasia; though if the prostate has been palpated within the previous two days this procedure has been claimed to disperse acid phosphatase into the circulation.

ALTERATIONS OF PLASMA CALCIUM AND PHOSPHATE

Hypocalcaemia

This is due either to deficient calcium intake and/or absorption, to hypoparathyroidism, or to excessive renal loss in tubular damage or acidosis. Hypocalcaemia is often part of the chronic renal failure syndrome. It is also sometimes seen in acute pancreatitis. In neonates it may be due to high-phosphate feeds, which bind calcium within the intestines. Hypocalcaemia causes hyperexcitability of the nervous system, which may present clinically as convulsions, and as tingling and numbness. The enhancement of neuromuscular irritability that gives rise to tetany may be caused not only by a low plasma calcium-ion concentration but also by a low plasma hydrogen-ion activity, and rarely by a low plasma magnesium-ion concentration. These factors are to a certain extent additive and if, e.g., a patient is suffering from tetany due to alkalaemia, raising the plasma ionised calcium level may to a limited degree restore normal sensitivity of the neuromuscular system and improve the tetany. Other effects of long-standing hypocalcaemia are cataracts, a prolonged coagulation time, and mental depression. Hypocalcaemia associated with hypoproteinaemia alone, when there is a normal ionised calcium, yields no metabolic abnormalities.

Hypercalcaemia

This is usually due to excess breakdown of bone, either from hyperparathyroidism, from malignant disease including myelomatosis, or occasionally from immobilisation: the commonest cause is osteolytic metastases in bone. It only results from excess absorption when there is overdosage of, or hypersensitivity to, vitamin D, or excess dietary intake of alkali-with-calcium. Hypercalcaemia causes muscular weakness, gastrointestinal symptoms, giddiness, extreme thirst, and marked lassitude – and renal damage with polyuria. If the plasma phosphate is normal or raised, there may be deposition of calcium phosphate at various sites as metastatic calcification. The initial symptom of renal calcification is a polyuria due to tubular damage, and renal failure develops if hypercalcaemia is prolonged. Hypercalcaemia leads to hypercalciuria and often to renal calculi. Severe hypercalcaemia carries the risk of a cardiac arrest.

Abnormal plasma phosphate

A high plasma phosphate, typically seen in renal failure, affects bone largely through effects on calcium distribution: hyperphosphataemia may also be due to excess cell breakdown. A low plasma phosphate is typically seen during imperfect fluid and electrolyte replacement, especially in previously malnourished patients; but is also present in primary hyperparathyroidism and in renal tubular syndromes. It causes weakness of skeletal and cardiac muscle, through depletion of ATP, when below about 0.5 mmol/l.

DISEASES AFFECTING THE METABOLISM OF BONE

Hypoparathyroidism

Idiopathic (autoimmune) atrophy of the parathyroid glands is sometimes seen, but hypoparathyroidism is usually caused by accidental vascular damage to the glands, or their complete removal, during thyroidectomy, or sometimes by irradiation or iron overload. The biochemical findings are due to deficiency of PTH. There is a low plasma calcium level which may be below 1.5 mmol/l principally due to a fall in ionised calcium, and a high plasma phosphate which may exceed 2 mmol/l. There is decreased withdrawal of calcium from bone causing thick bones of increased density, and osteoblast activity and bone formation may also be reduced. The plasma alkaline phosphatase level is normal or low. A low plasma calcium may lead to absence of calcium from the urine.

The clinical features are caused by the low plasma ionised calcium concentration. Treatment by calcium and 'vitamin D' must be controlled by serial estimations of the plasma calcium concentration, and examination of urinary calcium may be useful occasionally. There are risks of overdosage causing a high plasma calcium, and nephrocalcinosis with renal failure.

Pseudohypoparathyroidism. In this rare familial disorder the syndrome of hypoparathyroidism is associated with abnormal body build. It is caused by diminished tissue (bone and kidney) receptor-system sensitivity to PTH. Plasma PTH values are normal, or raised due to secondary hyperparathyroidism. Urinary cyclic AMP excretion (p. 137) does not increase after PTH injection, in contrast to the response in normal subjects and in patients with hypoparathyroidism. The conditions responds to calcium and 'vitamin D'.

Primary hyperparathyroidism

Primary hyperparathyroidism may be caused either by benign or malignant tumours of one or more parathyroid glands, or by hyperplasia of all the glands. Certain tumours may produce an ectopic PTH-like substance (p. 170). The autonomous adenoma that follows stimulation by prolonged hypocalcaemia is called tertiary hyperparathyroidism.

The biochemical findings are due to excess of PTH. There is a raised plasma calcium concentration which may exceed 4 mmol/l but which may only manifest when provoked by a low phosphate diet: less regularly the plasma phosphate is low, sometimes below 0.5 mmol/l. The urinary phosphate excretion is high and the urinary calcium excretion is high. If there is secondary renal damage the plasma phosphate level may be above normal, with a raised plasma urea. There is increased drain of calcium from the bones and increased osteoclastic activity; some compensatory increase of calcium deposition in the bones is associated with increased osteoblastic activity. In half of the cases, usually those of longer duration, there is a high plasma alkaline phosphatase and increased urinary hydroxyproline excretion, and these abnormal findings depend on the degree of bone involvement. There is a tendency to an alkaline urine, and to a hyperchloraemic metabolic acidosis.

If the plasma calcium rises above about 3 mmol/l signs of hypercalcaemia may appear, of which the earliest are loss of appetite and muscular hypotonicity. There may be abdominal pains, and even duodenal ulcer from increased secretion of gastrin and acid. When the bones are affected they show a generalised rarefaction, and in very advanced cases the cyst formation, fibrosis, deformities, pain, and fractures, of osteitis fibrosa cystica (von Recklinghausen's disease). A marked degree of hyperparathyroidism may be present without any demonstrable clinical or radiological changes in the bones. The high urinary calcium and phosphate cause an osmotic polyuria, which leads to polydipsia. Tubular damage due to calcium deposition furthers the polyuria. Formation of calcium phosphate and calcium oxalate stones is a common presenting symptom, though in such cases there is very often no obvious bony disease especially when there is a high calcium intake. In all cases of renal calculi (p. 226) the plasma calcium and phosphate should be estimated on more than one occasion, as perhaps about 5 per cent of cases are due to primary hyperparathyroidism. In long-standing cases renal damage may raise the plasma phosphate level.

Measurement of PTH in blood obtained by selective catheterisation of the neck veins may help in locating an adenoma. After removal of an enlarged parathyroid by surgery there may be a dangerous fall in the plasma calcium, and occasionally in the plasma magnesium (p. 40).

Investigations. The diagnosis can usually be made on the clinical and biochemical signs. When hyperparathyroidism is suspected, repeated estimation of plasma calcium (with plasma proteins) is usually as valuable a method of diagnosis as are more complex investigations – when hypercalcaemia is marginal, correction for possible hypoproteinaemia may be necessary to show a raised plasma calcium (p. 172). Measurement of calcium excretion may sometimes be useful: on a low calcium diet (2.5 mmol: 100 mg daily) a normal subject excretes less than 1.5 mmol (60 mg) per 24 h, whereas when there is excessive breakdown of bone *from any cause*, and normal renal function, the excretion exceeds 5 mmol (200 mg) per 24 h. Satisfactory measurement of phosphate clearance, or other phosphate excretion indices, is difficult, and the results are not easy to interpret.

The mechanism of the valuable *glucocorticoid suppression test* is unknown. When a patient with hypercalcaemia due to primary hyperparathyroidism is placed on a high dose of hydrocortisone (40 mg 3 × daily for 10 days), the plasma calcium, corrected for protein, is unaltered: whilst hypercalcaemia due to metastases or sarcoidosis, and often to ectopic PTH, is usually significantly reduced.

Multiple endocrine adenomas. Hyperparathyroidism may be a part of two distinct familial syndromes. In type I it is associated with the Zollinger-Ellison syndrome (p. 242; pancreatic gastrinomas) and pituitary chromophobe adenomas; in type II it is associated with medullary carcinoma of the thyroid and phaeochromocytoma. These may be related to the distribution of different APUD cells (p. 242).

Rarefaction of bone

Rarefaction of the skeleton may be diagnosed clinically or radiologically, and can be due to many types of metabolic disturbance. *Decalcification* strictly implies loss of calcium without loss of matrix.

Obvious radiological presentation of decalcification requires loss of about a quarter of the calcium of the bones.

For the investigation of doubtful cases of decalcification a 5-day calcium balance may be necessary, and for research purposes this can be associated with a phosphate and nitrogen balance. Tracer studies with labelled calcium may be used in special circumstances.

Excessive breakdown of bone

Either metabolic or destructive disorders can cause excessive bone breakdown. Bone formation is normal, or may be slightly increased in compensation for the excess breakdown.

Hyperparathyroidism produces a varying degree of decalcification. In chronic acidosis (possibly because the solubility of calcium phosphate is increased) and in hyperthyroidism, there may also be excessive dissolution of bone salts. Destructive lesions in bone, such as primary and secondary malignant disease of bone, and myelomatosis, may lead to widespread decalcification: there is a tendency to an alkalaemia. In certain types of malignant disease, particularly carcinoma of the bronchus and also occasional sarcomas, bone decalcification with biochemical features resembing primary hyperparathyroidism may be due to synthesis and release of a PTH-like substance, and sometimes of a prostaglandin, by the tumour.

In all these conditions the plasma calcium level and the urine calcium excretion are increased; renal deposition of calcium salts may occur. The plasma phosphate level is often raised, except in hyperparathyroidism uncomplicated by renal damage.

Osteoporosis

In osteoporosis there is reduction of normal bone mass, both matrix and calcium. This is probably never primarily a disorder of mineral balance, though the subject is controversial.

Osteoporosis develops when matrix formation is imperfect, even though plasma calcium and phosphate concentration are adequate for calcification: this is seen if there is defective function of the osteoblasts, or in certain disorders of protein metabolism. When there has been prolonged calcium deficiency, bone destruction may be increased and the resultant bone disorder may resemble osteoporosis. Where there is prolonged immobilisation of a limb, or in prolonged decubitus, disuse atrophy of the osteoblasts takes place and there is osteoporosis. However, dangerous hypercalcaemia may develop following immobilisation of bones and consequent dissolution of bone salt, especially if there is renal damage.

Senile or post-menopausal osteoporosis is associated with declining secretion of the oestrogens. When there is general protein deficiency (p. 93) e.g. due to malnutrition, or if negative nitrogen balance has developed (in Cushing's syndrome including prolonged corticosteroid administration, or in other hormonal disturbances; or in the post-operative period), then there may be defective matrix formation and osteoporosis. Defective matrix formation may also occur in vitamin C deficiency.

In chronic osteoporosis the plasma calcium, phosphate, and alkaline phosphatase levels are generally normal. The excretion of calcium in the urine may be increased.

Osteoporosis is common clinically. In the treatment a high protein diet, possibly with extra vitamin C and calcium, has been used. Oestrogens and androgens, which stimulate protein anabolism, are sometimes given, but their therapeutic effect is disputed.

Osteomalacia and rickets

In osteomalacia there is deficient calcification of a normal mass of bone matrix. It is a disorder of mineral balance. Defective calcification of the matrix develops when there is deficiency of calcium or phosphate at the bone-forming surface (the plasma calcium-phosphate product is usually less than 1.6) and also directly due to deficiency. The result of the deficient formation of calcified bone, with relatively normal bone destruction, is rarefaction.

In general it is deficiency of calcium that is important, and this may be due either to defective absorption or to increased excretion.

Absorption. A reduced amount of calcium enters the circulation if there is an absolute calcium deficiency in the diet. This is rarely seen if the general standard of nutrition is good, but there will be calcium deficiency on an apparently normal calcium diet if the body's needs for calcium are increased, as in lactation. Calcium and phosphate absorption are deficient when there is insufficient available 1,25-dihydroxycholecalciferol: this can result from dietary deficiency of the vitamin, or deficient skin synthesis, or decreased absorption, or impaired hydroxylation in hepatic or renal disease.

In Britain osteomalacia is usually due to a combined effect of malnutrition (generally from poverty) leading to deficient intake, and of the low-sunshine climate leading to deficient synthesis in the skin. In dark-skinned immigrants synthesis of cholecalciferol in the skin may be particularly deficient. Poor children who live in a sunny climate are less likely to develop vitamin D deficiency. In *rickets*, the special name given to vitamin D deficient osteomalacia in children, in addition to rarefaction there is disordered growth of cartilage and bone with characteristic pathological changes at the epiphyseal lines.

When osteomalacia is found in old people it is due principally to vitamin D deficiency. In disturbances of fat absorption there is deficient absorption of vitamin D, and consequent deficiency. The osteomalacia and hypocalcaemia that often develop in patients on anti-convulsant drugs (e.g. phenytoin) is probably due to altered calciferol metabolism from hepatic enzyme induction. Calcium absorption is decreased by a high concentration in the intestine of any anion which forms an insoluble calcium salt. If there is excess of phosphate in the gut (as is found in uraemia), then insoluble calcium phosphate will be precipitated and less calcium will be absorbed. Fatty acids, present in excess in steatorrhoea, likewise form insoluble calcium soaps within the lumen of the intestine.

Phytic acid (inositol hexaphosphoric acid), which is present in many cereals, gives rise to insoluble calcium salts. A high dietary phytic acid contributes to the calcium deficiency of some Asians, especially vegans, in Britain. In the steatorrhoea caused by coeliac disease absorption of calcium is deficient also because of the flattened mucosa, and absorption of phosphate may also be impaired: with the osteomalacia there is usually also osteoporosis. In other chronic gastrointestinal diseases, after gastrectomy, and occasionally in patients who are receiving ion-exchange resin therapy, calcium absorption may be impaired. Many patients with cirrhosis develop a multifactorial osteomalacia.

Excretion. In patients with renal tubular acidosis, whether as an independent defect or as part of many of the renal tubular syndromes, osteomalacia may be found. In children this must be distinguished from renal rickets. If acidaemia is severe there is increased loss of calcium in the urine leading to a low plasma calcium level. The acidaemia also directly diminishes the rate of calcification, or promotes decalcification. Phosphate loss (which may also be an independent disorder) occurs regularly in renal tubular osteomalacia, and the resultant picture may mimic true rickets. These patients are often resistant to vitamin D.

Secondary effects. Deficiency of calcium initially causes a low plasma calcium concentration: the plasma phosphate level is normal, and the alkaline phosphatase level usually raised, because stresses applied to the weakened bones stimulate osteoblastic activity. The urinary calcium is low unless the disorder is of renal origin. In osteomalacia the low plasma calcium often appropriately causes some *secondary hyperparathyroidism* which may restore the plasma calcium level to normal (but not above) and lower the plasma phosphate level: the calcium × phosphate product remains low. In rickets, because of this effect and because of defective absorption of phosphate, the plasma phosphate level is always low, and the plasma calcium low or normal. In severe steatorrhoea the plasma calcium usually remains low, with a low or normal plasma phosphate. The parathyroid hyperactivity associated with osteomalacia is insufficient to cause a hypercalcaemia unless an autonomous parathyroid adenoma develops (*tertiary hyperparathyroidism*) and in these patients osteitis fibrosa cystica does not develop.

Treatment of osteomalacia is treatment of its cause. Extra vitamin D and calcium should be given in all cases, and if necessary parenterally.

Some other disorders of calcium and phosphate balance

Renal osteodystrophy

Chronic uraemia is associated with this syndrome: the bone disorder is multifactorial. The primary biochemical disorder is phosphate retention (due to glomerular damage) and consequent deficient calcium absorption and acidaemia may play a part: there is also impaired renal 25-hydroxylation of vitamin D. The resultant low plasma calcium causes secondary parathyroid hypertrophy, and this will return the plasma calcium towards normal: alkaline phosphatase values are variable. Osteomalacia and other bone dystrophies also can develop in renal failure.

After long-term dialysis, phosphate *depletion* contributes to the bone disease.

Renal rickets is the bone disorder in children with chronic renal failure, due both to impaired vitamin D metabolism and to phosphate retention causing gut loss of calcium: the bone changes are associated with epiphyseal changes as in rickets.

Fanconi syndrome

This often presents in infants as vitamin D-resistant rickets and failure to thrive, or in adults as osteomalacia, and is due to deficiency (often congenital but sometimes secondary to a wide variety of disorders) of renal tubular reabsorptive mechanisms (p. 225). There are both functional enzyme deficiencies and structural defects ('swan-neck' lesion) in the proximal tubules. The commonest biochemical abnormalities are aminoaciduria, glycosuria, and phosphaturia: loss of uric acid, potassium, and bicarbonate may occur. There is a low plasma phosphate with normal plasma calcium and alkaline phosphatase levels.

Paget's disease (osteitis deformans)

There is disseminated irregular bone destruction and a marked tendency to new bone formation. The plasma calcium and phosphate levels are normal, but the alkaline phosphatase level is extremely high, often over 700 U/l. The plasma acid phosphatase activity may also be increased.

Idiopathic hypercalcaemia of infants

In this rare disorder there is a raised plasma calcium level, secondary renal damage with a raised plasma urea, and a normal plasma phosphate, alkaline phosphatase, and bicarbonate. The cause is probably excessive calcium absorption from the gut due to hypersensitivity to vitamin D. Clinically there is failure to thrive and often mental retardation.

Absorption hypercalcaemia and hypercalciuria

Hypercalcaemia due to excessive absorption of dietary calcium is occasionally seen without overdosage with vitamin D, but associated with alkalaemia and renal damage. Some cases are known as the milk-alkali syndrome – this used to be seen in patients who received, for long periods, excessive absorbable alkalis and milk for the treatment of peptic ulcer.

There is sometimes, from an unknown cause, increased absorption of calcium (and possibly slight hypercalcaemia) which leads to hypercalciuria and renal calculi (p. 226).

Sarcoidosis

A biochemical pattern identical to that in chronic hyperparathyroidism with renal damage may be seen. The cause of this rare hypercalcaemic syndrome is probably hypersensitivity of the intestine to vitamin D. The hypercalcaemia and hypercalciuria of sarcoidosis returns to normal after high doses of *hydrocortisone*, which does not affect the hypercalcaemia of hyperparathyroidism.

CHELATING AGENTS

Certain soluble organic compounds inactivate metals, e.g. by including them within ring structures in their molecules.

Sodium edetate (EDTA), given intravenously, will reduce the plasma ionised calcium by being a more powerful binding agent than the plasma proteins. The calcium chelate which is formed is excreted in the urine, and the low plasma ionised calcium leads to depletion of skeletal calcium. Chelating agents are important for the treatment of lead poisoning and for removing fissile materials from the body: to prevent depletion of skeletal calcium the calcium complex of sodium EDTA is used. Other chelating agents are desferrioxamine, used for the removal of iron in haemochromatosis (p. 135); D-penicillamine, used for the removal of copper in Wilson's disease (p. 136) and for complexing cystine to a soluble form in cystinuria (p. 225), and dimercaprol (BAL) used for the removal of heavy metals.

Further reading

MacIntyre I, Evans, JMA, Larkins RG. Vitamin D. *Clin Endocrinol* 1977:6:65–79.
O'Riordan JLH. Hormonal control of mineral metabolism. In: O'Riordan JLH, ed. *Recent Advances in Endocrinology and Metabolism 1*. Oxford: Blackwell Scientific Publications, 1978:189–217.
Paterson CR. *Metabolic Disorders of Bone*. Oxford: Blackwell Scientific Publications, 1975.

CHAPTER 12

THE LIVER

FUNCTIONS OF THE LIVER AND THEIR INVESTIGATION

The principal functions of the liver may be summarised.

1 The parenchymal cells of the liver (hepatocytes), which comprise 60 per cent of its mass, are responsible for the conjugation of bilirubin and for its excretion into the biliary tract.

2 The liver is the centre of metabolic activity for carbohydrate, protein, and lipid.

Carbohydrate. Sugars, and carbon residues from protein and fat, are converted to glycogen. Glycogen is stored as a carbohydrate réserve, being reconvertible to glucose.

Protein. Amino acids are deaminated, the nitrogen residues (and ammonia from the gut) being converted to urea.

Immunoglobulins are synthesised in the cells of the reticulo-endothelial system (though this is mainly outside the liver). Albumin and the other globulins, including coagulation factors, are synthesised in the parenchymal cells. Normal albumin synthesis is about 10 g/24 h, and this can increase to 15–20 g/24 h.

Lipid. The liver contains a store of triglyceride, some being derived from endogenous synthesis. Cholesterol, and from it bile salts, are synthesised. Cholesterol and other lipids are esterified, and vitamin D is hydroxylated. Bile salts are secreted into the biliary tract.

3 The liver detoxicates many metabolic products and drugs and toxins, often prior to their excretion in the urine. The detoxication process involves a chemical change, and/or conjugation principally with glucuronic acid, glycine, or sulphate.

4 The liver excretes many natural and foreign substances into the biliary tract.

5 The liver stores a variety of compounds, including iron and vitamin B_{12}, and vitamin A.

6 The Kupffer cells take part in the overall activities of the reticulo-endothelial system.

When the liver is diseased one or more but not necessarily all of its functions are impaired, though not always in the same order. The various 'liver function tests' are tests of derangement of individual or related functions of the liver (or of secondary derangements elsewhere in the body), and there can be no test for 'liver function' as a whole. It may be possible to extend a conclusion drawn from a single test to an appreciation of the activities of the liver as a whole, because many tests give similar abnormal results in particular diseases of the liver.

The results of liver biopsy are not necessarily comparable with the results of chemical tests, as many measured functional changes are not mirrored by visible structural changes in the liver cells and vice versa. In addition histopathological changes are rarely uniform throughout the liver in disease.

The adult liver has considerable functional reserve. An isolated part may be removed or severely damaged by a localised disease (for example by carcinoma), and if the remainder is healthy, liver function may remain apparently normal when tested biochemically in the resting state – and there can be regeneration of functional cells. On the other hand, in a disease such as infective hepatitis, in which there is diffuse damage to the majority of liver cells, detectable derangement of liver function is always present.

The metabolism of bile pigments

Erythrocytes at the end of their life-span are destroyed in the reticulo-endothelial system: this amounts to about 1 per cent of the total haemoglobin per day. Globin is separated from haem, and the porphyrin ring is opened (p. 125). Iron is released and becomes bound to transferrin: it is not excreted but enters the iron stores or is used for further haemoglobin synthesis. Most of the haemoglobin becomes bilirubin. Most of the bilirubin is derived from haemoglobin, though about 20 per cent comes from the breakdown of tissue cytochromes, myoglobin and other haem proteins, and some from erythrocyte precursors destroyed in the bone marrow. Bilirubin circulates in the plasma bound to albumin. In the liver, this (unconjugated) bilirubin enters the hepatocytes and is there conjugated primarily with glucuronic acid by a mechanism involving bilirubin-UDP glucuronosyltransferase. The pigment excreted in the bile is not the lipid-soluble and relatively water-insoluble unconjugated bilirubin but mainly the water-soluble conjugate, bilirubin glucuronide – usually referred to as conjugated bilirubin, or bilirubin esters.

The liver of an adult has the reserve capacity to conjugate and excrete 5–10 times its normal load of bilirubin, which is about 500 μmol/24 h. The enzymes responsible for conjugation are not fully active at birth (for example full activity of glucuronosyltransferase takes three weeks to develop), and even less so in prematurity, so the neonatal liver barely has the capacity to excrete its normal bilirubin load, and this load may be increased due to excessive breakdown of erythrocytes. Jaundice before 24 hours of age is abnormal, but a moderate hyperbilirubinaemia (<80 μmol/l) within the first week may not be pathological – 'physiological jaundice'.

Excretion of bile pigments (bilirubin and urobilinogen)

Conjugated bilirubin is secreted into the bile duct and passes to the intestines where it is deconjugated. In the large intestine it is reduced by bacterial action to various pigments and pigment precursors including urobilinogen (this is a collective name given to a group of colourless chromogens one of which is stercobilinogen, though other terminology is used). Most of the urobilinogen is excreted in the faeces where it is oxidised by the air to the pinkish-brown urobilin pigments. Urobilin, with many other compounds both known and unidentified, forms the colouring matter of faeces: stercobilin, which is strictly one of the components of urobilin, is sometimes used as an alternative name for the urobilin group of pigments. A small fraction of the urobilinogen is absorbed into the portal circulation, and in the liver some of this urobilinogen is re-excreted into the bile, whilst the remainder is excreted by the kidneys. When urine is exposed to air urobilinogen is oxidised to urobilin, though this makes up a negligible part of the colouring matter of normal urine. Most of the pigments that produce the colour of urine are unidentified, and they are known collectively as urochrome.

There is no bilirubin in the faeces of a normal adult. In the new-born, bilirubin is found in the faeces and there is no urobilinogen in the faeces or urine, as the bacterial reduction mechanism for conversion of bilirubin to urobilinogen takes some months to develop fully. Bilirubin is found in the faeces of adults whose gut has been sterilised by antibiotics.

Biliverdin, a green oxidation product of bilirubin and intermediate in haemoglobin breakdown (p. 125), has little importance in the study of human liver disease. The diagram (Fig. 12.1) summarises the normal metabolism of bilirubin in an adult.

Amniotic fluid

Bilirubinoid pigments are released into the amniotic fluid in small amounts when erythroblastosis has become severe in cases of isoimmunised pregnancy, particularly rhesus incompatibility. When measured, at about 32 weeks, the result can be used as a guide for early induction of labour or for intrauterine transfusion. The upper limit of normal for amniotic fluid pigment, expressed as bilirubin, is 2 μmol/l; however the usual method of assay is differential spectrophotometry to eliminate interference from haemoglobin. The reference values, and indications for treatment, depend on the time of gestation and on the laboratory method.

Plasma bilirubin and the van den Bergh reaction

Bilirubin (unconjugated) and conjugated bilirubin, which are both bound to protein (mainly albumin), can be distinguished chemically in plasma by their rate of reaction with diazotised sulphanilic acid to form azobilirubin (the van den Bergh reaction). Conjugated bilirubin reacts rapidly and a mauve colour appears within a few minutes (positive direct van

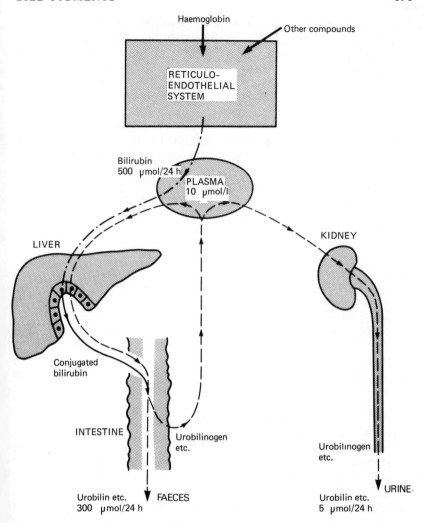

FIG. 12.1. Diagram of main pathways of the origin, circulation, and excretion of bilirubin and principal related compounds in a normal adult.

den Bergh reaction). Unconjugated bilirubin does not give this immediate colour (negative direct van den Bergh reaction), but a colour develops after adding alcohol, caffeine, or other special reagents (the indirect van den Bergh reaction). Biliverdin does not react. The intensity of the direct and indirect van den Bergh reactions is used as a measure of the plasma conjugated bilirubin and total (unconjugated plus conjugated) bilirubin respectively, the unconjugated bilirubin being calculated by difference. This separate estimation has taken the place of the simple van den Bergh reaction when it is necessary, as in certain types of haemolytic jaundice, to measure both bilirubin fractions. In the investigation of most cases of jaundice the total plasma bilirubin gives sufficient information.

The reference range for plasma total bilirubin in adults is 5–17 μmol/l, and normal plasma, containing a small proportion of conjugated bilirubin, does not give a positive direct van den Bergh reaction.

Bilirubin is slowly destroyed by ultraviolet or blue light, and phototherapy may be used for treatment of neonatal hyperbilirubinaemia.

Icterus index. This is an outdated simple measure of the yellowness of the plasma, which includes carotenoids as well as bilirubin. This assay can now be made relatively specific for total bilirubin by using a commercial meter, and this is very useful for rapid assessment of neonatal jaundice.

Jaundice

Jaundice can be detected clinically when the plasma total bilirubin exceeds about 35 μmol/l. When jaundice is receding bile pigments may remain in the skin and the patient appear more jaundiced than the plasma total bilirubin level would warrant.

No single classification of jaundice is satisfactory for all purposes. It is possible to consider primarily (a) the anatomical site of the pathological lesion causing the jaundice (pre-hepatic, hepatic, post-hepatic), or (b) the pathological causes (infective, toxic, etc.) or (c) the nature of the alteration in bilirubin metabolism.

Jaundice and altered bilirubin metabolism

Haemolytic causes. In haemolytic jaundice the rate of production of bilirubin is greater than the rate at which liver cells can excrete bilirubin. In adults the plasma bilirubin rarely exceeds 80 μmol/l, and the patient's skin is coloured orange-yellow. There is no excess conjugated bilirubin unless anaemia has caused secondary liver damage, or pigment stones obstruct the biliary tract. In infants excessive haemolysis and delayed formation of conjugating enzymes may lead to a plasma bilirubin in excess of 350 μmol/l. Kernicterus develops because the excess bilirubin is soluble in the lipid of the basal ganglia of the brain. Administration of sulphonamides may displace enough bilirubin from its albumin-binding to cause kernicterus.

Hepatocellular causes. Abnormalities at a hepatocellular level may be a defect of transport of bilirubin into the cell, defective conjugation, or defective excretion into the bile canaliculi. Cholestasis, or reduction of bile flow, may be the latter in the context of liver cell necrosis (e.g. infective hepatitis), or as specific failure of excretion, or post-hepatic obstruction.

Of the rare metabolic failures of bilirubin conjugation or transport, the commonest is *Gilbert's syndrome* (familial non-haemolytic hyper-bilirubinaemia) in which, because of deficiency of the transport mechanism, there is a fluctuating benign mild jaundice due to non-conjugated bilirubin: however most cases are healthy, not 'diseased'. In the *Crigler-Najjar syndrome* there is congenital deficiency of the UDPglucuronosyltransferase. There are other rare conjugated hyperbilirubinaemias.

In the common jaundice due to hepatocellular damage from disease, with a resultant increase of plasma conjugated bilirubin rather than of bilirubin, the plasma total bilirubin may exceed 300 μmol/l.

Cholestatic causes. When cholestasis predominates, and especially when the cause is obstruction, the plasma total bilirubin (almost all conjugated) may exceed 500 μmol/l, and the patient may appear greenish-yellow due to the presence in plasma and skin of a little biliverdin. Kernicterus does not develop because the excess conjugated bilirubin is water-soluble and is therefore not deposited in the basal ganglia.

Bile pigments in the urine in disease

Bilirubin. No bilirubin can be detected in normal urine. Bilirubin (unconjugated) is not excreted by the healthy kidney because of its low water-solubility and of its firm binding to protein, so that in haemolytic jaundice, when there is only a high plasma bilirubin, none can be detected in the urine – hence the old name for adult haemolytic anaemia, 'acholuric jaundice'. Conjugated bilirubin, being water-soluble and with some of it more loosely bound to protein, is readily excreted; and 'bilirubin' found in the urine is always in the conjugated form. If this is present in the urine of a patient with jaundice due to haemolytic anaemia, then secondary liver damage must have occurred with a consequent failure to excrete conjugated bilirubin in the bile. When there is a high plasma conjugated bilirubin, then this pigment can be detected in the urine when the plasma total bilirubin level exceeds about 30 μmol/l, and the froth (due to excess bile salts) of shaken urine appears yellow when the plasma bilirubin level exceeds about 50 μmol/l: though the threshold is variable. The technique of tests for bilirubin in urine, by using a diazo reaction in a commercial preparation or by oxidising it to biliverdin (Fouchet-Harrison test), can be found in Appendix IV. There is a method for quantitative assay of urine bilirubin, but this is rarely required.

Urobilinogen. A small amount of urobilinogen can be detected in fresh normal urine (p. 273), though these semiquantitative tests are insensitive and of little diagnostic value. The normal 24 hour urinary excretion is 0.5–5.0 μmol. In haemolytic jaundice much of the excess bilirubin in the plasma passes to the intestines where an increased quantity of urobilinogen is formed. Much of this urobilinogen is absorbed, and excess urobilinogen is excreted in the urine. In the pre-icteric and recovery stages of infective hepatitis, and sometimes in cirrhosis without jaundice, excess urinary urobilinogen is found presumably due to impaired ability of the liver cells to re-excrete urobilinogen.

In severe hepatocellular or obstructive jaundice bilirubin reaches the intestine only in small amounts, little urobilinogen is formed, and urobilinogen is absent from the urine. Reappearance of urobilinogen in the urine is a sign of recovery from cholestasis. If post-hepatic obstruction is due to malignancy and is complete, urobilinogen is constantly absent, whereas if it is due to a stone and is incomplete, bilirubin may occasionally pass into the intestine and urobilinogen be found in the urine.

Bile pigments in the faeces in disease
No bilirubin can be detected in the faeces of normal adults, but it is present in the faeces of infants.

The normal 24 hour faecal excretion of urobilinogen in an adult is 100–500 µmol. The quantity of urobilinogen excreted in the faeces is increased in the haemolytic anaemias, but this estimation, even in relation to the amount of total circulating haemoglobin, does not accurately measure the rate of erythrocyte breakdown. In severe cholestatic jaundice, or due to many oral antibiotics which alter the intestinal flora, faecal urobilinogen excretion is greatly diminished. The quantity excreted also relates to the completeness of post-hepatic obstruction, faecal urobilinogen and urobilin being often undetectable (clay-coloured stools) when the obstruction is complete due to a tumour, and appearing when there is incomplete obstruction.

Summary of changes in bile pigment metabolism
The results found in investigation of bile pigment metabolism in the principal types of jaundice are summarised in the table. Haemolytic anaemia is associated with characteristic disturbances of bile pigment metabolism provided that it is uncomplicated by secondary liver damage. Tests based on other aspects of disturbed liver function must be used for the differentiation of hepatocellular jaundice from obstructive jaundice, and for the diagnosis and investigation of liver disease in the absence of jaundice.

Carbohydrate metabolism

Although the liver maintains the normal plasma glucose concentration (p. 55), obvious changes in carbohydrate metabolism are seen only in severe disease. When there is acute necrosis of the liver, hypoglycaemia usually develops. In chronic liver disease the capacity of the liver to convert glucose and other sugars to glycogen for storage is reduced. Tests which measure the utilisation of glucose are unsatisfactory as liver function tests because of the variable extrahepatic utilisation of this

Disease	Plasma		Urine		Faeces
	Total bilirubin	Excess conjugated bilirubin (direct van den Bergh)	Urobilinogen	Bilirubin	Urobilinogen
Normal	Present	–	Present	Absent	Present ·
Haemolytic (spherocytosis)	+	–	Increased	Absent	+ +
Hepatocellular (infective hepatitis)	+ +	+	Variable	+	Low
Obstructive (carcinoma of pancreas)	+ + +	+ +	Absent	+ +	Absent

sugar. Glucose tolerance curves in patients with severe liver damage are often abnormal: 'lag-storage' curves, or curves showing mild impaired tolerance, may be seen.

Galactose/fructose tolerance tests. These measure the capacity of the liver to convert galactose or fructose to glycogen. After oral or intravenous administration of the test sugar, serial plasma analyses are made – the plasma galactose or fructose rises higher in cases of diffuse hepatocellular damage than in normal subjects. The oral tests are now little used because of variations in intestinal absorption. As a semi-research procedure a single intravenous dose of galactose may be given, followed by repeated capillary plasma galactose estimations over a period of one hour to calculate the slope of the elimination curve.

Protein metabolism

Changes in general protein metabolism, apart from alterations in plasma proteins and enzymes, are only significant in severe liver disease. If liver damage is both acute and massive, as in acute hepatic necrosis, conversion of the amino acids to urea is greatly reduced, and the plasma and urine amino acid levels rise. A classical finding in severe acute hepatic necrosis is the detection in the urine of crystals of the less soluble amino acids, leucine and tyrosine, though this is no longer used for a diagnostic test. Abnormal urinary amino acid patterns may be determined by chromatography. The plasma urea concentration may be below 2.0 mmol/l in acute hepatic necrosis, but this is not the case if there are complicating factors. A moderate degree of aminoaciduria may be found in cirrhosis of the liver, though without any diagnostically abnormal patterns; the plasma urea tends to be about 2.5 mmol/l due to deficient formation and to haemodilution.

The ammonium ions that are absorbed into the portal vein from the gut are normally almost completely metabolised by the liver, and little ammonia is present in peripheral blood (p. 103). When there is severe parenchymatous liver disease or cirrhosis, blood ammonia is increased. This is due to portal blood by-passing healthy liver cells in a collateral circulation (which may be marked after a porto-caval shunt), and to impaired liver cell metabolism.

Plasma proteins

In chronic liver disease, when large numbers of parenchymal liver cells have been destroyed, synthesis of albumin is impaired. In the absence of other known causes of hypoproteinaemia a plasma albumin concentration below 30 g/l indicates liver damage, and a value below 20 g/l is serious: haemodilution due to water retention (p. 202), and possibly decreased catabolism, may also play a part. The plasma concentrations of all other proteins that are synthesised in the parenchymal cells of the liver are also reduced. However the total plasma globulin level is raised, due to increase of the immunoglobulin fractions synthesised generally in the reticulo-endothelial system including the Kupffer cells. In acute hepatitis these changes may not be detectable by simple quantitative analysis.

Clotting factors

A low plasma fibrinogen may be found when there is extensive parenchymal cell damage, and the plasma concentration of prothrombin and of most other clotting factors is also reduced, giving a prolonged prothrombin time – see haematology texts. Alterations in blood coagulability must therefore be borne in mind if liver biopsy is proposed for the diagnosis of chronic liver disease – measurement of the prothrombin time and clotting time are essential preliminaries to liver biopsy.

Synthesis of prothrombin, and of several other clotting factors, depend upon the amount of vitamin K_1 that is reaching the liver cells, as well as on the functional state of those cells, for which the prothrombin time is a sensitive test. In obstructive jaundice, absence of bile salts from the intestine causes diminished absorption of vitamin K_1 and the prothrombin time is therefore prolonged. Intramuscular injection of vitamin K_1 will restore the prolonged prothrombin time to normal in 24 hours in a case of obstructive jaundice: it will not affect a prolonged prothrombin time which has been caused by hepatocellular damage, as there is then a defect in structural synthetic capacity for clotting factors.

Flocculation tests

Simple tests have been devised in which the patient's serum is added to a suitable colloidal system – the colloidal gold, thymol, cephalin-cholesterol, and zinc sulphate reactions. Normal albumin and the α-globulin mucoproteins stabilise such systems. Excess immunoglobulins destroy the stability of the system and precipitation or flocculation results.

These tests are of theoretical and historical importance, but have now been replaced almost everywhere for differential diagnosis of infective hepatitis from obstructive jaundice by the plasma enzyme tests, and for the measurement of excess γ-globulins by electrophoresis and quantitative immunoglobulin assay. Strongly positive results are typical of acute viral hepatitis, and are also seen in Hashimoto's disease and various acute collagen diseases; in an acute post-hepatic obstruction without secondary liver damage the flocculation reactions are normal.

Enzymes

Enzyme essays can be used principally in three different ways in the assessment of liver function. Some enzymes synthesised in the liver, e.g. cholinesterase, show a fall in their plasma activity when there is hepatocellular damage, Some membrane-bound enzymes synthesised in the liver, and also found in the bile, e.g. alkaline phosphatase, have a rise in their plasma activity when there is cholestasis. Many cell-active enzymes which are present in high concentration in liver parenchymal cells, especially in the cytosol, e.g. alanine transaminase, have a rise in their plasma activity when there is active hepatocellular damage.

Cholinesterase (formerly called pseudocholinesterase)
This estimation is now rarely used as a liver function test: reference values 2–5 U/l at 37 °C. A low plasma value is regularly found, proportional to the mass of remaining active cells, in chronic hepatitis – as is found with plasma albumin.

Alkaline phosphatase and related enzymes
The reference values in adults are 20–95 U/l: 3–13 King-Armstrong units/dl (see p. 178 for age and sex variation). A raised plasma alkaline phosphatase, particularly to more than 180 U/l (and usually in association with a raised plasma bilirubin) provides a measure of extrahepatic or intrahepatic biliary obstruction e.g. primary biliary cirrhosis. The increase is due mainly to stimulation by the cholestasis of excess enzyme synthesis in the liver cells lining the bile canaliculi: the part played by possible impaired secretion into the bile is controversial. Moderate increases, generally to about 150 U/l, are characteristically found in viral hepatitis. A raised plasma alkaline phosphatase with little increase in plasma bilirubin is also seen when there are primary or metastatic malignant deposits in the liver, and a similar increase is found in cirrhosis even in the absence of obstruction. An increased plasma alkaline phosphatase is an early sign of cholestatic liver damage due to certain drugs such as chlorpromazine.

In children or adolescents the physiological increase in alkaline phosphatase due to bone growth may mask changes due to hepatobiliary disease. There may also be possible confusion of increased bone and liver alkaline phosphatase when there is cirrhosis with osteomalacia, or multiple metastases. Electrophoresis can be used to distinguish liver and bone alkaline phosphatases in plasma (p. 178).

The related enzyme 5'-nucleotidase (reference values 2–15 U/l at 37°C), is generally increased in plasma in the same hepatobiliary disorders as is alkaline phosphatase, but is unaltered in bone disease.

Transaminases (aminotransferases)

The enzymes assayed most commonly in liver disease are alanine transaminase (ALT) – reference values 5–25 U/l (or alanine aminotransferase, formerly called glutamic-pyruvic transaminase) or aspartate transaminase (AST: p. 120). In general somewhat higher values of plasma alanine transaminase (which is solely cytoplasmic) than of aspartate transaminase (cytoplasmic and mitochondrial) are found in acute liver disease, and somewhat lower values in cirrhosis: the differences are not usually great, and it is probably not worth measuring both enzymes as a routine for clinical diagnosis. In viral hepatitis the transaminases rise above normal during the prodromal period. Peak values (of about 500–2000 U/l) are found at the time of maximum illness and the value returns to normal in about four weeks unless subacute liver disease develops. A similar but less marked pattern (with values rarely above 300 U/l) usually occurs in nonicteric hepatitis and in glandular fever. Hypersensitivity hepatocellular damage attributed to drugs may be shown by a continuing rise in plasma transaminase on repeated testing. Alcohol raises the plasma transaminases in alcoholics, but not in normal subjects. Moderately raised plasma transaminase values (usually between 50 and 300 U/l) are found in cirrhosis in proportion to the degree of active cell damage, but unrelated to coma or decompensation. In malignant disease involving the liver and in obstructive jaundice the plasma transaminase values are usually moderately raised owing to hepatocellular damage, but rarely exceed 300 U/l.

γ-Glutamyltransferase

This enzyme (GGT: reference values: male 10–50, female 7–30 U/l at 37 °C) provides a sensitive but non-discriminating assay for a variety of hepatobiliary disorders. In cholestatic disease it behaves like alkaline phosphatase, with particular sensitivity for hepatic metastases – there is no change in osteoblastic bone disease. In hepatocellular disease changes are similar to those of the transaminases.

The assay is particularly useful in the detection of microsomal enzyme induction by drugs, the most important of these being alcohol in the chronic drinker.

Other enzymes

It is possible to detect and measure the mitochondrial isoenzyme of AST in plasma in severe hepatocellular damage.

Other enzymes have slightly different applications. Isocitrate dehydrogenase seems to be slightly more sensitive to early hepatocellular damage. Some workers like to measure 'hepatic' LD, namely LD-4 and LD-5 (p. 120). In haemolytic jaundice plasma LD activity is increased due to release of erythrocytic LD-1 (p. 122). Iditol (sorbitol) dehydrogenase, though less sensitive than the transaminases, being absent from erythrocytes can be used to measure liver cell damage in the presence of severe haemolysis.

Lipid metabolism

Bile salts

The liver synthesises per 24 hours from cholesterol about 1.3 mmol (0.5 g) of bile acids: these are principally cholic acid and chenodeoxycholic acid, conjugated with glycine and taurine. The bile salts are excreted into the intestine where they are essential for the adequate absorption of fats (p. 77) and of vitamin K; bacterial reduction produces deoxycholic acid and lithocholic acid respectively. Only a small quantity of bile salts is lost in the faeces, most being reabsorbed in the terminal ileum and resecreted in the bile. In obstructive jaundice or severe hepatocellular damage the flow of bile salts to the intestine is reduced and there may be steatorrhoea (p. 239).

Bile salts cannot be detected in normal urine. The historic Hay's test (sprinkling flowers of sulphur on to the surface of urine) depends on the property of bile salts, excreted as sulphates, to lower surface tension: it is very insensitive and has no clinical value. The place of the recently introduced assay of plasma bile salt concentration as a test for cholestasis is not yet established: bile salt clearance tests are a further refinement.

Other lipids

Although the liver is active in many metabolic processes involving cholesterol and other lipids, the alterations which occur in disease are not studied as routine liver function tests because of lack both of sensitivity and of specificity.

In cholestasis, whether due to drugs, or as post-hepatic obstructive jaundice or the obstructive phase of hepatitis, the plasma free cholesterol level is greatly increased, and there is some increase in plasma ester cholesterol and in the phospholipids: lipoprotein X (p. 86) is always present. When there is parenchymal cell damage the free cholesterol level is variable (depending on a balance between retention and diminished synthesis) and there is a marked fall in the ester cholesterol and usually in the phospholipids. A low total plasma cholesterol is found in acute hepatic necrosis, or in the terminal stages of chronic hepatitis.

In biliary cirrhosis and obstruction there is a marked increase of all plasma lipid fractions including the phospholipids, and the increase in β-lipoproteins (p. 86) may be identified by electrophoresis: free fatty acids are often also increased. The biochemistry of fatty deposition in the liver (p. 87), and of cholesterol in relation to gall-stones (p. 205), are discussed elsewhere.

Hepatic detoxication

Although the liver conjugates a great many metabolic products besides bilirubin, liver function tests utilising only this principle are not at present used.

In the *hippuric acid test*, sodium benzoate was given intravenously, and the excretion of hippurate depended on the efficiency of the conjugation process – but was also very dependent on renal function.

Hepatic transport and excretion

A *bilirubin excretion test* has been devised which is sometimes valuable in the investigation of obscure mild hyperbilirubinaemias.

Porphyrins are excreted in the bile as well as in the urine. In many types of liver disease (particularly in acute hepatitis and cirrhosis), and in obstructive jaundice, biliary excretion of porphyrins is diminished and excess coproporphyrins can be found in the urine (p. 130).

The liver removes many dyes from the plasma, by uptake into the parenchymal cells, at a rate which depends on the plasma flow to the liver and on the functional capacity of the cells; then excretes them into the bile canaliculi, this being affected by cholestasis. It is feasible to investigate the functional competence of parenchymal cells by measuring the removal from plasma of a suitable dye. Bromsulphthalein has been widely used, and it is normally more than 80 per cent excreted into the bile after conjugation: its excretion is therefore similar to that of bilirubin but is more sensitive to damage of cell function. Indocyanine Green, which is excreted without conjugation, may also be used and is claimed to provide a more sensitive test: the dye is more expensive, but is non-toxic whereas bromsulphthalein occasionally produces reactions.

The *bromsulphthalein test* involves injection of 5 mg of dye per kg body weight, and measuring the plasma concentration 45 minutes later. In health the 45 minute value is less than 5 per cent – zero time taken as 100 per cent. The test is sensitive for assessment of diffuse hepatocellular damage in the absence of jaundice, but is non-specific and has largely been replaced by more specific tests. It gives positive results in heart failure or in cholestatic jaundice. For specialised studies in the investigation of transport disorders more frequent blood sampling over a longer period can be used, or clearance studies (which involve catheterisation) performed.

BIOCHEMICAL CHANGES IN LIVER DISEASE

Neonatal jaundice

The two main causes of jaundice in the new-born are excess production of bilirubin as a result of haemolytic disease (usually from blood-group incompatibility), and delayed formation of the enzymatic conjugating capacity of the liver, principally bilirubin-UDPglucuronosyltransferase. Because of the latter, premature infants may have a plasma unconjugated bilirubin up to 250 μmol/l at 5 days, which returns to normal as the glucuronosyltransferase is synthesised. When there is haemolysis, the unconjugated bilirubin may exceed 300 μmol/l. As, at this concentration and above, the deposition of the lipid-soluble bilirubin in the basal ganglia is likely to lead to the dangerous kernicterus, the level of 300 μmol/l is taken as the indication for exchange transfusion or phototherapy.

Biliary atresia produces a cholestatic jaundice with increased conjugated bilirubin, but the plasma alkaline phosphatase is usually normal in the early stages, as the immature liver cells cannot synthesise excess enzyme.

Viral hepatitis

Mild preicteric hepatocellular damage can be detected by raised plasma transaminases and by an increased excretion of urobilinogen in the urine. When the disease is established there is moderate jaundice with a raised plasma total and conjugated bilirubin, and bilirubin in the urine without urobilinogen, and pale stools. The plasma transaminases are markedly increased. The plasma albumin concentration may be slightly lowered, the α-globulin is variable, β-globulin may be raised, and there is an increase in γ-globulins. The flocculation reactions are strongly positive, and there is usually a moderate rise in the plasma alkaline phosphatase. The prothrombin time is prolonged.

During recovery from the acute attack bilirubin disappears from the urine and urobilinogen reappears. The plasma proteins, enzyme values, and flocculation reactions return to normal.

If the hepatitis becomes subacute the plasma proteins remain abnormal with a definite fall in albumin and persistently raised γ-globulin; the plasma alkaline phosphatase is raised, but bilirubin and transaminases may be only slightly raised.

In non-icteric hepatitis the changes are similar, but less marked, except that the plasma bilirubin remains within normal limits.

Alternatively the disease may progress in the early stages to acute hepatic necrosis, or in the subacute stage to chronic hepatitis.

Especial precautions must be observed in handling blood specimens from patients with hepatitis because of the risks of infection to laboratory staff (p. 256).

Chronic active hepatitis

This condition is marked by continuing destruction of liver cells, and most tests therefore give abnormal values. There is a low plasma albumin with much increased γ-globulins (IgG), and a marked increase in bilirubin. High values are found for both plasma alkaline phosphatase and for the transaminases. Smooth muscle antibodies and antinuclear factor can be usually detected in serum.

Cirrhosis

The biochemical alterations of function are the same whatever the pathological type of the disorder. There is variable and dissociated damage to the functions of the liver. The plasma total bilirubin level may be normal or slightly raised, and there is often excess urobilinogen in the urine but no bilirubin. The plasma albumin level is progressively decreased as healthy liver cells are replaced, and there is a rise in the γ-globulins. A typical electrophoretic pattern is usually found, for the excess immunoglobulins which are present have a high mobility and there is β-γ fusion (p. 115). The plasma transaminases may be only moderately raised unless there is a flare-up in cytolysis. The plasma alkaline phosphatase and γ-glutamyltransferase are usually slightly raised. There is early impairment of bromsulphthalein clearance. Plasma cholesterol tends to be low, with diminished esterification. Type I coproporphyrinuria is usually present. There is often impaired glucose tolerance. Alcoholics tend to have IgA excess.

There is almost always hyponatraemia that is largely dilutional, and a multifactorial potassium deficiency.

The damaged liver fails to metabolise hormones, including ADH. Feminising changes in men, and the spider naevi often found in this condition, have been ascribed to excess of circulating oestrogens.

Ascites. Causes of the ascites of cirrhosis are local factors, particularly portal hypertension, and systemic factors. These are mainly the low circulating albumin concentration, and the sodium retention with excessive water retention (causing a low plasma sodium concentration) accompanying secondary aldosteronism (p. 158).

Ascites may be due to many primary disorders. Ascitic fluid in cirrhosis and in congestive heart failure is usually a transudate, whereas that associated with peritoneal infections or malignancy is usually an exudate (p. 117).

Primary biliary cirrhosis

There is a mild and late cholestatic jaundice with a raised plasma total and conjugated bilirubin, and bilirubin in the urine. The plasma albumin level falls slightly and late in the disease; and there is a rise in the γ-globulins, due mainly to IgM. Antimitochondrial antibodies can be usually detected in serum. Marked alteration of lipid metabolism develops; plasma cholesterol and phosphilipids are increased, and electrophoresis shows lipoprotein X and excess β-lipoproteins, and xanthomatosis is common. The plasma alkaline phosphatase is often greatly raised. The plasma transaminases increase when there is active hepatocellular damage, but parenchymal cell function may be only slightly impaired. Steatorrhoea may develop in long-standing cases.

Post-hepatic (large bile duct) obstruction

There is a cholestatic jaundice, with a markedly raised plasma (conjugated) bilirubin, and bilirubin in the urine. Urobilinogen will be found in the urine and faeces only if the obstruction is incomplete or intermittent. The plasma alkaline phosphatase and total cholesterol levels are generally markedly raised, with an increase in α_2- and β-globulins. Unless the obstruction is long-standing, parenchymal cell function is not severely damaged; the plasma transaminases are usually only moderately raised, and the plasma albumin level is normal.

Prolonged obstruction may cause secondary biliary cirrhosis, which is biochemically indistinguishable from primary biliary cirrhosis. However the positive reaction for mitochondrial antibody of (autoimmune) primary biliary cirrhosis is negative in other forms of cholestasis.

Acute hepatic necrosis

All functions of the liver are profoundly altered. There is usually severe jaundice, with a high plasma total and unconjugated bilirubin, and bilirubin (but no urobilinogen) in the urine. The plasma transaminases are very greatly increased during the active phase and the alkaline phosphatase may be slightly increased. Failure of conversion of amino acids to urea leads to an increase in total plasma amino acids and increased urinary amino acids without specific changes on chromatography. The plasma urea is usually low, but if there is severe dehydration a normal and even slightly increased level may be found. The concentrations of all plasma proteins, except γ-globulins, are decreased, in particular the clotting factors. Hypoglycaemia may be profound, and the blood pyruvate and lactate concentrations are high, with an acidosis.

Hepatic coma

This is a frequent end-stage of hepatitis or of cirrhosis. The wide variety of abnormal laboratory findings are, in the case of the standard liver function tests, related to the stage of the underlying liver disease and not to the coma. Other altered biochemical values are related to secondary factors such as poor renal function, or diuretics, or vomiting.

The nature of the toxins affecting the central nervous system has not been elucidated, though a role for ammonia seems certain. Cerebral metabolism may be disturbed due to the excess ammonia accelerating the conversion of oxoglutarate to glutamate, and thus depriving the tricarboxylic acid cycle of oxoglutarate. There is an increased blood concentration of lactate, and of pyruvate and other keto acids, giving a metabolic acidosis often accentuated by renal failure: there may also be respiratory alkalosis due to hyperventilation. The distinctive odour, the foetor hepaticus, is due to mercaptans which are thought to arise from excess circulating methionine. Though there is often slight proteinuria the plasma urea is usually only slightly raised: however acute renal failure may develop.

Drug effects

Many drugs can cause jaundice, some by affecting bilirubin metabolism and some producing liver disease by a toxic effect on the cells. Examples of the first mechanism are the sulphonamides which may produce haemolysis, and novobiocin which may inhibit the conjugation of bilirubin. On the other hand, some drugs can *induce* the microsomal glucuronosyltransferase, and phenobarbitone is thus used for the treatment of unconjugated hyperbilirubinaemia by promoting conjugation and therefore excretion of the excess bilirubin.

There are many types of toxic reaction. Carbon tetrachloride is an example of a directly toxic drug, which produces acute hepatic necrosis: the similar effects of paracetamol are dose-related. Hypersensitivity is blamed for a clinical and biochemical picture resembling mild or severe infective hepatitis due to halothane: sensitivity to some other drugs, such as rifampicin or monoamine oxidase inhibitors, produces only a transient rise in plasma transaminase, and only rarely hepatitis. Susceptibility to methyltestosterone or oral contraceptives produces cholestasis (with an early rise in plasma alkaline phosphatase, and also in transaminases) which is usually transient; but hypersensitivity to chlorpromazine, with cholangiolitis, occasionally progresses to resemble biliary cirrhosis.

Malignant disease

Primary hepatoma is commonly marked by an increased plasma concentration of the oncofetal antigen, α-fetoprotein (p. 116). Jaundice may be late, and is preceded by increased bromsulphthalein retention, and increased plasma values for alkaline phosphatase and γ-glutamyltransferase.

In the far more common metastatic carcinomatosis, α-fetoprotein is normal, and there is (with the other biochemical changes of primary hepatoma) a likely increase in serum transaminases.

Gall-stones

The major component of most gall-stones is cholesterol, and they usually also contain variable amounts of calcium carbonate and phosphate and of bile pigments. In the bile, cholesterol is held in solution in micelles with the aid of phospholipids (mainly lecithin) and bile salts: the ratio of the concentrations of phospholipids plus bile salts to that of cholesterol determines its solubility. Amongst the factors that promote stone formation are alteration of this ratio by an abnormality in the secretion of hepatic bile, and stasis or infection in the gall-bladder which can provide sites for the initiation of cholesterol precipitation.

Pigment stones may be formed in haemolytic states when there is greatly increased bilirubin excretion in the bile. Their main individual component is bilirubin, with much amorphous material.

Choice of liver function tests

A single liver function test has little diagnostic value when done in isolation. A suitable selection of tests should always be performed and the choice of biochemical liver function tests depends on the purpose of the investigation. Multichannel analysers can be programmed (p. 5) to perform all the tests mentioned on all patient samples.

Probably the most frequent uses of liver function tests are in the differential diagnosis of jaundice of clinically uncertain origin, and in the assessment of residual function in chronic disease.

For differential diagnosis of jaundice separate estimation of plasma total and conjugated bilirubin (or if not available then the van den Bergh reaction) must be done, and the urine examined for bilirubin and urobilinogen. As well as these tests of pigment metabolism, estimation of the levels of a plasma transaminase and of alkaline phosphatase (or equivalent enzymes) are usually necessary when the differential diagnosis lies between acute hepatitis ('medical') and post-hepatic cholestatic ('surgical') jaundice. The results of these tests, in combination with clinical evidence, will in more than 90 per cent of patients indicate the nature and intensity of the lesion which is causing the jaundice. Determination of total and differential plasma proteins, of cholesterol, and of electrolytes, are not at this stage usually diagnostically valuable.

The other frequent use of liver function tests is for the detection and measurement of impairment of function in known or suspected chronic liver disease, even in the absence of jaundice. For this purpose, in addition to the total bilirubin, the estimation of total and differential plasma proteins (with electrophoresis, and including prothrombin time), and occasionally the bromsulphthalein retention test, are most useful: the -globulins represent the intensity of the reactive process. The plasma transaminases are used to measure active cell breakdown. The plasma alkaline phosphatase estimation is particularly useful for the evaluation of biliary cirrhosis and of carcinomatosis of the liver especially in the absence of jaundice. γ-Glutamyltransferase assay is valuable for the early detection of alcoholic liver damage. Electrolyte determination is usual when there is cirrhosis, and essential in the assessment and management of ascites.

It is important to measure plasma alkaline phosphatase and transaminase to check for possible cholestatic or hepatic toxicity of many drugs.

Analysis for various circulating autoantibodies is becoming of increasing importance in the investigation of chronic disease.

Further Reading

Murray Lyon I. Liver failure. *Medicine* 3rd series 1978; 18:912–916.

Price CP, Alberti KGMM. Biochemical assessment of liver function. In: Wright R, Alberti KGMM, Karran S, Millward-Sadler GH, eds. *Liver and Biliary Disease*. London: W.B. Saunders, 1979.

Sherlock S. Hepatic function in disease: bilirubin and protein metabolism. *Br J Hosp Med* 1971; 6:785–792.

CHAPTER 13

THE KIDNEYS

PATHOPHYSIOLOGY

The formation of urine

In a healthy adult about 650 ml of plasma (1200 ml of blood) pass through functioning renal excretory tissue every minute, and about 125 ml of glomerular filtrate is formed. Water passes freely from the plasma through the glomeruli, and those unbound constituents of the plasma that have a molecular weight of less than about 70 000 are present in the glomerular filtrate at about the same concentration as in the plasma. Substances of a higher molecular weight than about 70 000 do not pass freely through the glomeruli and are present in the glomerular filtrate at a lower concentration than in the plasma – though molecular size is not the only determinant for filtration. In man, excretion of the end-products of metabolism is almost wholly glomerular; tubular excretion of metabolites is of little importance except for potassium, urate, and creatinine at high plasma levels; however tubular excretion of many drugs (e.g. penicillin) is significant. The renal tubules conserve water and the soluble constituents of the body by reabsorption using both passive and active transport from the glomerular filtrate. Glucose, protein, amino acids, and most of the water and ions, are reabsorbed in the proximal portion of the tubules. In the distal portion of the tubules the remainder of the water and ions are reabsorbed, acidification of the urine takes place, and ammonia may be formed.

The urine that is finally secreted has an entirely different composition from the glomerular filtrate from which it is derived.

Constituent	Daily excretion	
	Glomerular Filtrate	Urine
Water	180 000 ml	1500 ml
Sodium	20 000 mmol	150 mmol
Albumin	4 g	0.04 g
	(60 μmol)	(0.6 μmol)
Urea	900 mmol	400 mmol

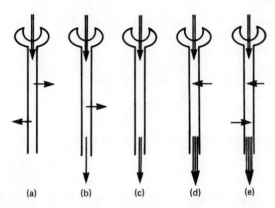

Fig. 13.1. Simplified diagram showing different ways in which the renal tubules can handle substances freely filtered through the glomeruli. (a) Glucose – virtually completely reabsorbed, (b) Urea – partly reabsorbed, (c) Inulin – unaltered, (d) Creatinine – partly secreted into the tubules, (e) p-Aminohippuric acid – wholly secreted into the tubules.

Different ways in which the renal tubules handle substances which have been freely filtered through the glomeruli are shown in Fig. 13.1.

(a) Glucose is present in urine in extremely low concentration, and the glucose in the glomerular filtrate may be considered to be completely reabsorbed by the tubules.

(b) Urea diffuses back from the tubules into the plasma to a limited extent.

(c) and (d) Inulin and p-aminohippuric acid (PAH) are foreign substances used in studies of renal function. (c) Inulin in the plasma, after being excreted into the glomerular filtrate, passes through the tubule without either secretion or reabsorption; no endogenous substance behaves exactly in this way. (d) PAH is excreted into the tubule, as well as into the glomerular filtrate, and the renal plasma is virtually freed ('cleared') of PAH in its passage through the nephron unit; the 8 per cent that is not cleared has passed through kidney tissue that is not excretory.

Clearance

These different types of excretion can be expressed quantitatively by using the concept of clearance. The clearance of any substance from the plasma is, in theoretical terms, the volume of plasma which a given volume of urine (usually a one minute excretion) 'clears' of that substance. It is calculated (as ml/min; or sometimes as ml/s) as

$$\frac{\text{Urine concentration} \times \text{Urine volume (ml/min)}}{\text{Plasma concentration}}$$

The units of concentration are irrelevant, as long as they are the same for plasma and for urine – they are now usually expressed as mmol/l.

In practice the kidneys do not clear one unit volume of plasma completely of an excreted substance, and have no effect on other unit volumes of plasma – hence clearance can be more conveniently defined as the minimum volume of plasma which is needed to provide the quantity of a substance which is excreted in the urine in one minute (or in one second). The renal clearance of any substance may be measured by comparing the urinary excretion of that substance over a given period with its average concentration in the plasma during that period, and the more constant is the plasma concentration the more reliable is the result. The average clearance, in adults, of glucose (assuming absence of glucose from the urine) is 0, of urea is 75, of inulin is 125, and of PAH is 650, all expressed as ml/min. These figures are corrected to standard surface area, 1.73 m^2, and surface area is used as the conventional standard of comparison because it correlates reasonably well with the functional mass of the kidneys.

Because of the way in which it is excreted by the normal kidney, the clearance of inulin (and sometimes of ^{51}Cr-EDTA) is taken as a measure of the glomerular filtration rate, namely 125 ml/min. The clearance of PAH (and sometimes of diodone) is taken as a measure of the effective renal plasma flow, namely 650 ml/min. These are all *exogenous* substances that require intravenous infusion. The filtration fraction (the proportion of the plasma that is filtered at the glomeruli, normally about 20 per cent) can be calculated as inulin clearance/PAH clearance × 100.

It is possible, by measurement of PAH excretion at high plasma PAH levels, to calculate a factor termed the tubular excretory maximum for *p*-aminohippuric acid (Tm_{PAH}). This is a measure of proximal tubular secretory function. By measurement of glucose excretion at high plasma glucose levels, a factor termed the tubular reabsorptive maximum for glucose (Tm_G) can be calculated; this is a measure of proximal tubular reabsorptive capacity though it is not independent of the glomerular filtration rate. All these clearance investigations are research procedures and, because they require infusion, not suitable for routine clinical work.

Clinical procedures. The simple measurement of *endogenous* creatinine clearance is often used as an estimate of glomerular filtration rate. It gives slightly higher results than inulin clearance as creatinine is secreted by the tubules at all levels of renal function. However in general the results of creatinine clearance determination are proportional to the true glomerular filtration rate until renal function becomes grossly impaired. Urea clearance measures principally, but not wholly, glomerular filtration, and gives a result lower (by about 30 per cent) than the glomerular filtration rate because urea is partly reabsorbed.

Such concepts and calculations assume that all nephrons have identical functional capacity, though this is not true in health or in disease.

Excretion of water and ions

The water and sodium that have been filtered through the glomeruli are largely reabsorbed in the tubules, principally by a counter-current mechanism involving the loop of Henle. The potassium in the glomerular filtrate is reabsorbed, and the urinary potassium is derived from tubular secretion in exchange for sodium. Filtered bicarbonate is normally all reabsorbed. A normal adult excretes about 1200 mmol of solutes per day, of which about 700 mmol are ionic, and the rest mainly urea.

Glucocorticoids control water and sodium excretion principally through their effect on the glomerular filtration rate (p. 155), mineralocorticoids exert an influence by controlling the ion-exchange of sodium in the distal tubules (p. 154), and antidiuretic hormone acts on the distal tubular reabsorption of water (p. 169).

Threshold

The threshold of a given constituent of the plasma is that concentration in the plasma above which, assuming normal glomerular and tubular function, it is excreted in the urine. A threshold substance is one which is normally present in the plasma at a concentration less than that necessary for it to be excreted in the urine. The threshold of glucose is about 10 mmol/l. As the plasma concentration of glucose is normally below this, glucose can be called a threshold substance. Tubular reabsorption of glucose removes from the glomerular filtrate practically all the glucose that is filtered through the glomeruli at plasma glucose levels below 10 mmol/l. The threshold level of urea is zero, i.e. urea is excreted in the urine however low its concentration in the plasma, and urea can be called a non-threshold substance. The threshold of any substance may be altered by physiological or pathological changes in the renal plasma flow, the glomerular permeability, or the tubular reabsorptive capacity.

Other functions of the kidney

The main function of the kidney is the maintenance of the *milieu intérieur* by changes in the rate of excretion of the different constituents of the plasma (including water).

Investigation of the changes which take place in the homoeostatic and excretory powers of the kidney in disease is the principal purpose of renal function tests. Other properties of the kidney must not be forgotten. The juxtaglomerular apparatus produces the enzyme renin, which acts on angiotensinogen in plasma to form the vasoconstrictor substance angiotensin, which is also the most potent stimulator of aldosterone secretion (p. 154). The kidney produces a specific stimulus to erythrocyte production, erythropoietin (p. 132) and converts 25-hydroxycholecalciferol to 1,25-dihydroxycholecalciferol (p. 176). The tubular cells have independent metabolic activities. The distal tubules produce ammonia from glutamine and amino acids, and hydrogen ions from carbonic acid, for exchange with sodium: their functions in the control of acid-base balance are discussed in chapter 4.

Renal damage and renal function

The effects of renal impairment depend to a great extent on whether the impairment is mainly of glomerular function or mainly of tubular function: all nephrons are not usually impaired to the same extent.

Glomeruli. Damage to glomerular function leads to a reduction in the glomerular filtration rate. Pre-renal disorders, such as haemo-concentration, or a fall in the peripheral arterial blood pressure, or passive venous congestion of the kidney, reduce the filtration pressure, hence there is a fall in the glomerular filtration rate: post-renal obstruction also reduces glomerular filtration by back-pressure. This fall, whether due either to pre-renal or post-renal causes or to renal disease, leads to retention of nitrogenous excretion products (either 'pre-renal' azotaemia or 'renal' azotaemia). There is some retention of water, phosphate, and potassium; a tendency to sodium loss, hypocalcaemia, and an acidosis in chronic cases; and a lowering of clearance values. Oliguria, usually of high osmolality and specific gravity, is present when the glomerular filtration rate falls. Pathological damage to the basement membrane of the glomeruli allows both plasma and erythrocytes to leak through the affected glomeruli: there is therefore both a mild proteinuria (more severe with membranous lesions) and a haematuria (more severe with proliferative lesions). The nephrotic syndrome is a particular dis-order of increased permeability that allows excessive loss of certain proteins.

Tubules. Damage to tubular function leads to failure of reabsorption and to loss of renal compensation for changes in body fluid volume, osmotic pressure, and acid-base status. The constituents of glomerular filtrate which are affected may be many, and include water, electrolytes, protein, and many non-ionised substances. Alternatively renal tubular syndromes may affect only one or a few reabsorbable substances.

It is possible to contrast renal insufficiency with renal failure. Renal insufficiency may be considered to be present when the plasma levels of excreted end-products are still normal, whilst in renal failure (usually when clearances have fallen below 50 per cent) these plasma concentrations, e.g. of urea, are above normal.

RENAL FUNCTION TESTS

Renal function tests have two main purposes. Either they detect possible renal damage in a patient who has a disorder that may involve the kidneys, or they determine the degree of functional damage of kidneys that are known to be diseased. Examination of the urine for protein, cells and casts checks for an 'active lesion', whilst clearance studies and related tests investigate loss of function. Once renal damage has been detected, renal function tests may reveal the principal site and degree of the disturbance in the nephron, but rarely the cause of the renal injury. About two-thirds of the renal tissue must be functionally damaged for renal function tests to show any abnormality, and renal failure develops when there is inability to maintain homoeostasis. A person who through hereditary misfortune or surgical necessity possesses only one healthy kidney will show a normal response to renal function tests. As with liver function tests, partial damage to most of the nephrons (as in nephritis), with the healthy remainder overworked, is more likely to show disturbed renal function than will complete destruction of some nephrons when the major remainder of the kidney remains healthy (as in carcinoma of the kidney). Even if renal function appears to be satisfactory when the patient is taking a normal dietary load, tests for adaptability of the kidney to abnormal circumstances may reveal failure of function when there is renal insufficiency.

Simple examination of the urine

Volume

The normal 24 hour urine volume of an adult is between 750 and 2000 ml. This depends on the fluid intake (which is usually a matter of habit) and on the loss of fluid by other routes (primarily sweating which, in absence of fever, depends on physical activity and on the external temperature). A marked alteration in the output of urine may be a prominent sign in disease of the kidneys.

Oliguria develops also in any non-renal disease in which there is a deficient intake of water, or excessive loss of fluid by other routes, for example by haemorrhage, or as diarrhoea and vomiting. Polyuria is a characteristic sign of chronic renal insufficiency. Polyuria of low osmolality is also found in diabetes insipidus, in hysterical polydipsia, or after mobilisation of fluid from ascites or oedema. Polyuria occurs as an osmotic diuresis in any disease where there is an increased excretion of metabolites, notably in diabetes mellitus.

The minimal 24 hour output of urine needed to remove the waste products of normal metabolism is about 500 ml. A patient may be said to have oliguria when the urine volume is below 400 ml in 24 hours, and anuria when the 24 hour volume is below 100 ml, but these terms are loosely used.

Quantitative measurements of urinary volume are of limited value unless measurements are also made of fluid intake and of fluid losses by other routes. The 12 hour day output and the 12 hour night output should be measured separately. Normally the day urine is of greater volume than the night urine. The night urine equals or may exceed the day urine in severe glomerulotubular disease (p. 223), if there is a disturbance of intestinal absorption (p. 241), or in Addison's disease (p. 158).

Urine concentration: osmolality and specific gravity

Osmolality is the physiologically significant measure of urine concentration. But this analysis requires laboratory apparatus, whereas measurement of specific gravity (which depends on the mass of solutes present and not on their osmotic activity) can be done in the side-room. Osmolality and specific gravity are usually affected in disease in the same direction, but because of variation in the nature of the solutes the one value cannot be calculated from the other.

In health urine contains between about 1500 and 700 mmol of solutes per 24 hours; the maximum and minimum values over that period are about 1000 and 3000 mmol/kg. The normal specific gravity (correctly called relative density) of a pooled 24 hour urine sample is between 1.025 and 1.010: the maximum and minimum values are usually about 1.030 and 1.005. Under normal circumstances the urine concentration varies inversely with the urine volume. The concentration of urine is highest in the first morning specimen (overnight urine), and is lowest in a specimen passed an hour after much fluid has been taken. Fixation of the specific gravity at about 1.010, or the osmolality at about 300 mmol/l, being the values of protein-free plasma, occurs in severe chronic renal disease. Disorders associated with oliguria usually produce a concentrated urine. Polyuria tends to lead to a urine of low concentration. In diabetes mellitus there is polyuria with urine of *high* concentration: even when the specific gravity of the urine has been corrected for the presence of glucose (p. 271) the specific gravity of the urine is still raised because of the high concentration of salts in the urine. A correction must also be applied when interpreting the urine specific gravity in the presence of marked proteinuria (p. 271), whilst protein has a negligible effect on osmolality. Oliguria with a low specific gravity (after correction for the proteinuria) and low osmolality occurs in acute tubular necrosis because the tubules do not concentrate the limited amount of glomerular filtrate.

pH

On a normal mixed diet the urine is usually acid, generally varying in pH between about 5.5 and 8.0. A vegetarian diet, which causes a tendency to alkalosis (p. 43), thereby produces an alkaline urine. The pH of the urine in disease may reflect both the acid-base status of the plasma, and the function of the renal tubules. It may also be grossly altered by bacterial infection of the urinary tract, or deliberately by acid- or alkali-forming drugs.

Appearance

If no coloured abnormal constituents are present, then the higher the concentration of urine the deeper is its colour. The rate of excretion of the normal urinary pigments ('urochromes') is constant, and a pale urine has a low specific gravity, a dark urine has a high specific gravity.

Coloured urines occur in certain diseases or metabolic disorders, and after the administration of many drugs (p. 215).

Smell

Urine which is infected with Gram-negative organisms often has a distinctive unpleasant smell. In addition, urine infected with urea-splitting organisms has an ammoniacal smell. If urine which had a normal odour on arrival at the laboratory develops such a smell, this indicates bacterial decomposition and the specimen is unfit for most chemical analyses. Certain drugs, for example paraldehyde, impart a typical odour, as does the rare maple syrup urine disease (p. 102).

Protein

The glomerular filtration of a protein is inversely proportional to its size, which in general varies with its molecular weight, and the shape and charge of the molecule also influences filtration. In general proteins with a molecular weight greater than 70 000 are not filtered. Normal urine contains a very small quantity of protein (40–120 mg/24 h), and this concentration cannot be detected by simple tests. The proteins present mainly arise from the plasma proteins. The albumin-globulin ratio of this normal urinary protein, which contains relatively more low molecular weight globulins than does plasma, is approximately 1:1. The trace of protein present in normal urine contains remnants of the 8 g of protein (about 4 g of which is albumin) which has passed daily into the glomerular filtrate at a concentration of about 40 mg/l, most of which has been absorbed and catabolised in the proximal tubules; and also consists of protein excreted from the tubules and lower urinary tract. Haemoglobin has a threshold at about 1 g /l plasma: haemoglobin released into the plasma is first bound to haptoglobins; when these are saturated the remaining free haemoglobin is filtered through the glomeruli (p. 128).

Tests for proteinuria. It is easier to test urine for dissolved protein (p. 271) if it is clear, and cloudiness can usually be removed from urine by filtering or centrifugation. The classical tests for urinary protein depend on denaturation and precipitation of the protein. This can usually be brought about by boiling the urine after acidification, or by adding to the urine an organic acid of high molecular weight; 25 per cent salicylsulphonic acid is commonly used. The salicylsulphonic acid test is slightly less sensitive than the boiling test, but much more convenient. No endogenous substance in solution in urine other than protein precipitates on boiling and remains insoluble after the urine has been acidified. Certain drugs of high molecular weight precipitate with salicylsulphonic acid, and false positive reactions are found when the urine contains radio-opaque diagnostic agents or tolbutamide. Uric acid in high concentration, e.g. in the urine of infants, precipitates with salicylsulphonic acid, but the precipitate dissolves on warming the mixture to 60 °C.

Colour of urine	Direct cause	Indirect cause
Red-brown	haemoglobin methaemoglobin	intravascular haemolysis crush syndrome
Red	rifampicin phenindione beetroot	antibiotic therapy anticoagulant therapy food
Reddish-purple Reddish purple (on standing)	porphyrins porphyrins	erythropoietic porphyria acute intermittent porphyria
Pinkish-brown (on standing)	urobilin	haemolytic anaemia
Orange (green fluorescence)	eosin riboflavin	colouring agent, e.g. in sweets vitamin therapy
Yellow	mepacrine tetracyclines	malaria therapy antibiotic therapy
Green-yellow	bile pigments	cholestatic jaundice
Green-blue	pyocyanin methylene blue	*Ps. aeruginosa* infection colouring agent
Blue (especially on standing)	indigo compounds	indicanaemia in intestinal disease or suppuration
Purple	phenolphthalein (in alkaline urine: the urine becomes clear on acidification)	purgatives
Brown-black (on standing)	melanin homogentisic acid	malignant melanoma alkaptonuria (inborn error of metabolism) ochronosis associated with phenolic poisoning
Black	iron sorbitol	parenteral iron therapy
Cloudy	bacteria and leucocytes bacteria (in acid urine) urates (pink), oxalates (in alkaline urine) phosphates	urogenital tract infection *in vitro* infection usually normal usually normal
Smoky	erythrocytes	glomerular damage or slight urinary tract haemorrhage

The commercial strip tests, which are colour reactions based on the protein error of indicators, are popular because of their convenience. They are simple, do not require clarification of the urine, and are very roughly quantitative; but may give false weak positives in alkaline urine. They are relatively insensitive to proteins of low molecular weight, such as Bence Jones protein and β_2-microglobulin.

If quantitative analyses are required, they should be done by laboratory methods, and not by the very imprecise ward Esbach's test.

Differential urinary protein excretion. The protein present in the urine in renal disease is a mixture of albumin and globulins. When there is glomerular damage the major urinary protein becomes albumin, and in nephritis the albumin-globulin ratio of the urinary protein is typically about 5:1. In renal tubular syndromes and to some extent in upper urinary tract infections a particular excess of low molecular weight α-globulins and of β_2-microglobulin is found: separation can be performed by polyacrylamide electrophoresis.

It is possible by immunological methods or by gel filtration of plasma and urine to measure the clearances of specific proteins of known and different molecular weights. Proteins commonly used are, in order of increasing size, β_2-microglobulin, albumin or transferrin, IgG, and α_2-macroglobulin. If low molecular weight proteins are cleared much more readily than those of high molecular weight, the proteinuria is described as selective, indicating relatively less damage to basement membrane and a better prognosis. The opposite is non-selective proteinuria, with a low ratio between the clearances (e.g. IgG/transferrin) indicating greater damage. Increased clearance of β_2-microglobulin in relation to albumin is an indication of tubular damage.

Casts. The tubules secrete an α_1-glycoprotein called Tamm-Horsfall protein, of molecular weight about 80 000. In the presence of albumin it comes out of solution in gel form as casts. Various types of casts have different inclusions; e.g. granular casts contain degenerated tubular cells.

Mucus protein. This may be found in urine when there is disease of the lower urinary tract, or it may be derived from semen, when spermatozoa will be present in the urinary deposit, or from vaginal discharge. Mucus protein is precipitated from urine in the cold on adding 33 per cent acetic acid dropwise.

Bence Jones protein. This low molecular weight protein is a light chain of myeloma globulin and is synthesised in excess in multiple myeloma (p. 111). Electrophoresis of concentrated urine is the most sensitive test; and Bence Jones protein may also be detected by layering urine on concentrated HCl (Bradshaw's test), or by salting out. The classical test for Bence Jones protein is that it precipitates when acidified urine is heated to 40–50 °C (whereas normal urinary protein does not begin to precipitate until 60 °C) and redissolves on heating the urine to boiling point, to reappear on cooling, at about 70 °C: this now is only of historical interest. Indicator strip tests for proteinuria are relatively insensitive to Bence Jones protein.

Haemoglobin and haemoglobin derivatives. These are proteins and give the normal tests for urinary proteins. These compounds can be detected and identified by spectroscopic and chemical examination (p. 128).

Causes of proteinuria

An anatomical way of classifying proteinuria is as pre-renal, renal, and post-renal.

Pre-renal. This is caused by a general disease which affects the kidneys, and is an indication of renal damage (as increased glomerular permeability) in such conditions as essential hypertension and eclampsia. The proteinuria of severe anaemia is due to renal anoxia, and that of heart failure is due to anoxia and to congestion. The often transient proteinuria of fever, exercise, and of cerebral vascular accidents may be from secondary 'toxic' glomerular damage. Slight proteinuria may often be found in severe malignant disease. The 'benign' proteinuria which occasionally occurs in pregnancy, and 'orthostatic albuminuria', have been thought to be due to mechanical pressure on the renal veins which causes renal vascular congestion, but may be due to other causes of altered renal circulation. Orthostatic proteinuria may be found in many presumably healthy young men, especially with lordosis, at routine medical examination; in this condition, in contrast to patients with glomerulonephritis, a morning urine sample passed on waking is free of protein, and erythrocytes are never found in excess. In all these types of pre-renal proteinuria the proteinuria rarely exceeds 2 g in 24 hours, and erythrocytes and casts are scanty.

True pre-renal proteinuria, without renal damage, is rare, and long-standing proteinuria will in itself cause renal damage. If there is haemoglobinaemia then there will be excretion of haemoglobin in the urine even where there is no renal damage. Bence Jones proteinuria, myoglobinuria (p. 127), and haemoglobinuria are pre-renal proteinurias.

Renal. Primary disease of the kidneys is almost invariably associated with proteinuria; and continuous proteinuria must be considered due to renal damage until the contrary is proved. Proteinuria may be the only sign of early renal damage from nephrotoxic drugs; or in disease, and diabetes mellitus is a frequent cause of this. Recovery from acute glomerulonephritis cannot be assumed whilst proteinuria is still present. In different types of renal disease different degrees of proteinuria are seen. In glomerulonephritis the proteinuria caused by leakage through the damaged glomeruli varies with the type of pathological disorder. The nephrotic syndrome is usually associated with 10–20 g proteinuria per 24 hours: such massive proteinuria may cause secondary tubular damage which then reduces tubular reabsorption of protein. An eventual fall in the plasma albumin level usually develops when urinary losses of protein continuously exceed 5 g in 24 hours. Proteinuria that is due to failure of tubular reabsorption is always slight (<2 g/24 h), and being of low molecular weight proteins may be missed by indicator strip tests (p. 271).

Proteins derived from the renal tract, particularly enzymes such as

β-N-acetylglucosaminidase, may be found in excess in the urine during rejection of a renal transplant.

Post-renal. Proteinuria of post-renal origin is always accompanied by cells, and is minimal. It is found in severe infection of the lower urinary tract, and is associated with haematuria when the renal pelvis or the ureter is irritated by stone or when there is local malignant disease.

Formed elements

The microscopical examination of fresh urine for erythrocytes, other cells, and casts is an important part of the tests of renal function: the finding of more than an occasional leucocyte, erythrocyte, or granular cast points the way to further investigations. The Addis count is an enumeration of the erythrocytes, leucocytes, and casts in a 12 hour urinary sample collected under standard conditions. Collection for so long a period permits degeneration of cells, and a 2 hour morning collection is preferred. This estimation, though tedious, is a useful non-biochemical procedure when it is performed serially for progress, as it eliminates variations in the urine cell and cast content due to changes in water excretion.

The commercial strip tests for free haemoglobin in urine (which utilise its peroxidase activity) are also a test for erythrocytes (p. 274).

Crystals

In urine crystals are usually not pathological. Uric acid and calcium oxalate may be found in health in acid urine, and phosphates in alkaline urine. However cystine crystals are pathological, and are an indication of the inborn error of metabolism, cystinuria (p. 225).

Complex tests of function

If the clinical findings or simple urine examination indicate that renal damage may be present, assessment of glomerular or of tubular damage is then indicated.

Glomerular function

Creatinine clearance test

The value of this test is that of a roughly quantitative measure of glomerular damage when simpler tests have already demonstrated renal impairment. Although it is often so performed, the test is not usually suitable, because of lack of sensitivity, as the first diagnostic test for impairment of renal function. The creatinine clearance may be normal when early renal damage has been demonstrated by (tubular) failure to concentrate urine in the water deprivation test, or by the presence of proteinuria – as in hypertension. This test may be done over 4 hours, but a 24 hour period is recommended. The results are independent of the rate of urine flow.

Method. A careful and accurate 24 hour collection of urine is made. At some time during the day (but not within 1–3 hours after a large meal) a blood sample is taken for plasma creatinine analysis; this and the whole 24 hour urinary collection are sent to the laboratory.

Interpretation. Endogenous creatinine clearance is a rough measure of the glomerular filtration rate and is normally 100–130 ml/min (1.7–2.1 ml/s) in an adult of normal size. Correction is necessary for surface area (p. 209) in children, or in adults of abnormal build.

Values below 90 ml/min (corrected to normal surface area) are indicative of diminished glomerular filtration rate. The test has particular value in the general assessment of renal function in cases when plasma analyses are invalid, e.g. after dialysis, or when the plasma urea (but not the plasma creatinine) has been lowered by a low protein diet. Because there is considerable tubular secretion of creatinine when the plasma creatinine is high, the test is not then quantitative for glomerular filtration rate. In such advanced renal failure, the urea clearance may give a more quantitative measure of overall renal function.

Urea clearance test (Van Slyke)

This formerly popular test measures overall renal damage, mainly in respect of glomerular function. It has now largely been replaced by the creatinine clearance test, because of the latter's greater ease of performance and closer relation to the glomerular filtration rate. Shorter periods of collection are required here because of diurnal fluctuation of plasma urea, in contrast to relative constancy of plasma creatinine concentration.

The urea clearance test requires accurate collection of two successive complete 60 minute urine specimens, and a blood sample is taken during the test. The clearance is calculated as the mean of that of the two successive hours, and is traditionally expressed as a percentage of the average normal clearance in adults, 75 ml/min. A urea clearance of less than 70 per cent is abnormal. Because of back-diffusion, the clearance of urea falls when there is a low urine volume, and the results are invalid when this is <2 ml/min.

Tubular function

The response to these concentration tests is impaired early in tubular damage, or in any severe renal disease with a fall in glomerular filtration rate. The tests are invalid if the patient is receiving diuretics, or on a very low protein diet.

Urine concentration test

The simplest screening test is to measure the osmolality of every urine specimen passed over a 24 h period of normal activity. If the osmolality of any sample exceeds 800 mmol/kg, or the specific gravity is above about 1.020, then concentrating activity is unimpaired.

Vasopressin test

This is less unpleasant for the patient than is full water deprivation, and depends only on renal tubular function.

Method. The patient has nothing to drink after 18:00. At 20:00, five units of vasopressin tannate is injected subcutaneously. All urine samples are collected separately until 09:00 the next day with the patient taking normal food and fluid.

Alternatively 2 μg of the synthetic analogue, DDAVP (Desmopressin), is injected intramuscularly, or 40 μg given intranasally, at 09:00 without overnight fluid restriction, and all urine samples collected for the next 12 h.

Interpretation. Satisfactory concentration is shown by at least one sample having a specific gravity above 1.020, or an osmolality above 700 mmol/kg (reached between 5 and 9 h in the DDAVP test). The test may be combined with measurements of plasma osmolality: the urine/plasma osmolality ratio should reach 3, and values less than 2 are abnormal.

Water deprivation test (24 hours)

Although this test is simple and sensitive, it is unpleasant for the patient, and many investigators prefer a vasopressin test. However this test differs in that it depends both on the posterior pituitary response to water deprivation, and on the renal tubular response to antidiuretic hormone. The test is contraindicated if there are biochemical or clinical signs of renal failure. It is also used in the differential diagnosis of hysterical polydipsia and diabetes insipidus (p. 169).

Method. Day before test. No fluid is permitted after breakfast until the conclusion of the test, and normal meals are otherwise taken.

Day of test. After waking the patient empties his bladder, and the urine is kept. Further samples are collected at 60 min and 120 min.

Interpretation. If any of the three specimens has an osmolality above 900 mmol/l, or a specific gravity (corrected for protein) above 1.025, the renal concentrating capacity is unimpaired and the ADH response is normal.

Urine dilution (water load) test

This simple test, of measuring the rate of excretion of a water load, is no longer performed as it is very insensitive for alteration of renal tubular function.

Urinary acidification test

This procedure tests the ability of the renal tubules to form an acid urine and to excrete ammonia. It is useful if there is doubt whether a patient's acidosis (confirmed by plasma analysis) is due to a pre-renal cause, or to kidney damage as in renal tubular acidosis.

Method. The patient fasts from midnight until the conclusion of the test.

Zero time. The patient empties his bladder completely – the urine is collected.

The patient takes 0.1 g (1.9 mmol) of ammonium chloride/kg body weight and drinks a litre of water – a standard dose of 5 g is sometimes used. In children the dose should be proportional to the body surface area.

At 2 hours, 4 hours, and 6 hours: complete urine specimens are collected – the laboratory may require use of special containers.

Interpretation. In a normal subject the urine will be acidified to pH 5.3 or less, and will contain more than 1.5 mmol of ammonia per hour, in at least one of the specimens. If there is marked damage to the renal acidifying powers the pH of the later specimens of urine will be unaltered from that of the resting specimen, and less than 0.5 mmol of ammonia per hour will be excreted. The pH results are more significant than the ammonia results, as 3 days are needed for full development of extra ammonium ion excretion.

There is a more sensitive 5 day test: this requires the patient to be in hospital and is rarely needed.

Dye excretion tests for combined glomerulotubular function

Many dyes are excreted by the kidneys, and measurement of their concentration in the urine after parenteral injection can be used as a measure of renal function.

Phenolsulphonphthalein (phenol red) is filtered by the glomeruli, and mainly secreted by the proximal tubules. Its excretion essentially tests for renal plasma flow, and is therefore impaired early in conditions such as heart failure. After intramuscular or intravenous injection of 6 mg of dye to a normal subject, 40–60 per cent of the dose will be excreted in the first hour, and another 20–25 per cent in the second hour: less than 50 per cent excreted over the 2 hours is abnormal.

Indigo-carmine is sometimes used in surgical practice. During cystoscopy both ureteric orifices may be observed, and after intravenous injection of 100 mg dye, colour should be seen issuing from both ureters, in about equal concentration, in 15 minutes, whilst maximum excretion is normally reached in 45 minutes.

Plasma analyses as renal function tests

Analyses of blood plasma are frequently helpful in the assessment of known renal disease. There is no plasma constituent whose concentration depends solely on the functional state of the kidneys. In renal failure all non-protein nitrogen constituents of the plasma are retained. Plasma (or blood) urea estimations are frequently performed as a test of renal function, but the causes of a raised plasma urea are many (p. 96) and it is not possible to detect renal damage by a raised plasma urea or creatinine until renal function has fallen by about 50 per cent as measured by the creatinine clearance test. Analyses of plasma creatinine are now preferred to that of urea as a quantitative measure of known glomerular damage. A low protein intake, or dialysis, invalidates the use of plasma urea as a measure of glomerular filtration rate, whilst plasma creatinine is much less affected by diet; severe muscle wasting invalidates the use of plasma creatinine. This estimation is most useful for the assessment of the severity and progress of renal failure in acute tubular necrosis, acute glomerulonephritis, chronic renal diseases, and in post-renal obstruction.

Other plasma analyses, e.g. measurement of electrolytes and acid-base state, or of proteins, although valuable and often necessary in the assessment of known disease, show alterations in a variety of other disorders.

BIOCHEMICAL CHANGES IN RENAL DISEASE

Acute renal failure

Pre-renal failure. This is caused by any major decrease in renal perfusion, such as acute circulatory failure as in shock. Glomerular filtration falls, and there is oliguria with a plasma/urine osmolality ratio of about 1.5. The urine contains a trace of protein, and less than 10 mmol/l of sodium. The plasma urea concentration rises rapidly as the reduced amount filtered is largely reabsorbed; whereas creatinine, not being reabsorbed, shows much less increase in plasma concentration.

Intrarenal failure. This is caused by prolonged renal ischaemia, or by a variety of toxins (including incompatible blood transfusion) producing acute tubular necrosis. Decreased glomerular filtration, and possibly tubular obstruction by debris, contribute to the renal failure. In the first phase there is anuria or marked oliguria, and any urine that is passed has an osmolality similar to that of plasma, and contains more than 30 mmol/l of sodium. The urine also has an apparently high specific gravity because of the high protein content; however the corrected specific gravity is about 1.010. There is a profusion of all types of casts, and the urine may contain haemoglobin or myoglobin if this high tubular concentration of the pigment is the cause of the disorder. The clinical and biochemical features of uraemia rapidly develop; there may also be features of tubular syndromes, such as aminoaciduria.

Should the patient recover, with or without dialysis, there is a diuretic phase, partly because the recovering tubules have a low reabsorptive power. In this phase there may be a polyuria of 3–5 litres per day, continuing mild proteinuria, and loss of salts. Return of concentrating ability and fall of plasma urea heralds recovery. Water, sodium, and potassium balance must be carefully monitored, by plasma and urine analyses, throughout the course of the disease.

Acute glomerulonephritis

In the acute phase of a glomerulonephritis there is oliguria, haematuria (a 'smoky' urine), and proteinuria of up to about 5 g/24 h. Moderate numbers of casts are present in the urine. Glomerular filtration is impaired, the creatinine clearance is lowered, and there is retention of non-protein nitrogen, sodium, and water. Renal plasma flow is unaltered: there is a low filtration fraction. Tubular function is slightly impaired. The plasma albumin level may be slightly lowered, and there is often a decrease in the total protein concentration because of haemodilution. Retention of sodium and water leads to dilution of the extracellular fluids, and this dilution in combination with general capillary damage gives rise to oedema. Hypertension is common. The condition may progress to anuria, azotaemia, acidosis, and hyperkalaemia, whilst uraemic symptoms may or may not be present.

The onset and degree of recovery may be assessed by examination of the urine for protein, and quantified by clearance measurements. Persisting nephritis is accompanied by a proteinuria of up to 0.5 g/24 h, and occasionally by haematuria. Proteinuria disappears when recovery is complete.

Compensated chronic renal failure

Chronic bilateral renal disease, due to various pathological causes, leads to renal failure as the disease progresses. The concentrating power of the kidney is lost and this proceeds until only a urine of fixed osmolality (about 300 mmol/kg) and specific gravity (1.010) can be formed. There is an osmotic mild polyuria (more marked at night) which leads eventually to dehydration. There is progressive loss of clearance values, and the renal failure is no longer termed compensated when the plasma urea rises above normal. This occurs when glomerular filtration falls below about 50 per cent, depending somewhat on dietary protein. The other plasma non-protein nitrogen constituents, particularly creatinine and uric acid, also rise. Proteinuria is rarely above 5 g/24 h as the severely damaged glomeruli may lose their ability to excrete protein. Excretion of casts is variable.

Metabolic acidosis develops because of retention of the hydrogen ions of acid phosphates and sulphates and of organic acids, and also because of failure of the damaged tubules to produce hydrogen ions and ammonia. The high plasma phosphate concentration and failure to metabolise 25-hydroxycholecalciferol (p. 176) are usually associated with a fall in the plasma calcium level, which can cause secondary hyperparathyroidism. Demineralisation is seen and 'renal rickets' can develop in children: in adults various types of osteodystrophy, aggravated by acidosis, may be seen (p. 185). The hypocalcaemia does not usually lead to tetany because of the counteracting acidosis (p. 179). As a rule there is a moderate degree of potassium retention, especially when there is oliguria; and excessive urinary loss of sodium which leads to sodium depletion. Potassium deficiency is occasionally seen. Glucose tolerance is often impaired. Plasma amylase is increased due to retention. The usual lipid abnormality is a Type IV hyperlipidaemia (p. 86) due to increased synthesis of triglycerides, but an increase in plasma cholesterol (Type IIb) may develop.

Chronic pyelonephritis. In this type of chronic renal disease tubular damage predominates. Concentrating power is therefore lost early and there is polyuria, whilst the plasma urea and creatinine may be still normal: later all features of chronic renal failure develop. The urine contains many leucocytes but very little protein, generally less than 2 g/24 h.

Uraemia (end-stage renal failure)

As renal failure progresses and glomerular filtration falls below about 10 per cent of normal the clinical syndrome of uraemia begins to appear. The patients shows symptoms of irritation of the gastrointestinal tract, mental and neurological disorders, haematological and vascular changes and muscular twitching, and has a foetid or ammoniacal odour of the breath. These symptoms, and the eventual death in coma, are only slightly due to the raised level of urea in the plasma, for the effects of solely a raised plasma urea are a diuresis, headache and sedation, and possibly gastrointestinal irritation (due to conversion of urea to ammonia). Hypertension, anaemia, and circulatory failure; and sodium depletion with dehydration, acidosis, hypocalcaemia, and potassium retension, may all play a part. Phenols, guanidines, indoles, abnormal amino acids, and undetermined 'toxic retention products' including 'middle molecules' of molecular weight 500–5000 (but not creatinine), have all been blamed as the cause of the symptoms. Calculations based on the plasma electrolyte concentrations (p. 52) often show a low 'anion gap' due to undetermined cations, possibly organic bases.

Haemodialysis. The treatment of chronic renal failure by repeated dialysis requires close and specialised biochemical control, but anomalous biochemical ill-effects may nevertheless develop. Phosphate deficiency may be seen. Osteodystrophy can worsen, and metastatic calcification is a risk. Over-rapid dialysis produces a low extracellular osmotic pressure: the *disequilibrium syndrome* involves cellular overhydration due to urea being too rapidly removed from the e.c.f., but still tending to remain in the cells, with a consequent osmotic imbalance. If the plasma creatinine is normal whilst the plasma urea continues to rise, this reflects increased protein intake or catabolism, and not ineffective dialysis.

The nephrotic syndrome

The syndrome of nephrosis, whatever the initial pathological cause of the disorder, is accompanied by typical biochemical changes. The primary disorder is proteinuria, usually of 5–30 g/24 h, due to excessive glomerular permeability – in severe cases secondary tubular damage may reduce reabsorption of protein. Excessive albumin catabolism has also been suggested. The urinary proteins are those of molecular weight less than about 200 000; they are mainly albumin, with the low molecular weight metal-binding globulins and γ-globulins. The extent and 'selectivity' of the protein leakage can be investigated by differential clearances (p. 216). These proteins are decreased in the plasma, and this change, with an increase in pre-β and β-lipoproteins (and fibrinogen), gives the characteristic electrophoretic pattern (p. 114). Urinary copper and iron are increased; plasma iron, copper, and total calcium and protein-bound hormones, are decreased. The low plasma albumin, and sodium retention due to secondary aldosteronism, gives rise to oedema – which tends to develop when proteinuria exceeds 10 g/24 h. Haematuria, nitrogen retention, and depression of clearance values only occur when there are complications. The cause of the considerable increase in most plasma lipid fractions is not certain, but is related to the hypoalbuminaemia (p. 81). There is often lipaemia and the plasma cholesterol level may reach 25 mmol/l.

Renal tubular syndromes

Disorders of the renal tubules, whether congenital or acquired, affect one or many of the functions of the tubule – namely reabsorption of nitrogenous compounds, principally amino acids (p. 101); reabsorption of glucose; reabsorption of water and electrolytes; production of ammonia and hydrogen ions. When there are congenital tubular transport defects, there are often parallel intestinal transport defects.

Of the many proximal tubular defects renal glycosuria (without other abnormalities) is not uncommon (p. 59), and there can be specific loss of phosphate causing a rickets-like disturbance (p. 185).

Fanconi syndrome (p. 103). This includes disorders that combine generalised aminoaciduria and loss of glucose, phosphate, urate, potassium, and protein of low molecular weight: often there is an acidosis. The proximal tubules may show pathological damage.

Cystinuria. There is diminished reabsorption of the related basic amino acids cystine, ornithine, arginine, and lysine: in homozygotes the 24 hour excretion of cystine may be increased from the normal 0.05 mmol to become above 2 mmol, and calculi form because cystine is relatively insoluble.

Renal tubular acidosis. There is a distal tubular defect of failure of ion-exchange with consequent hyperchloraemic acidosis (and failure to excrete a urine more acid than pH 6.0) and eventual osteomalacia. There is urinary loss of calcium and phosphate, sometimes with nephrocalcinosis, and also of potassium causing hypokalaemia. In the rarer proximal tubular acidosis, often seen in a Fanconi syndrome, the primary disorder is failure to reabsorb bicarbonate. Other types have been identified.

Loss of tissue

When renal tissue is lost, e.g. due to calculi, glomeruli and tubules are as a rule equally removed and the remainder of the kidney is healthy. No symptoms occur unless the greater part of the renal tissue is destroyed. There is no proteinuria. Gross tissue damage leads to a fall of the creatinine clearance, and nitrogen retention with acidosis may be seen as in chronic renal failure.

Post-renal obstruction

If obstruction to the outflow of urine is prolonged, due for example to prostatic enlargement or to spreading carcinoma of the cervix, the patient may become uraemic from the effects of the back-pressure, and may have tubular damage leading to sodium loss. Unless the obstructive cause leads to bleeding, the only urine abnormality may be a trace of protein. The level of the plasma urea or creatinine can be taken as a measure of the degree of obstruction. When slow decompression of the urinary tract is performed before prostatectomy, a levelling-out of the progressive fall in the plasma creatinine may be taken as an indication that surgery should proceed.

Ureteric transplantation

The ureters may be transplanted into the colon or into an isolated loop of ileum. In either case severe hyperchloraemic acidosis may develop. This is due to differential reabsorption of urinary chloride more than of urinary sodium from the bowel, and possibly also to renal tubular damage from pyelonephritis. Potassium deficiency is often present. Urea and excess ammonia may also be reabsorbed from the bowel, and there can be mild uraemic symptoms.

Renal calculi

The components of renal calculi comprise low molecular weight crystalloids which make up most of the stone, and high molecular weight matrix substances which are partly mucoprotein. A calculus cannot form unless at some time the urine was saturated in respect of the crystalloids of the calculus.

The largest number of calculi consist either of calcium oxalate, or of mixtures of calcium phosphate and magnesium ammonium phosphate, sometimes with calcium carbonate or calcium oxalate – these are whitish. The aetiology of most of these calcium-containing calculi is unknown. Abnormalities such as a continually concentrated urine (e.g. due to excessive sweating by unadapted Europeans in the tropics), bacterial infection (particularly when this makes the urine alkaline), or 'stasis' (due to congenital abnormalities or acquired obstruction) are often predisposing factors: the contribution of initiators and inhibitors of crystallisation is uncertain. Calcium calculi are less soluble in alkaline urine. Hypercalciuria is present in many cases, and excess gut absorption of calcium (e.g. idiopathic hypercalciuria, p. 186) may often be the cause. Renal tubular acidosis produces hypercalciuria and an alkaline urine. Of the many causes of hypercalcaemia with hypercalciuria (p. 180), primary hyperparathyroidism is probably the most important specific disease as the calculi may be the presenting feature (p. 181). In osteoporosis (p. 183) there can be hypercalciuria with a normal plasma calcium.

Oxalate crystals may also arise from a rare inborn error of metabolism, *primary hyperoxaluria*. In hyperuricaemia, usually due to gout (p. 97), uric acid calculi (which are brown) are common; these are less soluble in acid urine. Cystine calculi (which are yellow) are usually the presenting feature of cystinuria.

Biochemical investigations. Any stones already passed by the patient should be analysed for the constituents named above. Essential investigations on the patient's plasma are for calcium, phosphate, and alkaline phosphatase, for urate, and also for urea and bicarbonate. A 24 hour urine is examined microbiologically; and chemically for cystine, calcium, and often oxalate. Further investigations may be necessary to establish the cause of any hypercalcaemia.

Other calculi

Prostatic calculi. These contain calcium phosphate and carbonate, but no oxalate.

Bladder calculi. These are usually renal calculi that have passed into the bladder and enlarged. They may originate in the bladder in infected urine, as calcium-magnesium-ammonium phosphate.

Choice of renal function tests

Examination of the urine is the most important initial test for suspected renal damage, particularly if glomerular; and this need not require sending a sample to the chemical pathology department. Search must be made for protein, erythrocytes, and casts. The creatinine clearance is quantitative for glomerular impairment, until this is severe, and need rarely be done unless simpler tests are abnormal. The estimations of plasma urea or creatinine, though often used as an early test for renal damage, are best employed as a guide to progress and prognosis once the presence of renal disease is established. Special tests are required for the nephrotic syndrome and for the renal tubular syndromes. The concentration test is sensitive, and is possibly the most useful single simple test of function for confirming that renal tubular impairment is present.

These investigations are relevant whether performed for the identification of the cause of a proteinuria, for determining if non-renal symptoms are due to primary renal disease, or to detect the effects on the kidney of a primary non-renal disease.

Changes which may occur in other body constituents during renal disease have been described under the headings of the respective diseases: these changes refer not only to the renal damage but also to the effects of the primary renal damage on the body as a whole.

Further reading

Berlyne GM. *A Course in Renal Diseases.* 5th ed. Oxford: Blackwell Scientific Publications, 1978.

Peacock M, Robertson W. Renal calculi. *Medicine* 3rd series 1978; 27:1372–1381.

Pitts RF. *Physiology of the Kidney and Body Fluids.* 3rd ed. Chicago: Year Book Medical Publishers, 1974.

Wills MR. *Metabolic Consequences of Chronic Renal Failure*, 2nd ed. Aylesbury: Harvey Miller and Medcalf, 1978.

CHAPTER 14

THE ALIMENTARY TRACT

SALIVARY GLANDS

The salivary glands secrete about 1000 ml of saliva every 24 hours, mainly from the parotid glands. The electrolyte composition of saliva is variable, and is on average Na^+ 15 mmol/l, K^+ 20 mmol/l, Cl^- 20 mmol/l, HCO_3^- 10 mmol/l. The saliva contains amylase, and if there is acute obstruction to the outflow of the secretions from the parotid glands amylase is retained and regurgitated into the blood stream. The obstruction may be intraglandular, due to swollen cells as in acute parotitis and particularly in mumps; or extraglandular, if there is a salivary duct stone. The plasma amylase level may rise during the acute phase of the obstruction to over 1000 U/l (reference values 70–300 U/l or 40–160 Somogyi units). The estimation may be useful in the differential diagnosis of facial swelling, or of meningoencephalitis possibly due to mumps virus. When there is pancreatitis as a complication of mumps, the plasma lipase increases as well.

STOMACH AND DUODENUM

Every 24 hours the normal stomach produces about 1000 ml of gastric juice when the subject is fasting, whilst the stomach of a subject who is taking a normal diet secretes 2000–3000 ml of juice per 24 hours. Gastric juice is a mixture of secretions. Parietal cells secrete hydrochloric acid and intrinsic factor, and zymogen cells (chief-cells) secrete the pepsinogens, and other enzymes: other cells produce an alkaline mucus. The average pH of mixed gastric juice is about 1.5, and the average concentration of the principal electrolytes is H^+ 80 mmol/l, Na^+ 50 mmol/l, K^+ 15 mmol/l, Cl^- 130 mmol/l. The principal physiological stimulants to gastric secretion are the vagus nerve impulses and the polypeptide hormone gastrin(s) released from specialised antral cells in response to food, and finally both stimulation and inhibition of this secretion by intestinal hormones stimulated by food in the duodenum.

In diseases of the stomach and duodenum alterations of gastric secretion often occur. Analysis of gastric secretions has a limited but specific value in the diagnosis and assessment of disorders of the upper gastrointestinal tract.

Simple examination of the resting juice

The resting juice is obtained by emptying the stomach through a nasogastric tube after the patient has fasted for 12 hours overnight.

Appearance. Gastric juice should be clear and colourless; a trace of bile from duodenal reflex has no significance. If there is delay in gastric emptying, food residues may be present. A trace of fresh blood may be seen in the normal resting juice sample, and this is due to trauma caused by the passage of the tube. A large quantity of digested blood (the 'coffee-grounds' appearance) shows that there has been oesophageal or intragastric bleeding; this is abnormal and usually indicates that cancer of the stomach or a bleeding gastric ulcer is present. A small amount of mucus may be present normally mainly from swallowed saliva: excessive quantities of mucus may be found when there is gastritis.

Volume. The volume of the resting juice averages about 50 ml, less than 100 ml being normal. A resting juice volume of more than 150 ml is abnormal, and indicates delay in gastric emptying due to pyloric obstruction, or gastric atony.

Acidity. The possible measurements of gastric acidity are as hydrogen-ion activity with a pH meter, and as titratable acidity by titration with alkali to within the range pH 7.0 (physicochemical neutrality) to pH 7.4 (physiological neutrality). The concentration of acid is expressed as millimoles per litre, and this has the same numerical value as the old 'units' per 100 ml.

Pepsin(s). Pepsins, produced from pepsinogens by acid, are normally present in gastric juice, and are secreted in parallel with gastric acid.

A small amount of the pepsin is secreted into the plasma and excreted into the urine as uropepsinogens. Its excretion very roughly follows the peptic secretory activity of the stomach. Measurements of pepsinogen in gastric juice, plasma, and urine are not used routinely.

Tests for gastric acidity

The original stimulus applied to the stomach to test its capacity to secrete acid was a simple meal such as tea and toast: hence the term 'test meal'. Oral stimulants are unsatisfactory as they do not produce maximum secretion of acid, they mix with and dilute the gastric secretions, and give variable results. If gastric secretory response is to be measured, a stimulus must be used which gives maximum stimulation to the gastric secretion of acid by all the parietal cells (parietal cell mass). Histamine was formerly used, especially as the augmented histamine test with its unwanted effects blocked by an antihistamine, or by using an analogue (ametazole: Histalog). These have now been replaced by a synthetic gastrin: this is a better stimulant and more pleasant for the patient.

Pentagastrin test

Pentagastrin (Peptavlon; ICI) is a synthetic pentapeptide which contains the key C-terminal portion of the gastrin molecule (cf. tetracosactrin, p. 159).

Method
(i) The test is preceded by a 12 hour overnight fast.
(ii) Pass a wide bore stomach tube (a Levin or a Ryle's tube, size 12–16 French) into the stomach, and check the positioning of the tube by fluoroscopy.
(iii) Aspirate the resting juice completely. This may be examined for volume and general appearance.
(iv) Collect the basal spontaneously secreted gastric juice quantitatively by continuous suction for a period of 60 minutes, at a subatmospheric pressure of 30–50 mmHg (4.0–6.5 kPa).
(v) Inject intramuscularly 6 µg pentagastrin/kg body weight.
(vi) Continuously aspirate the stimulated secretion for the next 60 minutes, dividing this collection into four separate specimens representing 0–15, 15–30, 30–45, and 45–60 minute samples.
The five collections of gastric secretion (basal and four stimulated) are sent to the laboratory in separate containers, each clearly labelled with the times of collection.

Interpretation. In normal subjects the total basal acid output (BAO) is less than 5 mmol/h, and the maximum acid output (MAO) in the 60 minutes after pentagastrin is about 20 mmol in a man and 10 mmol in a woman.

The average outputs of patients with duodenal ulcer are about twice normal and about one-third of the patients have diagnostic hyper-secretion. The peak acid output (PAO) is calculated as twice the secretion in the highest two consecutive 15 minute periods, and is normally less than 45 mmol/h in a man and 30 mmol/h in a woman.

A high BAO (more than 5 mmol/h) and/or a high PAO suggest a duodenal ulcer, whereas a PAO less than 15 mmol/h is evidence against a duodenal ulcer. Patients with gastric ulcer generally have a normal acid secretion. Patients with carcinoma of the stomach may have achlor-hydria or may secrete normally.

Absolute achlorhydria (anacidity) exists if none of the specimens has a pH less than 7. This occurs regularly in pernicious anaemia, occasionally in gastric carcinoma, and rarely otherwise: absolute achlorhydria excludes any form of peptic ulcer. Hyposecretion, with no 'free acid' (pH 3.5–6.5) and less than 1 unit change in pH after pentagastrin, is a non-specific finding that is seen in a variety of conditions, e.g. hypochromic anaemia or gastritis.

Insulin test

This is used to investigate the completeness of a vagotomy which has been performed for the treatment of peptic ulcer. Insulin-induced hypoglycaemia causes (via the hypothalamus) vagal stimulation of gastric acid secretion if the vagus nerves are still intact.

Method. Pass a gastric tube and collect a 1 hour basal secretion. Inject soluble insulin (0.2 units/kg) intravenously and collect complete samples of gastric juice every 15 minutes for 2 hours, and of blood for glucose estimation every 30 minutes.

The patient must be closely observed, and intravenous 50 per cent glucose kept available, because of the risk of severe hypoglycaemia.

Interpretation. An increase of acid secretion of less than 20 mmol/l above the basal activity is taken as indicating that vagotomy has been complete, provided that (i) adequate hypoglycaemia (less than 2 mmol/l) has been produced, (ii) the stomach has been found capable of secreting hydrochloric acid in response to pentagastrin stimulus, which may follow directly after the insulin test. As vagotomy is rarely absolutely complete, the acid response to insulin is a function of residual innervation.

Tubeless tests

These were devised to enable free acid in the gastric secretion to be detected without submitting the patient to the discomfort of the passage of a gastric tube, and of an injection, and without sending specimens to the laboratory.

The test material consists of a dye linked to a resin, and caffeine as a stimulant to acid secretion. When the reagents are swallowed, dye is released if hydrochloric acid is present in gastric juice, and this dye can be detected in the urine. If there is achlorhydria, the dye is not released from the resin and therefore does not appear in the urine. These tests are very unreliable, and give both false positive and false negative results.

Role of gastric secretion tests

In general all the tests of acidity show the same pattern of responses. Patients with gastric ulcers have the same range of acid secretion as do normal subjects, so there is little point in testing them routinely. The only disease consistently associated with achlorhydria is Addisonian pernicious anaemia, though this finding is rarely needed for diagnosis (p. 133). Achlorhydria is sometimes found in patients with gastric carcinoma or mucosal atrophy (e.g. in severe hypochromic anaemia), though gastric function tests are rarely needed.

Hyperchlorhydria usually accompanies a duodenal ulcer, though there is no consensus relating degree of secretion to choice of treatment.

After partial gastrectomy or vagotomy, tests are necessary to investigate the completeness of the operation or the cause of recurrent ulceration.

Biochemical effects of disease of the stomach and duodenum

The biochemical assessment of a patient who is suffering from a long-standing disease of the stomach, e.g. carcinoma or ulcer, or after surgery, must be concerned with the effects of malnutrition and of loss of secretions. The extent of malnutrition is best estimated by measurement of the blood haemoglobin, and of the plasma albumin concentration which often falls below 25 g/l in cases of carcinoma of the stomach. If the albumin is below 35 g/l restorative measures should, if possible, be undertaken before the patient is submitted to surgery. The protein deficiency is caused both by a low intake, and by loss from the surface of the ulcer or cancer (protein-losing enteropathy). Vomiting causes loss of secretions. Because of the acidity of gastric juice, prolonged vomiting leads to a severe hypochloraemic alkalosis (p. 49) and often to ketosis, as well as to water and potassium depletion: this alkalosis will not develop if there is vomiting in a patient with achlorhydria. The alkalosis may be accentuated by medication with alkali, or caused by prolonged alkali treatment without vomiting. Bleeding from gastric or duodenal disease gives rise to a high plasma urea (p. 96).

After gastrectomy or gastroenterostomy the patient may develop either the 'dumping syndrome", or post-gastrectomy hypoglycaemia, or both. The *dumping syndrome* is seen shortly after a meal, associated with the osmotic effect of food rapidly entering the duodenum. The cause of all the symptoms is not known, but there is hypovolaemia and a temporary fall of the plasma potassium level. *Post-gastrectomy hypoglycaemia* occurs about two hours after a carbohydrate meal: it is due to the reaction that follows temporary hyperglycaemia, which is caused by rapid gastric emptying and consequent over-rapid absorption of carbohydrate. These patients show a 'lag storage' glucose tolerance curve (p. 69).

PANCREAS

The pancreas is an organ that is relatively inaccessible to biochemical study. In acute pancreatic disease changes can be found in the blood, and often in the urine, which are relatively diagnostic. In chronic pancreatic disease indirect biochemical evidence of disordered function is difficult to obtain in the early stages, and the analysis of pancreatic secretions, which is the direct test of pancreatic function, is difficult because of the necessity for duodenal intubation.

Acute pancreatitis

Swelling of the acinar cells in an acutely inflamed pancreas leads to regurgitation of pancreatic enzymes into the blood stream. Of the main pancreatic enzymes, amylase, lipase (triacylglycerol lipase), and trypsinogen and chymotrypsinogen, amylase is more frequently estimated than is lipase: an immunoassay for trypsin *concentration* in plasma has recently been introduced. Pancreatic and salivary amylases are closely related isoenzymes; the salivary glands do not secrete a lipase or a proteolytic enzyme.

Amylase

During an attack of acute pancreatitis the plasma amylase level rises rapidly, often to over 2000 U/l. A level of over 1000 U/l, in a clinically suspicious case, is usually diagnostic of acute pancreatitis. It is important to perform the estimation within the first 24 hours as the enzyme rise may be transient, and the level usually falls to normal within two or three days as the acute attack resolves.

Other disorders of the upper gastrointestinal tract, particularly perforated duodenal ulcer, intestinal obstruction, and peritonitis affecting the exposed surface of the pancreas, may be accompanied by a raised plasma amylase. The probable causes are leakage of pancreatic juice into the peritoneal cavity whence the enzymes can be absorbed into the circulation, or involvement of the ampulla in the inflammatory process associated with a duodenal ulcer which blocks the secretion of pancreatic juice into the duodenum. Administration of morphine also raises the plasma amylase by contracting the pancreatic duct sphincter. In such cases, however, the plasma amylase level usually does not increase above 1000 U/l, and the slow rise and fall of plasma enzyme concentration may take a week or more. Tubal pregnancy may show a high plasma amylase, arising from the fallopian tube. Amylase is sometimes measured in fluid from an abdominal fistula to see whether this arises from the pancreas.

As the molecular weight of amylase is only 48 000, it is readily excreted; urine amylase is less than about 3000 U/24 h. In all these cases of raised plasma amylase, unless there is glomerular failure (which itself causes amylase retention), there is a slow rise and fall of urine amylase. In acute pancreatitis the value may be 10 000 U/l: the estimation may be useful after the peak of the acute episode has passed.

Macroamylasaemia is a rare harmless congenital condition in which a high plasma amylase is caused by a binding to an abnormal globulin, and urine amylase is normal.

Other biochemical changes

Plasma lipase has a similar but probably slower pattern of rise and fall in pancreatitis than amylase; the peak activity is at about 48 hours and the level usually remains high for about a week. Lipase assay is particularly valuable if a case of pancreatitis is not seen until after 48 hours of onset. The reference range by the usual olive-oil hydrolysis method is 0–1.5 units, and in a typical case of pancreatitis a value above 6 units is found: however the method for rapid emergency assay is not as good as for amylase. Leakage of lipase from the inflamed pancreatic surface in acute pancreatitis causes hydrolysis of fat in the peritoneal cavity. Calcium may be fixed as calcium soaps on these patches of fat necrosis, and partly for this reason the plasma calcium may be low (even low enough to cause tetany) between about 2 and 10 days from the onset of the acute attack. However hyperparathyroidism and pancreatitis sometimes coexist. Plasma trypsin values increase over the same period.

In acute pancreatitis there is often a transient hyperglycaemia and glycosuria. Methaemalbuminaemia develops in acute haemorrhagic pancreatitis due to absorption of altered haemoglobin (p. 128).

Chronic pancreatitis

In the investigation of non-acute disease of the pancreas estimation of plasma or urine enzyme in the resting state rarely yields information of diagnostic value: the very slow cell destruction does not release enzyme at a sufficient rate to raise the plasma activity, and in the long-term both pancreatic isoamylase and trypsin values in plasma are lowered. The only reliable biochemical tests are those based on investigation of duodenal aspirate (pancreatic secretion), after injection of the physiological stimulants which are secretin (acting primarily on the intralobular ducts) or pancreozymin/cholecystokinin (acting on the acinar cells), or after stimulation by a standard 'meal'. The starch tolerance test, which investigates amylase secretion indirectly by measuring changes in plasma glucose after a starch 'meal', as compared with a glucose 'meal', is specific but very insensitive.

Hormonal stimulation tests

Method. After an overnight fast a double lumen tube is passed, and its position checked radiologically. Continuous suction (by water-syphon or electric pump) is applied both to the stomach and to the duodenum. All duodenal samples are collected into iced bottles to preserve the enzymes.

There is 10 minutes preliminary suction, to ensure complete emptying of the gut. Two successive 10 minute samples of pancreatic juice, which are the resting controls, are collected from the duodenal tube. An injection of a pancreatic stimulant is then made. Secretin – Boots (1 unit/kg body weight) is given as an intravenous injection, and this causes an increase in the secretion of bicarbonate and in the volume of juice. Following the injection, samples are collected over three successive 10 minute periods.

There are many varieties of procedure. An enzyme stimulation test may directly follow the secretin test, with injection of pancreozymin-Boots (1.5 units/kg), and further collection of three 10 minute samples.

Interpretation. The volume of a 10 minute control sample is normally about 10 ml: the pH is about 7.5 and the bicarbonate content 25 mmol/l. All enzymes are present, but only amylase is usually measured.

The injection of secretin into a normal subject causes an increase in the volume of aspirate to at least 2 ml/kg body weight calculated over an hour, the secretion rate usually being maximal in the first 10 minutes.

There is a rise in the bicarbonate concentration to a peak of above 90 mmol/l; and in the pH to above 8.

Pancreozymin injection causes little change in the volume or alkalinity of the juice, but there is a doubling of the activity of the enzymes.

Maximal stimulation. The above simple procedures give submaximal stimulation. Tests have been devised that involve continuous intravenous infusion of high doses of secretin + pancreozymin, and these achieve a peak bicarbonate output in normal subjects of 30 ml/h. Their diagnostic indication is uncertain.

In chronic inflammatory pancreatic disease there may be diminished resting values of volume, alkalinity, and enzymes; the typical effect of secretin stimulation is a failure of the bicarbonate to exceed 60 mmol/l with a normal volume response: loss of enzyme response to pancreozymin is late. When there is destruction of pancreatic tissue with obstruction, e.g. due to malignant disease, then the typical effect is loss of volume and enzymes, with only a late fall of bicarbonate response.

Lundh meal

This tests the trypsin response of the pancreas to a protein stimulant: it is simpler than the hormone stimulation tests, but not so discriminating.

Method. After an overnight fast a single lumen Levin 12 tube is passed, and positioned fluoroscopically in the duodenum. The patient is given a standard meal which contains 18 g corn oil, 15 g Casilan (casein hydrolysate) and 40 g glucose, in 300 ml water. A complete 2 hour duodenal aspirate is collected by continuous suction, and stored on ice. There are many varieties of procedure.

Interpretation. The normal stimulated pancreatic juice has a trypsin activity, in the pooled sample, of 25–80 µmol/ml min (TAME method). In chronic pancreatic disease or carcinoma the activity is usually below 20 units.

Pancreatic cystic fibrosis (mucoviscidosis)

This disease, which is probably the commonest inborn error of metabolism in Caucasians, is a general hereditary dysfunction of the exocrine glands. Cysts may be found in the lungs (and also the liver) as well as in the pancreas, and these produce viscid secretions rich in glycoprotein. It presents in children as failure to thrive, and there is often steatorrhoea, and bronchitis with obstructive pulmonary disease. The diagnostic feature is a high content of sodium and chloride in the sweat, the concentrations tending towards those found in the plasma, and may be more than twice those found in the resting sweat of control children. In this disease even moderate sweating may cause serious sodium depletion. In healthy children the sweat sodium rarely exceeds 50 mmol/l, and a sweat sodium of more than 65 mmol/l is highly suggestive of pancreatic cystic fibrosis: in adults the sweat sodium is more variable, but a value exceeding 90 mmol/l is suggestive of cystic fibrosis. A palm-print screen-ng test for a similar critical level of sweat chloride in children is available, but for the detection of doubtful cases it is necessary to collect sweat with care and assay its sodium concentration. Changes in salivary electrolytes, though similar to those found in sweat, may not be diagnostic: a rapid test has been devised which involves placing a sodium ion electrode (p. 22) in the child's mouth.

Owing to obstruction, in the early stages there is often a high plasma trypsin: as secretion of trypsin is generally deficient, this often leads to there being excess albumin in the meconium of the newborn.

Pancreatic enzymes in the faeces

Up to 20 g of pancreatic enzyme protein is secreted daily, and almost all is digested and reabsorbed: trypsin is the only pancreatic enzyme that is assayed in the faeces. The estimation of faecal trypsin is no longer performed for the diagnosis of chronic pancreatic disease in adults as the range of normal is very wide, and because of the presence of similar bacterial enzymes. In steatorrhoea normal faecal chymotrypsin excludes chronic pancreatic disease. In children complete absence of trypsin from *fresh* faeces is suggestive of pancreatic cystic fibrosis.

Biochemical effects of pancreatic disease

Faecal fat

The processes of normal digestion of fat, and the excretion of the end-products of fat digestion, have been discussed in chapter 6. In chronic pancreatic disease, fat digestion is impaired because lipase secretion is deficient. The percentage of fat which is absorbed falls from the normal 90–95 per cent of the total output, to become within the range 20–70 per cent, and fat globules are seen on microscopical examination of the faeces. Excretion of more than 30 mmol (8 g) is definitely abnormal. The demonstration of increased fat, most of which is unsplit, in a dried faeces sample, is no longer used for diagnosis because of lack of specificity. The effects of the high excretion of fat in chronic pancreatic disease are similar to those which develop in steatorrhoea from any cause, and are discussed below (p. 239).

Faecal nitrogen

The processes of normal digestion of protein and the excretion of the end-products of protein digestion have been discussed in chapter 7. In chronic pancreatic disease protein digestion is impaired because trypsin secretion is deficient. Undigested muscle fibres are found in microscopical examination of the faeces, and the 24 hour faecal nitrogen output is greatly raised (creatorrhoea) from the normal 1–1.5 g (70–110 mmol) to be within the range 3–9 g (200–600 mmol): these investigations are no longer used for diagnosis. When it is important to establish whether there is sufficient digestion of protein (or deficient absorption of amino acids, or excess protein loss in the gut), a nitrogen balance test can be done (p. 94).

Loss of secretions

Pancreatic secretions may be lost (with bile and intestinal secretions) through an ileal fistula or in diarrhoea, or by themselves through a pancreatic fistula. About 2000 ml/24 h of an alkaline fluid, with an average electrolyte concentration of Na^+ 140 mmol/l, K^+ 10 mmol/l, HCO_3^- 70 mmol/l, Cl^- 70 mmol/l, may be lost from the body. If this loss of secretions is prolonged there will be sodium and water depletion and a metabolic acidosis (p. 50): there may also be potassium deficiency. Loss of enzymes and of bile salts gives rise to protein maldigestion and malabsorption, and to steatorrhoea.

Other effects

Chronic disease of the pancreatic acinar tissue does not initially involve the islet tissue, and carbohydrate metabolism is not affected in the early stages of the disease. However, in patients who have had pancreatic carcinoma or severe chronic pancreatitis for some time, or following total pancreatectomy, impaired glucose tolerance with hyperglycaemia and glycosuria are often seen (p. 62). Deficient digestion of protein leads to a negative nitrogen balance; protein malnutrition and a low plasma albumin result. Sufficient amylase is usually secreted for starch digestion to be unaltered. The plasma calcium, vitamin B_{12}, and iron, are usually normal, because mucosal absorptive capacity is little altered.

INTESTINAL TRACT

Loss of intestinal secretions

A healthy subject secretes every 24 hours about 3000 ml of intestinal secretions. Their electrolyte content depends on the site of secretion, but an average value for ileal secretions is Na^+ 130 mmol/l, K^+ 15 mmol/l, HCO_3^- 35 mmol/l, Cl^- 100 mmol/l. Almost all the water and electrolytes that are secreted are reabsorbed, and faecal loss of electrolytes in health is negligible: similarly about 50 g of mucosal and enzyme protein altogether passes into the gut and is digested and reabsorbed daily. Intestinal secretions may be lost as vomit or diarrhoea (especially from high intestinal obstruction), through a fistula or ileostomy, or by suction. Loss of intestinal secretions may be very severe in diarrhoea. The very alkaline pancreatic juice and bile are usually lost at the same time as are the intestinal secretions.

Such losses lead to gross water and sodium depletion, with metabolic acidosis and potassium deficiency. Diarrhoea has a high potassium content (often 30 mmol/l); it is also particularly dangerous in infants, because they have a low intracellular fluid reserve and more easily become water-depleted (p. 28). Acidosis and potassium deficiency tend also to be more marked in infants. Purgation causes potassium depletion and acidosis.

When, as in the *blind loop syndrome*, there is pooling of intestinal secretions and alteration of the bacterial flora, then there is excess indole synthesis with high urinary indican secretion (reference values 0.1–0.4 mmol/24 h), and deficiencies of vitamin B_{12} and of folic acid. Steatorrhoea may be present.

Protein loss

In severe chronic intestinal disease, such as ulcerative colitis (which does not cause steatorrhoea), there is excessive loss into the bowel of nitrogen as well as of water and electrolytes. This nitrogen loss can also occur due to specific protein exudation through the mucosa in a variety of conditions with increased permeability of the gut mucosa, when albumin and globulins are lost (*protein-losing gastroenteropathies* p. 93). Faecal nitrogen need not be grossly increased if the disorder is high in the gastrointestinal tract, for much of the protein is digested to amino acids which are absorbed and metabolised, and excess nitrogen is lost in the urine. The rate of loss exceeds the reserve capacity of the liver for the synthesis of albumin, and this leads to depletion of the body protein, a negative nitrogen balance, and a low plasma albumin. The condition may be diagnosed by intravenous injection of a substance that is treated by the mucosa similarly to albumin, e.g. ^{131}I-polyvinyl pyrrolidine of molecular weight about 40 000. This is therefore excreted into the gut in the gastroenteropathies, and the radioactivity in the faeces can be detected and measured.

Steatorrhoea

The term 'steatorrhoea' is applied to abnormal ill-formed stools that contain excessive quantities of fat. Both the daily volume and the total wet and dry weight of faeces are increased; they are pale, bulky, greasy, often frothy, and offensive – and may float. Simple diarrhoea usually causes a slight increase in the total faecal fat and there may be some deficiency of splitting though the stool does not appear greasy.

Steatorrhoea, as part of the malabsorption syndrome, occurs at the preabsorptive stage in chronic pancreatic disease and pancreatic cystic fibrosis due to lipase deficiency; in intra-hepatic or post-hepatic biliary obstruction, due to bile salt deficiency (with generally well-formed stools); after massive resection of the gut or severe disease of the small intestine, in gastrocolic fistula and sometimes after gastrectomy, partly due to inadequate mixing and rapid passage through the intestines and to secondary deficiency of pancreatic function. In primary malabsorptive disorders (which include tropical sprue, coeliac disease, and Whipple's disease) the pathological alteration of the small intestinal mucosa prevents the absorption of fat. Tropical sprue may be of dietary or infective origin. Coeliac disease in children, and usually also in adults, is caused by sensitivity to (or failure to detoxicate) the gliadin fraction of dietary wheat gluten, which leads to damage of the mucosa. There is a *heavy chain disease* (p. 111) of α-*chains* in which intestinal lymphoid infiltration causes steatorrhoea and diarrhoea. Conditions such as intestinal lymphadenopathies interfere with fat absorption at the post-absorptive stage.

Biochemical effects of steatorrhoea and of intestinal malabsorption

In all types of steatorrhoea the failure of fat absorption leads to deficient intake of energy. The total plasma cholesterol level is often low. There is also malabsorption of the fat-soluble vitamins A, D, and K, which may lead to clinical vitamin deficiencies, particularly in the sprue syndrome. There is a low fasting plasma carotene level. The plasma vitamin A level rises little after oral vitamin A administration (100 000 units) and this finding may be useful as a *screening test* in the investigation of steatorrhoea: the value would normally double in 6 h. Deficiencies of the B group vitamins develop when the intestinal bacterial flora is altered.

The biochemical effects of coeliac disease and related disorders are due to the multiple absorption deficiencies of the small intestine. The major abnormality is of fat absorption, not of fat digestion, and steatorrhoea is a prominent symptom. The percentage of absorbed dietary fat is usually within the range 45–85 per cent, and the stool can be seen microscopically to contain fat globules, fatty acid crystals, and soap plaques. Unsaturated fatty acids are more easily absorbed than are saturated fatty acids. The effects of the steatorrhoea have been described above. Digestion of protein is not affected, and absorption of amino acids is impaired only in severe or long-standing cases. The nitrogen content of the faeces may be moderately raised up to 4 g (250 mmol) per 24 hours, and the plasma protein concentrations may be normal or there may be a slight fall in the albumin level: the prothrombin time is prolonged, and the immunoglobulin concentrations may be reduced. Absorption of carbohydrates is diminished, and the patient may have attacks of hypoglycaemia, and a flat glucose tolerance curve (p. 65): there may also be secondary disaccharidase deficiencies (p. 73). The deficiency of calcium absorption, which is due to the mucosal defect, and partly to malabsorption of vitamin D and to excessive calcium excretion in the stools as calcium soaps, causes hypocalcaemia, osteomalacia and tetany. There may also be impaired absorption of phosphate, and hypophosphataemia (p. 171). There may be deficient absorption of vitamin B_{12}, iron, and folic acid (this particularly in tropical sprue). Tests using radioactive vitamin B_{12}, such as the Schilling test (p. 133), can be used to investigate ileal absorption.

In prolonged steatorrhoea, or if there is also diarrhoea, electrolytes are lost. The patient may have water and sodium depletion, hypokalaemia may be marked, and there is often phosphate loss. Delayed urinary excretion of an oral water load can be demonstrated, and the night 12 hour urine volume may be larger than the day 12 hour urine volume.

Vitamin C (ascorbic acid) deficiency. This occasionally develops due to malabsorption, but is usually nutritional. The biochemical confirmation of a mild nutritional deficiency is not entirely satisfactory. A common procedure is to give 700 mg of vitamin C orally daily until at least 70 mg are excreted in the 8 hour overnight urine: this occurs within 3 days in a normal subject, and may take more than a week if the patient is unsaturated. Analysis of 'buffy coat' (leucocytes + platelets) for ascorbic acid concentration provides a better index of tissue saturation than does analysis of plasma ascorbic acid, which reflects recent dietary intake.

Differential diagnosis of chronic pancreatitis and of coeliac disease

The commonest causes of steatorrhoea are biliary obstruction, chronic pancreatitis, and coeliac disease; the differential diagnosis of the second and third of these may not always be possible on clinical grounds alone. In theory distinction could be made on the degree of splitting of the excess fat in the stools directly or after giving ^{131}I-triolein, normal splitting signifying coeliac disease, and deficient splitting signifying pancreatic disease. In practice a moderate impairment of splitting may be found in many cases of either type of disorder and this investigation is no longer performed: the results of fat-absorption tests or of faecal fat analysis are not necessarily diagnostic.

The trypsin deficiency and impairment of protein digestion which is found in pancreatic disease, and the impairment of carbohydrate absorption which is found in coeliac disease (in contrast to the 'diabetic' impaired glucose tolerance of pancreatic disease), are more characteristic if present. If the facilities are available, more definite biochemical diagnosis of pancreatic disease can be obtained by duodenal intubation and examination of pancreatic juice after stimulation.

Xylose absorption test. The best test of carbohydrate absorption uses the partly metabolised pentose, D-xylose. After an oral dose of 25 g to adults, in the fasting state, a normal subject excretes 4.5–8 g (30–50 mmol) of xylose in the urine in the next 5 hours. In the sprue syndrome less than 4 g (28 mmol) is excreted; in pancreatic disease absorption and excretion are usually unaltered. The test is not valid in old persons or when there is impairment of renal function: in the latter case, when urine values are unreliable, a plasma xylose level less than 2.0 mmol/l at 90 minutes is considered abnormal.

As 25 g of xylose sometimes causes nausea, a 5 g dose is becoming popular though the test is not so discriminating. The critical level of excretion in 5 hours is then about 1.25 g (8 mmol).

Other tests

In the investigation of disease of the gastrointestinal tract (including the pancreas), non-biochemical modes of investigation may be more diagnostic than those described here.

Specific failures of intestinal function

The above disorders generally affect all aspects of intestinal function. There are a variety of specific alterations of the brush-border membrane, which may primarily affect digestion (e.g. alactasia, p. 54), or absorption (e.g. Hartnup disease, p. 102).

GASTROINTESTINAL HORMONES

The APUD concept

A variety of similar cells throughout the body, of presumed common embryological origin, are capable of producing peptides, of storing amines, and of amine precursor uptake and decarboxylation – and are therefore called APUD cells, and their tumours sometimes generically called apudomas. These cells produce the various hormones of the gastrointestinal tract, and also comprise the anterior pituitary, the parathyroid, and the thyroid C cells. The APUD cells exist in nervous tissue, and are thought to be present in the bronchi.

Knowledge of the physiology of the growing number of identified peptide hormones from diffuse endocrine cells in the gastrointestinal tract is advancing rapidly. Gastrin, and secretin and pancreozymin, have long been used as stimulants in tests of gastrointestinal function, and immunoassay is enabling certain plasma assays to become valuable in diagnosis. Glucagon and insulin are discussed in chapter 5.

Gastrin

The reference range for plasma gastrin is 5–50 pmol/l. Very high values are found in achlorhydria, particularly in pernicious anaemia.

The *Zollinger-Ellison syndrome* of severe peptic ulcers and hypersecretion is caused by a gastrinoma, usually of the islet cells of the pancreas but sometimes of antral G-cells: the massive basal secretion of acid (more than 200 ml of juice with an HCl content of more than 20 mmol/h) is little increased by pentagastrin. Immunoassay of plasma gastrin in cases of hyperacidity shows a diagnostic high value. A 100 per cent rise in plasma gastrin after secretin stimulation may be confirmatory. This may be part of a pluriglandular syndrome of multiple endocrine adenomas (p. 182).

Vasoactive intestinal peptide

This hormone (VIP), produced in excess by a pancreatic tumour (VIPoma), gives rise to the Werner-Morrison syndrome of very severe spasmodic watery diarrhoea, with water and salt loss, hypokalaemia, and achlorhydria. This can be diagnosed by finding a very high plasma VIP.

Argentaffin system

The argentaffin cells, which are scattered diffusely throughout the mucosa of the alimentary canal, produce as an internal secretion 5-hydroxy-tryptamine (serotonin) via 5-hydroxytryptophan (5-HTP) – this is not a polypeptide. Serotonin is carried by the blood platelets, and is also present in the nervous system. Its full physiological and psychological significance is at present not known, but it can cause capillary constriction and affect gastrointestinal motility.

The rare metastasising *malignant carcinoid tumour* produces excess serotonin, which leads to a syndrome characterised by flushing attacks, diarrhoea, and right heart valvular disease and heart failure. Pellagra, and even protein deficiency, may be caused by deviation of tryptophan to the excess hormone. The plasma serotonin level is increased, and the condition is usually diagnosed by the excessive urinary excretion of a serotonin metabolite, 5-hydroxyindolylacetic acid. This is normally 10–45 µmol/24 h, and is characteristically above 100 µmol/24 h, and may be raised above 1000 µmol/24 h in malignant carcinoid – ingestion of bananas gives a false positive result. A simple urinary screening test is available. Occasionally the precursor, 5-HTP, is produced in tumours and excreted in excess.

FAECAL OCCULT BLOOD

The nature of blood in the faeces depends on the quantity, and on whether it has been digested. Significant quantities of unaltered blood are bright red, and of altered blood produce a dark 'tarry' stool or melaena.

Occult blood is not identifiable by direct visual examination. It can be detected in faeces by similar methods to those used for detecting blood in urine. The usual methods are sensitive and will respond to a haemorrhage of 5–10 ml. For maximum sensitivity the patient must be taken off all meat for three days before collection of the specimen for analysis, as haemoglobin derivatives from ingested meat give a positive reaction to the test in the same way as haemoglobin derivatives which have originated from the patient's blood. Most iron preparations that are given by mouth, although they may colour the faeces black, do not interfere with the chemical tests. However, iron(II) [ferrous] sulphate tablets may *cause* gastrointestinal bleeding, and iron(II) carbonate and iron(II) fumarate can give false positive reactions with the sensitive tests. Simple and less sensitive commercial side-room tests are available (p. 274).

The occult blood test detects blood which may have come from any site in the gastrointestinal tract. The test is valuable in the investigation of obscure anaemias, and in the search for pathological lesions, such as malignant disease or peptic ulcer. If a sensitive technique gives a negative result on three consecutive daily samples of stool then bleeding from the alimentary tract may be excluded.

For accurate quantitative determination of gastrointestinal bleeding it is necessary to measure haemoglobin, in the faeces, that is derived from radioactively labelled erythrocytes which have been injected intravenously.

Further reading

Baron JH, Williams, AJ. Gastric secretion tests. In: Taylor S, ed. *Recent Advances in Surgery 9*. Edinburgh: Churchill-Livingstone, 1973:166–198.

Bloom SR. Hormones of the gastrointestinal tract. In: Baron DN, Compston N, Dawson AM, eds. *Recent Advances in Medicine 17*. Edinburgh: Churchill-Livingstone, 1977:357–386.

Davenport HW. *Physiology of the Digestive Tract*. 3rd ed. Chicago: Year Book Medical Publishers, 1977.

Losowsky MS. Small bowel disease and malabsorption. *Medicine* 3rd series 1978; 16:790–802.

Wormsley KG. Pancreatic function tests. *Clin Gastroenterol* 1972; 1:27–51.

CHAPTER 15

THE NERVOUS SYSTEM

Biochemical changes in the brain, spinal cord, or peripheral nerves have been found in many organic neurological disorders but at present their study is rarely of immediate diagnostic value, though they add greatly to our knowledge of the pathological processes. Nor have biochemical studies in primary psychiatric disorders yet yielded sufficient conclusive information to be an accepted guide to aetiology or diagnosis.

THE PSYCHOSES

Although certain abnormal biochemical findings are often present in some psychotic disorders, their relation to the aetiology or to the symptoms remains uncertain. With the exception of measurement of drug concentrations (e.g. lithium, p. 41) for control of therapy, analysis of blood or other body fluids is at present of no value for diagnosis or management.

Depression

There is some evidence of an abnormal metabolism of the cerebral monoamines, in particular noradrenaline and/or 5-hydroxytryptamine. It may be that the primary disorder is a cell membrane transport deficiency; due to this, during depressive phases there is retention of water and sodium.

Schizophrenia

It has been suggested that there may be an associated abnormal metabolism of dopamine and related compounds.

Secondary psychoses

Psychological symptoms may be present in a large number of somatic diseases in which there are biochemical changes, although the relation between the specific abnormal chemistry and the symptoms is usually unknown. However, appropriate biochemical investigations in suspected secondary psychoses may reveal such metabolic disorders as severe sodium or potassium depletion (p. 30, 38), magnesium deficiency (p. 40), hypercapnia (p. 49), beri-beri (p. 71), chronic alcoholism (p. 71), pellagra (p. 123), acute porphyria (p. 131), Wilson's disease (p. 136), thyrotoxicosis or myxoedema (p. 151, 152), toxaemia of pregnancy (p. 165), liver failure (p. 203), uraemia (p. 224).

ORGANIC DISEASES OF THE NERVOUS SYSTEM

The results of analysis of cerebrospinal fluid can be often correlated with certain primary disorders of the central nervous system; but biochemical analyses of blood or urine are, in most such diseases, of little diagnostic or prognostic value.

Specific abnormal findings in different disorders which secondarily affect the nervous system, and where chemical pathology investigation may be helpful, are described under appropriate headings elsewhere in this book. Some of these neurological end-results of biochemical disorders are summarised below.

Coma

This is an end-result of many severe metabolic disturbances such as water depletion (p. 28), hypercapnia (p. 49), uncontrolled diabetes mellitus (p. 63), hypoglycaemia (p. 64), panhypopituitarism (p. 140), myxoedema (p. 152), acute hypercalcaemia (p. 180), liver failure (p. 203), uraemia (p. 224). It is not known whether these very different biochemical abnormalities act through any final common pathway.

Drug coma. This is a separate problem, and is often very difficult to diagnose, both in excluding the organic causes listed above, and specifically for the offending drugs. Indeed about one-third of cases of drug coma admitted in emergency are due to multiple drugs, and combination with alcohol accounts for another one-third, and information from bottles of tablets and from friends cannot be relied on.

Most laboratories have facilities for the quantitative determination in blood of carboxyhaemoglobin, iron, paracetamol, salicylates, alcohol and barbiturates, and for the identification of the type of barbiturate by chromatography. Benzodiazepenes and tricyclic antidepressants are frequently taken; the identification of these, and many other drugs, in urine is usually feasible. Quantitative assay of the newer tranquillisers and hypnotics generally requires a specialised laboratory. Blood analysis is the most important, but if available samples of urine and gastric contents (including vomit and lavage) and necessarily of any medicines found, are to be sent to the laboratory.

Analysis is important medicolegally and for monitoring progress, as well as for diagnosis.

Mental retardation

In some cases this is due to specific biochemical abnormalities, especially inborn errors of metabolism, such as leucine sensitivity (p. 65), galactose or fructose intolerance (p. 73), and other chronic hypoglycaemias (p. 66), many mucopolysaccharidoses and lipidoses (p. 67, 87), phenyl ketonuria and certain other disorders of amino acid metabolism and organ cacidurias (p. 101), lead poisoning (p. 131), hypothyroidism (p. 152), pseudohypoparathyroidism (p. 181), infantile hypercalcaemia (p. 186), kernicterus (p. 201).

Peripheral neuritis

A wide variety of metabolic disorders, with known specific biochemical abnormalities, may have consequent symptoms and signs of generalised polyneuritis. This may be evident in diabetes mellitus (p. 63), chronic alcoholism (p. 71), thiamine deficiency (p. 71), organophosphorus poisoning (p. 122), pernicious anaemia (p. 132), lead poisoning (p. 131), acute porphyria (p. 131), and from many other external toxins.

Open neural tube defects

These abnormalities result in high concentrations of α-fetoprotein and acetylcholinesterase in amniotic fluid: this is important for prenatal diagnosis (p. 165).

CEREBROSPINAL FLUID

Formation and composition

Cerebrospinal fluid (CSF) is secreted into the sub-arachnoid space, principally through the choroid plexuses, by processes involving active transport: it is not just a plasma ultrafiltrate. In healthy adults the rate of production is 100–250 ml per 24 hours and the total volume of CSF is 100–200 ml.

The only chemical components of CSF that are commonly estimated are protein and glucose: chloride estimations are rarely required. The chemical composition of CSF from a normal subject depends on the site of withdrawal: the reference values for ventricular and lumbar CSF in an adult are:

	Ventricular	Lumbar
Total protein	50–100 mg/l	100–400 mg/l
Glucose	3.0–5.5 mmol/l	2.5–4.5 mmol/l
Chloride	120–130 mmol/l	120–130 mmol/l

Generally only lumbar CSF is examined. A sample of CSF submitted for chemical analysis should, if possible, be fresh and free from blood. It may be difficult to obtain an absolutely blood-free sample, but if only a small amount of blood is present which is merely sufficient to cause turbidity just visible to the naked eye the analytical findings will not be significantly altered. If the fluid cannot be analysed for glucose within half an hour of withdrawal, then to prevent glycolysis by any cells or bacteria present the CSF should be put into a bottle which contains sodium fluoride, such as that often used for blood glucose, Usually conditions requiring chemical and serological analysis of CSF also require examination of cells, and often microbiological analysis. Local procedures must determine the way such specimens are sent to different laboratories.

Alterations in the chemical content of CSF may not necessarily be caused by disease within the central nervous system, but can be a reflection of changes in the chemistry of the plasma and extracellular fluid from which the CSF is produced – e.g. in diabetes mellitus the high plasma glucose concentration leads to a high CSF glucose concentration.

The table shows a compilation of the more important changes in the composition of lumbar CSF in disease (p. 250).

Appearance

Normal CSF is clear, and any colour of CSF is usually due to oxyhaemoglobin or to bilirubin. Turbidity in fresh CSF may be due to erythrocytes, leucocytes, or bacteria. Colour can be seen when the erythrocyte concentration in the CSF sample exceeds about 50×10^6 cells/l, and opalescence can be seen when the leucocyte concentration exceeds $100-200 \times 10^6$ cells/l.

If there is blood in the CSF sample that was caused by the lumbar puncture it will disappear from the fluid after a few millilitres have been collected (using three consecutive bottles), and the supernatant fluid will be clear after centrifugation. If there is blood in the CSF that was caused by past haemorrhage, then it will be distributed uniformly throughout the fluid, and the supernatant fluid will usually be pale yellow. The erythrocytes of haemorrhage caused by the puncture have a normal shape: the erythrocytes of a pathological haemorrhage are usually crenated.

Xanthochromia, a yellow colouration in the CSF, can be due either to haemoglobin or to other pigments, usually bilirubin. After haemorrhage the xanthochromia is initially due to oxyhaemoglobin, which is then converted into bilirubin. Bilirubin can be detected in CSF about 6 hours after the haemorrhage, reaches a maximum concentration a week to 10 days afterwards by which time the erythrocytes have usually disappeared, and is no longer detectable after three weeks.

Both (unconjugated) bilirubin and conjugated bilirubin pass across into the CSF when the permeability of the blood-brain barrier is altered, or when there is a high plasma bilirubin – this also probably alters the permeability. A high CSF bilirubin is therefore found in chronic cholestatic jaundice and in icterus neonatorum. In premature infants there is increased permeability of the blood-brain barrier.

Carotenoids pass from the plasma into the CSF when the permeability of the blood-brain barrier is altered. This occurs in general disorders of the meninges or in the space below a spinal block. The term 'Froin's syndrome' is given to the yellow fluid of high protein concentration which coagulates spontaneously, and that can be withdrawn from below a spinal block; the xanthochromia results from capillary haemorrhage.

Protein

The total concentration of protein in CSF is usually approximately measured by turbidimetry. Quantitative electrophoretic analysis shows that albumin is the main protein, that pre-albumin is usually seen, and that about 10 per cent of the protein is γ-globulin: macroglobulins are not seen. During the first month of life the total CSF protein concentration may be as high as 800 mg/l, and there is a higher proportion of γ-globulin.

Changes in disease

In most diseases of the central nervous system, and occasionally in general toxic states such as uraemia, or after a myelogram, there is an increase in the CSF protein concentration. This increase may be due to an increased permeability of the blood-brain barrier to the plasma proteins (with no change in cells) or to release of protein from the nervous system (when there is usually an increase in the number of lymphocytes in the CSF). Marked increase in the CSF protein is seen in acute meningitis. In chronic conditions such as multiple sclerosis and general paresis there may be a slight rise in the total CSF protein and this is principally due to an increase in globulins. Very high CSF protein concentrations (up to about 10 g/l) are found in the space below a spinal block, and this is principally due to albumin which has leaked from the plasma. A spinal block is usually due to tumour, but arachnoid adhesions in pyogenic meningitis can also cause loculation of fluid. In cerebral tumours (except in acoustic neuroma, when high values are regularly found), the CSF protein may be normal, but this depends on the site of the tumour in relation to the subarachnoid space.

Because CSF is derived from plasma, the CSF proteins will also alter following marked changes in the plasma proteins, as in myelomatosis.

Globulins

Simple chemical tests for excess CSF globulin (e.g. Pandy reaction using phenol) are mainly sensitive to γ-globulins but are now rarely used: normal CSF gives negative reactions.

Accurate determination of the different globulins in the CSF is not usually required: it is performed by electrophoretic or immunological methods, and the important analysis is for the γ-globulins. Reference values depend on the method. The patient's blood must be analysed at the same time, because changes in plasma protein concentrations affect their concentrations in CSF.

When CSF contains proteins derived from plasma, as in acute meningitis, due to increased capillary permeability, albumin and γ-globulins are increased; in bacterial meningitis there is a particular increase in IgM. When CSF contains proteins derived from brain and spinal cord, then mainly the local immunoglobulins are increased. In multiple scle-

Disease	Protein g/l	Gold curve	Glucose mmol/l	Cells	Other points
Reference values	0.15–0.40	0–0	2.5–4.5	Scanty L ($0-4 \times 10^6$/l)	Clear
Acute Meningitis					
Pyogenic	1.0–10	M	0–1.5	P+++	Turbid with clot
Tuberculous	0.5–4.0	Weak M	1.0–2.5	L+P±	Clear with fine clot
Syphilitic	0.5–1.0	P or L	1.5–4.5	L++P±	
Virus	0.3–1.0	Normal	Normal	L++	In acute phase
Meningism in acute fevers	0.15–0.5	Normal	Normal	L+	
General paresis (G.P.I.)	0.3–1.0	P	Normal	L+P±	
Tabes dorsalis	0.3–0.8	Normal or Weak P or L	Normal	L+P±	
Epidemic encephalitis	0.15–1.0	Normal	2.5–7.0	L+	
Poliomyelitis					
Pre-paralytic phase	0.15–0.4	Normal	Normal	L+P+	
Early paralytic phase	0.4–1.0	Weak P or L	Normal	L+	
Multiple sclerosis	0.3–0.9	Weak P	Normal	L+	Oligoclonal γ-globulin bands
Cerebral tumour	0.15–1.0	Normal	1.0–4.0	Normal	High protein in acoustic neuroma
Spinal block (Froin's syndrome)	0.5–10	M	Normal	Normal	Opalescent with massive clot: yellow

Note: Gold curve: P = paretic; L = luetic; M = meningitic. Cells: L = lymphocytes; p = polymorphonuclears.

rosis there is an increase in IgG, both total and in relation to albumin or other CSF proteins; and oligoclonal γ-globulin bands, from lymphocytes or plasma cells, are often present.

Lange Colloidal Gold reaction. Serial dilutions of CSF are mixed with a colloidal gold sol: possible colour changes are 0 to 5. Normal CSF usually gives zero colour change at all dilutions. Colour change at low dilutions, known as the first zone or Paretic curve (e.g. 5555543100; weak reaction 2333210000), is seen when the total CSF protein is normal or slightly increased and there is increase of γ-globulin. Colour change at medium dilutions, known as a mid-zone or Luetic curve (e.g. 0123321000), is seen when the total protein is raised but γ-globulin is raised more than albumin. Colour change at high dilutions, known as the end-zone or Meningitic curve (e.g. 0001234454), is seen when total protein is greatly raised due to a rise in both albumin and globulin – the albumin has to be 'diluted out' to permit the precipitating action of the γ-globulin.

The Lange reaction was principally used in the investigation of neurosyphilis and of multiple sclerosis (see table opposite), but is now largely superseded by assay of immunoglobulins.

Fibrinogen

Normal CSF does not form a fibrin clot on standing. When there has been haemorrhage into the CSF, the fibrinogen from the blood may be sufficient for a clot to form in the fluid which has been withdrawn. If the total CSF protein is above 2 g/l, there is usually sufficient fibrinogen present to produce a clot. Fluid from below a spinal block contains a high concentration of fibrinogen. A delicate slowly developing coagulum, the 'spider-web' clot, is often seen in the CSF of acute tuberculous meningitis, but may occur in neurosyphilis or polio-meningitis. CSF must be examined for clot formation within 24 hours of withdrawal because autolysis destroys the fibrin.

Glucose

The glucose content of CSF may be estimated precisely by any technique used for plasma glucose estimation, and a rough screen may be performed by urine-glucose methods (p. 271).

The concentration of glucose in the CSF largely depends on the plasma glucose, and normally stays at about 60 per cent of its concentration in the plasma because of incomplete penetration of the blood-brain barrier. The CSF glucose changes slowly when the plasma glucose changes, and there is even a slight post-prandial rise. If the blood-brain barrier is damaged, it becomes more permeable to glucose, and the CSF glucose approaches the plasma glucose level. This is seen due to damage to cerebral capillaries, in encephalitis, general septicaemia, and following cranial injury. Infection of the meninges (except viral), with excess of polymorphonuclear leucocytes in the CSF, lowers the glucose level because the leucocytes and many types of bacteria are glycolytic, and in chronic cases there is also decreased permeability. In pyogenic meningitis the CSF glucose is very low, whereas in tuberculous meningitis the decrease is less and may be used as an index of the activity of the infection. Presence of malignant (including leukaemic) cells within the meninges also lowers the CSF glucose.

Rhinorrhoea of unknown origin can be tested for glucose. If it is present, then the rhinorrhoea is principally CSF; if glucose is absent, then the rhinorrhoea is principally nasal secretions.

Chloride

This analysis is rarely indicated as it gives no diagnostic information that is not provided by the CSF protein and glucose.

The concentration of chloride in the CSF is slightly higher than that in the plasma. Variation in the plasma chloride level, e.g. due to vomiting, will cause parallel variation in the CSF chloride level. In meningitis, and especially in tuberculous meningitis, the CSF chloride level is low – it is uncertain to what extent this depletion of chloride is due to general chloride loss from extracellular fluid, and to what extent to chloride shift into cells.

Other investigations

The non-protein nitrogen constituents of plasma (urea, uric acid, etc.) are present in CSF in concentrations which are 90–95 per cent of those in the plasma. When there is nitrogen retention due to chronic renal failure the CSF urea concentration rises in parallel with the plasma urea: this assay performed at autopsy may occasionally be valuable for retrospective diagnosis. In phenylketonuria the CSF phenylalanine is raised with the plasma phenylalanine, and similarly in other inborn errors of metabolism.

The pH of CSF is normally about 7.3, and becomes acid in pyogenic meningitis due to bacterial fermentation. In acid-base disorders there is a slower change in CSF pH than in blood pH; although, being almost free of protein and cells, CSF is poorly buffered. In respiratory acidosis, however, CSF pH changes in parallel with the blood pH; bicarbonate diffuses into the CSF much more slowly than does carbonic acid, and CSF pH is sensitive to changes in P_{CO_2}.

The CSF calcium level is 1.2–1.4 mmol/l, of which 95 per cent is ionised calcium. However (because CSF is a secretion) this does not strictly follow the changes in plasma ionised calcium in disease, and cannot be used to determine this fraction.

Intracellular enzymes are present in low activity in CSF (LD 5–40 U/l, AST 5–12 U/l: at 37 °C). Increases up to 10 times normal are found due to release of enzyme from damaged brain tissue when there has been an abscess, haemorrhage, or infarction, or in primary or metastatic malignant disease (even with a normal CSF protein), but such estimations are of little practical diagnostic value. Creatine kinase is present in high concentration in brain tissue: its rise in *plasma* after cerebral infarction is mainly derived from muscle CK-MM (p. 120) and not from brain (CK-BB), and has not been shown to have diagnostic value.

An immunologically measurable globulin, myelin basic protein, has been claimed to show an increase in *plasma* concentration, in proportion to the degree of cerebral damage, after head injury.

None of the above investigations are required for diagnosis or management.

Further reading

Davison AN, ed. *Biochemistry and Neurological Disease*. Oxford: Blackwell Scientific Publications, 1976.

Thompson EJ, Norman PM, Macdermot J. The analysis of cerebrospinal fluid. *Br J Hosp Med* 1975; 14:645–652.

SUBMISSION OF SPECIMENS FOR ANALYSIS

The most satisfactory relationship between a clinician (whether general practitioner or specialist) and a chemical pathologist is for the clinician to be able to discuss any problem for which he requires assistance and for the chemical pathologist to suggest how he can help most effectively, which investigations are advisable, and what specimens he requires. The laboratory specialist is also in a position to help assess the significance of the results. Consultation about unexpected results may also detect laboratory error. As the resources of the laboratory are limited, the chemical pathologist has to advise and warn the clinician when the tests requested, by their nature or number, are overstraining these resources.

The principles that underly the selection of tests have been discussed in chapter 1.

Organisation of work

In all laboratories, and for all types of analysis, it is important that the specimen should be delivered as early as possible so that the work can be dealt with and reported on the same day, and as soon as possible after collection to avoid artefactual change. If the clinician regards an analysis as particularly urgent, it is essential that he makes contact with the laboratory staff personally so that the relevant degree of priority can be given to the tests. This is particularly important when only one of a large number of tests requested at the same time on the same patient is in fact urgent. Because of automation, most analyses are done in batches at certain times of the day, and some complex and less urgent tests only on some days of the week. By knowledge of local arrangements delays can often be minimised. Most large laboratories now issue their own local list of tests that are done regularly, with particulars of the types of sample required, recommendations on procedures for the performance of complex tests of function, and their own reference values. The comments below and elsewhere in this book are meant only as a general guide.

Completion of request forms
Some laboratories no longer include a space for relevant clinical information on their request forms. Whenever possible this information should be provided, as it is often a guide to the interpretation of unusual results, to the instigation of further investigations, and to picking up mistakes. It includes relevant drugs, both for their physiological effect on

body chemistry, and because of chemical interference with methods – this technical problem may be soluble, if it is recognised, by modifying the method. Request forms should be signed (or legibly initialled) by an identifiable doctor who is prepared to take responsibility for the information given and for the tests requested on the form, and who can be contacted for further enquiries or for communication of results that may call for urgent clinical action.

The extreme importance of accurate patient and sample identification on the request form and on the specimen label cannot be over-emphasised. Surname, first name, date of birth (preferred to age) are all necessary; but a hospital number, or NHS number (in Britain), is or should be the only absolutely unambiguous factor, and is particularly relevant to avoiding confusion with names that are not in European style. This is especially important when the laboratory uses automatic data processing and cumulative reporting. The specimen, and the form, must also bear the date and time of collection. In hospitals the ward (or outpatient department) and consultant's name, and outside hospitals the general practitioner's name and address serve not primarily for identification, but mainly so that the result is returned in time to a doctor who can act on it. This is particularly applicable to the laboratory's responsibility for telephoning results that need rapid clinical attention.

Non-routine analyses

Emergency tests. Analyses should be requested as urgent only when the *immediate* management of the patient depends on the result, for example blood glucose in a patient with suspected diabetic coma. Out-of-hours analyses are not necessarily urgent, e.g. the daily plasma electrolytes of a patient on intravenous therapy measured on a Sunday morning. Both these types of non-routine investigations have to be analysed individually, at a cost about 10 times greater than that of the same analyses done in batches during the normal working day. This service is particularly open to abuse by over-enthusiastic junior clinical staff.

Unusual tests. Special investigations, not given in a laboratory's routine list, must not be requested on specimens sent without previous arrangement and consultation. They can often be done after special preparation by the laboratory staff. It may be possible for the local laboratory to send a specimen to another laboratory which specialises in the particular investigation – this centralisation of unusual or complex tests is necessarily becoming increasingly common. There is a Supraregional Assay Service for many individual hormones, proteins, and some other substances. Such special (and expensive) investigations are normally arranged between laboratories, and the local chemical pathologist should first screen the request to see if it is justified. These tests are not acceptable if sent directly by the clinician.

Avoidance of error

Errors can arise in the collection, labelling, and processing of specimens, in the actual analytical procedures, and in the recording and transmission of results; so care is required by the wards and by the laboratory. If a clinician suspects that a result is erroneous he must contact the laboratory as soon as possible because specimens, once analysed, are normally only stored for a limited period before being discarded. This contact enables the individual result to be checked, and provides an additional form of quality control.

Most laboratories prefer not to telephone results except in an emergency, because of the real risk that results are heard and copied wrongly. Seeking and telephoning results also takes up a lot of time for the laboratory staff.

Quality control

Laboratories monitor the reliability of their analytical work by a variety of quality control procedures. One method of internal quality control is to analyse the same stored sample day after day, and the results should not fluctuate outside a narrow range. One method of external quality assessment is to analyse a sample that has been sent to very many laboratories from a national source, and to examine how the local results fall within the national pattern. In general, the performance of a laboratory is worse if it handles only a small work-load, and if it is not supervised by a medical or scientific specialist.

Avoidance of health hazards

If the patient is known or suspected to be carrying the hepatitis B virus or equivalent infecting agent, special precautions **must** be taken in the transmission of specimens. Blood (or other) samples must be in screw-capped containers and placed in a sealed plastic bag: the request form must be separated from the sample; and both must be marked, e.g. with a red star. This procedure enables the laboratory staff to take special precautions against infection.

Urine and faeces samples that may be infected with pathogens must likewise be identified.

Blood

Most laboratories arrange to collect blood samples from outpatients by their own staff, and many have facilities for sending laboratory staff or special phlebotomists round the wards to collect the daily routine batch of non-urgent specimens whose request forms are received by a specific time. Otherwise the clinical staff usually have this responsibility for venous and arterial blood samples, but most laboratories prefer to do the collection of measured capillary blood samples themselves. The amount of blood required for any test, and the type of anticoagulant (if any), should be found from the local list. If in doubt, one syringe/tube full (about 10 ml) of blood, either clotted or with lithium heparin as anticoagulant, will serve for most of the common analyses except glucose (p. 58) and the acid-base components (p. 44). When large numbers of analyses are required on a single sample, it is usually not necessary to provide as much blood as would be needed if these were isolated analyses – the laboratory staff can advise. In general fasting samples are preferred, and when blood samples are required day after day for serial investigation, samples should preferably be taken under similar conditions in relation to drugs, meals, rest, recumbency, and time of day.

In the case of infants and children it is usually not desirable or possible to obtain a sufficiently large venous specimen for analysis by the usual laboratory techniques. Laboratories have available suitable micromethods, and arrangements may be made to analyse a capillary sample collected by heel prick into a special tube.

A particularly important feature in venepuncture is the avoidance of stasis, caused by a prolonged use of a tourniquet. This increases the concentration in plasma of proteins and protein-bound substances such as calcium (and similar changes may be produced by standing up after recumbency) due to shift of water from the vascular compartment. Stasis also increases the plasma concentration of substances present in high concentration in muscle, such as lactate due to tissue anoxia. It is also important to avoid both forcible ejection of blood through the needle into the tube (by first removing the needle), and also any contamination with water or antiseptic: these produce haemolysis, which invalidates potassium analyses and many other investigations. Another error is taking blood from the same arm that is receiving an intravenous infusion.

Urine

Qualitative tests on urine are generally performed in the side-room on an early morning sample (see Appendix II). For quantitative analyses a 24 hour collection is almost always needed. The need for a preservative varies with local preference, and according to the instability of the component to be analysed. If in doubt, a 24 hour sample collected without preservative, but refrigerated, will serve for most of the common analyses.

It is surprisingly difficult to collect an accurate 24-hour urine excretion from a ward patient unless he is in a metabolic ward with specially trained staff, and it is even more so from an outpatient. The following procedure is recommended. On rising, patient empties bladder. This specimen is discarded. *All* urine passed for the next 24 hours is collected into the special bottle: on rising the next morning the patient empties the bladder again, 24 hours after the first specimen, and this final specimen is added to the bottle, which is sent to the laboratory. For most investigations collection from 08:00 to 08:00 is recommended. The dates and times of starting and finishing the collection must be clearly stated on both the request card and the bottle.

Faeces

Qualitative tests, usually for occult blood, are generally performed in the side-room on a portion of a single stool. For quantitative studies (usually for fat) it is necessary to collect at least a complete three day excretion (p. 78) to allow for daily variation. Otherwise analyses of faeces are generally done as part of a balance test (p. 94).

Other fluids

The procedure for collection of CSF is described on p. 247: it must be remembered that samples of CSF often also require cytological and microbiological examination.

It is recommended that the laboratory be first consulted if other types of specimen (e.g. from ascites, joints, or fistulas) are to be sent, if other than the usual analyses, e.g. for protein, are required. The same precaution applies before sending specimens for new or unusual complex tests of function.

Further reading

Using the Laboratory. 2nd ed. London: Department of Health and Social Security, 1977.

SI UNITS

The Système International d'Unités (SI), which was approved internationally in 1960, has become generally accepted for scientific, technical, and medical use in Britain and throughout most of the world.

The application of SI to medicine involves the choice of units of measurement, and also of their mode of expression. There are special features that are particularly relevant to chemical pathology.

Volume

Because the base unit of length is the metre (m), the unit of volume becomes the cubic metre (m^3). This is often inconvenient and unfamiliar, so it has been accepted that the working unit for volume shall be the litre (l), which is an alternative name for the cubic decimetre (dm^3: $1000\,cm^3$). The litre and submultiples of the litre are used in chemical pathology for all measurements of volume.

The decilitre (dl), or 100 ml as it is traditionally expressed, is a non-standard unit of volume. However, so many measurements of body fluid components have been referred to this unit that its abandonment, and replacement by the litre, was not an early change, but has now been accepted (except for haemoglobin) throughout medicine. For example a serum total IgG of 150 mg/100 ml (150 mg/dl) has now become 1500 mg/l or 1.5 g/l.

Per cent (%) means 'per hundred parts of the same'. Thus 'mg %' means milligrams per hundred milligrams, and must *never* be used to mean 'milligrams per hundred millilitres', which differs by a factor of the order of one thousand.

Amount of substance

The base unit is the mole (mol). This unit is defined as the amount of substance of a system which contains as many elementary units as there are carbon atoms in 12 grams of carbon-12. It replaces the gram-molecule, gram-ion, gram-equivalent, etc. For example, one mole of hydrogen ions (H^+) has a mass of 1 g (strictly 1.008 g); one mole of hydrogen (H_2) has a mass of 2 g; one mole of water (H_2O) has a mass of 18 g; one mole of glucose ($C_6H_{12}O_6$) has a mass of 180 g. All chemical substances interact in proportions related to their relative molecular mass ('molecular weight'), ionic mass, etc.

The use of the equivalent and its submultiples (e.g. milliequivalent) has now been abandoned. Where monovalent ions are concerned (e.g. Na^+), 1 mEq is numerically identical to 1 mmol, and their analytical results are therefore expressed as mmol/l or mmol/24 h etc.

Because the activity of glucose, and other non-ionised substances, also is proportional to its molar concentration and not to its mass concentration, it is logical also to express its concentration in body fluids as mmol/l and not as mg/100 ml: a mass/volume concentration of 180 mg/100 ml becomes 10 mmol/l. The same argument applies to non-monovalent ions: for calcium the mass/volume concentration of 10 mg/100 ml becomes 2.5 mmol/l, which contains about 1.2 mmol/l of ionised calcium.

For some substances, particularly many proteins, the exact relative molecular mass is not known, and therefore mass concentration per litre is still used and not molar concentration. This also applies to mixtures.

Enzyme activity

Originally units for measurement of enzyme activity, particularly in body fluids, were arbitrary. They were usually named after the originators of the analytical method, such as the King-Armstrong unit for alkaline phosphatase and the Somogyi unit for amylase. International agreement led to a unit applicable to any enzyme, which is the amount that will catalyse the transformation of one micromole of substrate per minute, under defined conditions. This enzyme unit is used in chemical pathology now for most enzymes, and has the symbol U.

A recent recommendation for a unit of enzyme catalytic activity related to SI is that which produces an observed catalysed reaction rate of substrate transformation of one mole per second, under defined conditions. The unit is called the katal (kat). Conversion factor: $1 U \simeq 16.7$ nkat.

Pressure

The unit is the pascal (Pa). In medicine in general, pressure measurements actually made as the height of a liquid column (particularly arterial blood pressure) will continue for the present to be expressed in terms of that liquid, as millimetres of mercury (mmHg) or centimetres of water (cmH_2O): the appropriate measurement in pascals should also be given. Partial pressures of gases are expressed only in pascals. Conversion factors are (at s.t.p.): $1\,mmHg \simeq 133$ Pa, $1\,cmH_2O \simeq 98$ Pa.

Energy

The unit for all forms of energy is the joule (J).

The special unit for heat energy, the calorie, which is generally used in medicine and nutrition as the thermochemical kilocalorie (kcal; which is the same as the Medical Calorie, Cal) shall eventually be abandoned. Conversion factor: $4.2\ kJ \simeq 1\ kcal$.

Further reading

Baron DN, ed. *Units, Symbols, and Abbreviations*. 3rd ed. London: Royal Society of Medicine, 1977.

Baron DN, Broughton PMG, Cohen M, Lansley TS, Lewis SM, Shinton NK. The use of SI units in reporting results obtained in hospital laboratories. *J Clin Pathol* 1974; 27:590–597.

APPENDIX III

REFERENCE VALUES

The tables in this appendix list accepted reference ranges for the results of those laboratory investigations in chemical pathology that are at present most commonly required in clinical work. The principles underlying the concept 'reference values', and their alterations with age, sex, and other factors have been discussed in chapter 1. In these abbreviated tables no account is taken of the effects of these variations except for the hormones, and where necessary reference is made to the main text. The main tables are applicable to adults, and a separate table (III.4) lists certain reference values for children of different ages.

In the main tables the results are given both in SI units (with emphasis on moles) and in traditional units, with rounded-off conversions. Table III.4 for children gives results in SI units only.

TABLE III.1 *Plasma/Serum*

Constituent	Reference values		Conversion factor from SI to traditional units	Notes
	SI or other international units	*Traditional units*		
Aldosterone	100–500 pmol/l	3.5–18 ng/100 ml	0.036	
Amino acid nitrogen	2.5–4.0 mmol/l	3.5–5.5 mg/100 ml	1.401	fasting
Aminotransferases – see transaminases				
Ammonia (whole blood)	12–60 μmol/l	20–100 μg/100 ml	1.703	
Amylase	70–300 U/l	40–160 Somogyi units/100 ml		
Anion gap	6–16 mmol/l	6–16 mEq/l	1.000	
Bicarbonate	24–30 mmol/l	24–30 mEq/l	1.000	as CO_2 content
Bilirubin				
total	5.0–17 μmol/l	0.3–1.0 mg/100 ml	0.058	
conjugated	<3.0 μmol/l	<0.2 mg/100 ml	0.058	
Caeruloplasmin	0.3–0.6 g/l	30–60 mg/100 ml	00.0	
Calcium	2.1–2.6 mmol/l	8.5–10.5 mg/100 ml	4.000	1.0–1.2 mmol/1 is ionised as P_{CO_2}
Carbon dioxide (whole blood)	4.5–6.0 kPa	35–46 mmHg	7.502	
Carbonic acid	1.1–1.4 mmol/l	1.1–1.4 mEq/l	1.000	
Carotenoids	1.0–5.5 μmol/l	50–300 μg/100 ml	53.69	
Chloride	95–105 mmol/l	95–105 mEq/l	1.000	
Cholesterol – total	4.0–6.5 mmol/l	160–260 mg/100 ml	38.67	
Cholinesterase	2–5 U/l	2–5 iu/l		at 37°C: Dibucaine Number > 80
Copper	13–24 μmol/l	80–150 μg/100 ml	6.355	
Cortisol	200–700 nmol/l	8–35 μg/100 ml	0.036	marked circadian rhythm (p. 155): at 09:00
Creatine	15–60 μmol/l	0.2–0.8 mg/100 ml	0.0131	
Creatinine	60–120 μmol/l	0.7–1.4 mg/100 ml	0.0113	
Creatine kinase	3–100 U/l	3–100 iu/l		at 37°C: sex differences, p. 120

TABLE III.1 *Plasma/Serum continued*

Constituent	Reference values — SI or other international units	Traditional units	Conversion factor from SI to traditional units	Notes
Enzymes – see individual enzymes				
Fatty acids – free	0.3–0.6 mmol/l	0.3–0.6 mEq/l	1.000	fasting
Ferritin	15–250 µg/l	1.5–25 µg/100 ml	0.100	
Folate	5.0–20 µg/l	5.0–20 ng/ml	1.000	
Gastrin	5–50 pmol/l	10–100 pg/ml	2.100	
Glucose (whole blood)				
venous	3.0–5.5 mmol/l	55–100 mg/100 ml	18.016	fasting values; plasma concentrations are 10–15 per cent
capillary	3.2–5.7 mmol/l	60–105 mg/100 ml	18.016	higher at 37°C; sex differences
γ-Glutamyltransferase	7–50 U/l	7–50 iu/l		p. 198
Haptoglobins	5–30 µmol/l	30–180 mg/100 ml	6.446	(whole blood)
Hydrogen ion activity exponent (pH)	7.36–7.44	7.36–7.44		
Insulin	10–30 mU/l	10–30 µu/ml	1.000	fasting
Iron	11–34 µmol/l	60–190 µg/100 ml	5.585	marked circadian rhythm (p. 134); at 08:00: sex differences
Iron-binding capacity – total	45–75 µmol/l	250–400 µg/100 ml	5.585	p. 134.
Ketones	0.06–0.2 mmol/l	0.06–0.2 mEq/l	1.000	as acetoacetate
Lactate	0.75–2.0 mmol/l	0.75–2.0 mEq/l	1.000	fasting
Lactate dehydrogenase				
total	130–500 U/l	130–500 iu/l		
'heart specific'	120–260 U/l	120–260 iu/l		at 37°C; as 'hydroxybutyrate dehydrogenase'
Lead (whole blood)	0.5–1.7 µmol/l	10–35 µg/100 ml	20.72	
Lipase	18–280 U/l	0–1.5 Cherry-Crandall units		
Lipids – total	4.5–10 g/l	450–1000 mg/100 ml	100.0	fasting

TABLE III.1 *Plasma/Serum continued*

Constituent	Reference values		Conversion factor from SI to traditional units	Notes
	SI or other international units	*Traditional units*		
Magnesium	0.7–1.0 mmol/l	1.8–2.4 mg/100 ml	2.431	at 37 °C
5'-Nucleotidase	2–15 U/l	2–15 iu/l		
Osmolality	275–295 mmol/kg	275–295 mosmol/kg	1.000	as P_{O_2}
Oxygen (whole blood)	11–15 kPa	85–105 mmHg	7.501	
Phosphatases				
acid – total	0.5–5.5 U/l	0.3–3.0 KAu/100 ml		tartrate-labile
– 'prostatic'	0–1 U/l	0–0.5 KAu/100 ml		higher in adolescents: sex differences p. 178.
alkaline – total	20–95 U/l	3–13 KAu/100 ml		
Phosphate – inorganic	0.8–1.4 mmol/l	2.5–4.5 mg/100 ml	3.097	as phosphorus
Phospholipids	1.8–3.0 mmol/l	150–250 mg/100 ml	77.4	as lecithin
Potassium	3.8–5.0 mmol/l	3.8–5.0 mEq/l	1.000	
Protein				
Total	62–80 g/l	6.2–8.0 g/100 ml	0.100	
Albumin	35–52 g/l	3.5–5.2 g/100 ml	0.100	
Globulin (total)	18–32 g/l	1.8–3.2 g/100 ml	0.100	
γ-Globulin (total)	7–15 g/l	0.7–1.5 g/100 ml	0.100	
IgA	1.5–4.0 g/l	150–400 mg/100 ml	100.0	
IgG	8.0–16.0 g/l	800–1600 mg/100 ml	100.0	
IgM	0.5–1.5 g/l	50–150 mg/100 ml	100.0	
Fibrinogen	2–4 g/l	0.2–0.4 g/100 ml	0.100	
Pyruvate	50–80 μmol/l	0.4–0.7 mg/100 ml	0.0088	
Sodium	136–148 mmol/l	136–148 mEq/l	1.000	fasting

TABLE III.1 *Plasma/Serum continued*

Constituent	Reference values		Conversion factor from SI to traditional units	Notes
	SI or other international units	*Traditional units*		
Thyrotrophic hormone	0–5 mU/l	0–5 mU/l		
Thyroxine	60–130 nmol/l	4.5–10 μg/100 ml	0.0777	
Transaminases				
alanine	5–25 U/l	5–25 iu/l		at 37 °C
aspartate	5–35 U/l	5–35 iu/l		at 37 °C
Transferrin	1.2–2.0 g/l	120–200 mg/100 ml	100.0	
Triglyceride	0.3–1.8 mmol/l	25–150 mg/100 ml	87.5	fasting, as glycerol
Urea	3.0–6.5 mmol/l	18–40 mg/100 ml	6.006	
Urate	0.09–0.42 mmol/l	1.5–7.0 mg/100 ml	16.81	sex differences p. 97
Vitamin A	1.0–3.0 μmol/l	30–90 μg/100 ml	28.65	
Vitamin B_{12}	160–900 ng/l	160–900 pg/ml	1.000	
Zinc	12–17 μmol/l	80–110 μg/100 ml	6.537	microbiological assay

TABLE III.2 *Urine values per 24 hour excretion*

Constituent	Reference values		Conversion factor from SI to traditional units	Notes
	SI or other international units	Traditional units		
Aldosterone	15–50 nmol	5–18 μg	1.3605	
Amino acid nitrogen – free	4–20 mmol	50–300 mg	14.01	
Amylase	200–1500 U	10–7000 Henry-Chiamori units		
Ascorbic acid	0–45 μmol/8 h	0–8 mg/8 h	0.176	overnight sample
Calcium	2.5–7.5 mmol	100–300 mg	40.08	
Chloride	170–250 mmol	170–250 mEq	1.000	
Copper	0.2–1.5 μmol	10–100 μg	63.55	
Creatine	0–0.4 mmol	0–50 mg	131.1	
Creatinine	9–18 mmol	1.0–2.0 g	0.1131	
Glucose	0.1–1.0 mmol	20–200 mg	180.2	
Hydrogen ion activity exponent (pH)	5.5–8.0	5.5–8.0	1.000	range over 24 h
5-Hydroxyindoleacetic acid	10–45 μmol	2–8 mg	0.1912	
Hydroxyproline	80–250 μmol	10–35 mg	0.1311	
Indicans	0.1–0.4 mmol	20–80 mg	251.3	
Lead	0–0.3 μmol	0–60 g	207.2	
Nitrogen – total	0.7–1.5 mol	10–20 g	14.01	
Osmolality	700–1500 mmol	700–1500 mosmol	1.000	total solute excretion
Phosphate	15–50 mmol	0.5–1.5 g	0.031	as phosphorus
Porphyrins				
δ-Aminolaevulinic acid	1–40 μmol	0.1–5.0 mg	0.1311	
Porphobilinogen	1–12 μmol	0.2–2.0 mg	0.2262	
Coproporphyrin	0.15–0.3 μmol	100–200 μg	654.7	
Uroporphyrin	6–40 nmol	5–30 μg	0.8308	

TABLE III.2 *Urine values per 24 hour excretion continued*

| Constituent | Reference values | | Conversion factor from SI to traditional units | Notes |
	SI or other international units	Traditional units		
Potassium	40–120 mmol	40–120 mEq	1.000	
Protein (total)	40–120 mg	40–120 mg	1.000	
Sodium	100–250 mmol	100–250 mEq	1.000	
Steroid hormones				
Oestriol		$\mu g \times 0.0035 = \mu mol$	288.4	varies with time of
Pregnanediol		$mg \times 3.1 = \mu mol$	0.3205	menstrual period or pregnancy: see chapter 10
17-Oxosteroids: *men*	25–80 μmol	7–24 mg	0.2884	
women	15–60 μmol	4–17 mg		
17-Oxogenic steroids: *men*	20–75 μmol	6–22 mg	0.2884	
women	15–60 μmol	4–17 mg		
Urea	250–600 mmol	15–35 g	0.0601	
Uric acid	1.5–4.5 mmol	250–750 mg	168.1	
Urobilinogen	0.5–5.0 μmol	0.3–3.0 mg		
Vanilmandelic acid	10–35 μmol	2–7 mg	0.5907	
Volume	750–2000 ml	750–2000 ml	0.1982	

TABLE III.3 *Faeces values per 24 hour excretion*

| Constituent | Reference values | | Notes |
	SI or other international units	*Traditional units*	
Total wet weight	60–250 g	60–250 g	
Total dry weight	20–60 g	20–60 g	
Coproporphyrin	0.15–0.5 mmol	0.1–0.3 mg	
Fat – total	10–18 mmol	3–5 g	as stearic acid
Nitrogen – total	70–110 mmol	1–1.5 g	
Urobilinogen	100–500 μmol	60–300 mg	

TABLE III.4 *Infants and Children*

Constituent		Birth (full term)	1 week	1 Month	3 Years	6 Years	15 Years	Adult
Blood								
Glucose–fasting	(mmol/l)	1.2–4.5	2.5–4.7					3.0–5.5
Serum/Plasma								
Urea	(mmol/l)		1.5–4.0			2.5–6.0		3.0–6.5
Bicarbonate	(mmol/l)			18–24				24–30
Chloride	(mmol/l)			98–106				95–105
Potassium	(mmol/l)	3.5–6.5		4.0–5.8				3.8–5.0
Sodium	(mmol/l)			136–144				136–148
Calcium	(mmol/l)	1.8–3.0		2.2–2.8		2.2–2.7		2.1–2.6
Phosphate	(mmol/l)	1.2–2.8		1.5–2.3		1.0–1.8		0.8–1.4
Alkaline phosphatase	(U/l)	35–105		70–230		70–175	70–210	20–95
Aspartate transaminase	(U/l)			4–80		5–40		5–35
Bilirubin – total	(mmol/l)	10–110	20–140	5–17				5–17
Protein – total	(g/l)	50–70		55–70	60–75			62–80
Albumin	(g/l)	25–40		33–45	35–48			36–52
Cholesterol	(mmol/l)	2.2–5.2			3.0–6.2			4.0–6.5
Urine								
Creatinine	(µmol/kg·24 h)		45–120			90–160		130–220
17-Oxogenic steroids	(µmol/24 h)					3–20	10–45	15–75
17-Oxosteroids	(µmol/24 h)					0–7	10–30	15–80
Volume	(ml)		50–300		500–700	600–1000		750–2000

SIMPLE BIOCHEMICAL TEST PROCEDURES

The commercial introduction of rapid tablet and strip tests for abnormal constituents has greatly simplified the testing of urine and faeces in the wards and outpatient department, and by general practitioners, and has enabled patients to test their own specimens themselves. Nevertheless, care is still required, and as well as having individual snags described below, these test materials are sometimes less stable, especially in hot moist climates, than the classical solid and liquid chemical reagents. The theoretical bases of these tests are described in appropriate sections of the main text. The various combination strips, which carry multiple tests, are cheaper and more convenient than a multiplicity of single tests, but bear the risk of possible confusion in the readings. They also test only for glucose and not for reducing substances, and testing for the latter is of special importance in paediatrics for detection of galactose and fructose (p. 73).

The success of the commercial test materials for urine and faeces led to the development of similar tests for use on blood. So far only those for glucose have been successful: the semiquantitative tests for blood urea (p. 95) are not widely used.

New and modified tests are continually being introduced.

Urine

The results of testing urine for most soluble constituents are more satisfactory if the urine is fresh. For the classical wet chemical tests cloudy urine can usually be cleared by filtration, or by allowing it to stand and decanting the supernatant liquid.

If any unexpected abnormality is found the urine should be sent to the laboratory for confirmation of the result.

Specific gravity (p. 213)

The specific gravity (relative density) of urine is measured at room temperature with a floating urinometer, taking care to see that the urinometer is not in contact with the sides of the container when taking the reading. If the specimen is too small to float the urinometer, dilute the urine with an equal quantity of water and take the specific gravity of the mixture. Then specific gravity urine = 1.000 + twice 'last two figures' of specific gravity of mixture.

NOTE: The accuracy of the urinometer should be checked periodically, using distilled water, specific gravity 1.000.

The specific gravity can be corrected for the effects of dissolved glucose (0.004 per 10 g/l) or protein (0.003 per 10 g/l), but osmolality (p. 213) is then the more precise measurement.

pH (p. 213)

Dip a wide-range indicator paper into the urine, and compare with the standard colours shown on the maker's chart. The use of litmus paper is not advised because it is insufficiently sensitive.

Protein (p. 214)

(a) i. **Albustix (Ames)**/ii. **Albym-Test (Boehringer).** The end of the strip is dipped into the urine and removed immediately. A greenish-blue colour indicates the presence of protein – see makers' colour charts. This is a roughly quantitative test, and is sensitive to about 60 mg albumin/l: it is less sensitive to Bence Jones protein and other proteins of low molecular weight e.g. β_2-microglobulin. A faint positive must be checked by the salicylsulphonic acid or boiling test, as this may be a false positive produced by alkaline, strongly buffered urine.

NOTE: Urine containing traces of cetrimide or similar substances (used to disinfect urinals) will give a blue colour.

(b) **Boiling test.** Pour about 10 ml of clear urine into a test tube. Make slightly acid by adding, drop by drop, 33 per cent acetic acid solution. This prevents the precipitation of urinary phosphates. Heat to 100 °C, either by direct flame or preferably in a water bath. Compare with a test tube of untreated urine: a white cloud or precipitate indicates the presence of more than 100 mg protein/l.

(c) **Salicylsulphonic acid test.** To 5 ml of clear urine add 10 drops (0.5 ml) of 25 per cent salicylsulphonic acid solution. A white cloud (best observed by comparison with a control tube of the original urine against a dark background) indicates the presence of more than 100 mg protein/l.

NOTE. Urine containing tolbutamide, and certain X-ray contrast materials from intravenous pyelography, gives a false positive reaction.

Reducing substances and glucose (p. 72)

(a) **Clinitest (Ames).** This tablet test is a modified form of the Benedict's reaction, but is slightly less sensitive, detecting about 10 mmol/l (0.2 g glucose/dl). Place 5 drops of urine and 10 drops of water in a small test tube. Drop in one tablet; 15 seconds after boiling has stopped compare the appearance with the maker's colour chart. The colours produced are almost the same as those of the classical Benedict's test.

(b) **Benedict's test.** Add 0.5 ml (or 8 drops) of clear urine to 5 ml of Benedict's reagent, shake, and place in boiling water for 5 minutes. Allow to stand for 2 minutes. The presence of reducing substances is indicated by a precipitate varying from green through yellow to reddish-brown, depending on the quantity present. The test is sensitive to about 5 mmol/l (0.1 g glucose/dl), and full reduction occurs with about 100 mmol/l (2 g/dl).

(c) i. **Clinistix (Ames)/ii. BM-Test-Glucose (Boehringer)/iii. Tes-Tape (Eli Lilly).** These are specific tests for glucose. Dip the strip into urine and remove. When glucose is present the moistened end turns i. purple at 10 seconds/ii. brown at 60 seconds/iii. green at 60 seconds – see makers' colour charts. This test is sensitive to about 3 mmol/l (0.05 g glucose/dl) but is not quantitative.

NOTE: A high concentration of ascorbic acid will inhibit (by reduction) a weak positive reaction. Powerful oxidising agents such as hypochlorite may give a false positive reaction.

iv. **Diastix (Ames).** This similar test is sensitive to about 5 mmol/l (0.1 g/dl) and is semiquantitative: the colour change, read at 30 seconds, is through green to brown – see maker's colour chart. This formulation is used in Ames' multiple test strips. The reaction is inhibited by a high concentration of ketones.

Ketones (p. 74)

(a) i. **Acetest (Ames).** This tablet test is based on Rothera's test and is less sensitive. Place 1 drop of urine on to a table which is on a clear surface, and observe the top surface of the tablet. A purple colour, appearing within 30 seconds, indicates significant ketonuria, more than 0.5 mmol/l (5 mg acetoacetic acid/dl).

ii. **Ketostix (Ames)/iii. BM-Test-Ketone (Boehringer).** These are similar strip tests which are used by dipping into the urine, removing, and reading at 15 seconds: a purple colour indicates a positive reaction.

NOTE: These tests are roughly quantitative, and can be read against the makers' colour charts. They may also be used for the detection of ketoacids in plasma. They are less sensitive to acetone than to acetoacetic acid.

(b) **Rothera's test.** One-third fill a test tube with solid ammonium sulphate-sodium nitroprusside mixture (500:1). Saturate the powder with urine, add 1 ml of concentrated ammonia solution and allow to stand. A purple colour indicates the presence of acetone or acetoacetic acid.

NOTE: This test is now rarely used: it is too sensitive for routine ward use as it gives a positive reaction with acetoacetic acid at a concentration less than 0.1 mmol/l (1 mg/dl). Salicylates do not give a positive reaction.

(c) **Gerhardt's test.** To 5 ml of fresh, clear urine add about 1 ml of iron(III) [ferric] chloride reagent (10 per cent $FeCl_3$ in 2M-HCl): a plum-red colour indicates the presence of acetoacetic acid in concentration greater than 5 mmol/l (50 mg/dl).

NOTE: Salicylates give a purplish colour with $FeCl_3$. They can be distinguished from acetoacetic acid as follows: boil 10 ml of urine vigorously for 10 minutes, allow to cool, and then repeat the test as above. Salicylates remain in the urine and still give a positive Gerhardt test;

acetoacetic acid will have been decomposed and the urine will not give a
positive reaction. Chlorpromazine gives a mauve colour with FeCl₃ and
phenylpyruvic acid a green colour.

Bilirubin (p. 193)

(a) i. Ictotest (Ames). This is a tablet test, based on a diazo reaction
similar to the van den Bergh reaction. Place 5 drops of urine on 1 square
of the paper mat provided. Put a tablet on the square. Put 2 drops of
water on the tablet. If the test is positive the mat around the tablet turns
blue within 30 seconds: the sensitivity is 2 μmol/l (0.1 mg bilirubin/dl).

ii. Bilur-Test (Boehringer). This is a similar strip test which is used by
dipping into the urine, removing, and reading at 20 seconds: a pink-to-
violet colour indicates a positive reaction. The test is sensitive to 6 μmol/l
(0.3 mg bilirubin/dl).

iii. Ictostix (Ames). This is now only produced as part of a multiple test
strip: its use is as ii.

(b) Fouchet-Harrison test. To 10 ml of acidified urine add 5 ml of
10 per cent barium chloride solution, shake well and filter. To the barium
salt precipitate on the filter paper (which absorbs the bile pigment) add
1 drop of Fouchet's reagent (1 per cent FeCl₃ in 25 per cent trichloracetic
acid): a green or blue colour indicates the presence of more than 1 μmol/l
(0.05 mg bilirubin/dl).

(c) Froth test. Shake vigorously 10 ml of urine. Yellow tinged froth,
best detected in daylight in comparison with normal urine similarly
shaken, appears if bile pigments are present. This test is neither as
sensitive nor as specific as the two preceding tests.

Urobilinogen (p. 193)

(a) Ehrlich's test (Watson-Schwartz modification). To 1 ml of *fresh* clear
urine add 1 ml of 0.7 per cent *p*-dimethylaminobenzaldehyde in 60 per
cent HCl. Mix and allow to stand for 5 minutes. Add 2 ml of a saturated
solution of sodium acetate and mix. Normal urine gives a faint red
colour. If urobilinogen is absent, the mixture is yellow. Excess urobilinogen (or porphobilinogen) gives a deep red colour.

NOTE: The urobilinogen colour, but not the similar porphobilinogen
colour (p. 130), can be extracted by shaking the mixture with chloroform or
amyl alcohol. Ehrlich's aldehyde reagent also reacts with p-*aminosalicylic*
acid.

(b) Urobilistix (Ames). This is a strip test based on the Ehrlich
aldehyde reaction. It will detect normal or increased levels, but cannot be
used to show absence of urobilinogen: its sensitivity is 3 μmol/l (0.2
mg/dl). The test gives a similar positive reaction with porphobilinogen.

It is used by dipping into *fresh* urine, removing, and reading at 60
seconds: a yellow to brown colour indicates a positive reaction.

(c) Ugen-Test (Boehringer). This is a strip test based on a diazo
reaction. It is used by dipping into *fresh* urine, removing, and reading at

30 seconds: a pink-to-red colour indicates a positive reaction. The test is sensitive to 7 μmol/l (0.4 mg/dl).

Blood and haemoglobin (p. 214)

(a) **Hemastix (Ames)**. This is a strip test based on a peroxidase reaction with o-tolidine as the indicator, which is used by dipping into the urine, and reading at 30 seconds. A blue colour indicates a positive reaction and this is sensitive to 15 μg/dl of haemoglobin or to 5×10^6 r.b.c./l.

(b) **Sangur-Test (Boehringer)**. This is a similar test which uses a different peroxidase reaction. It is sensitive to 30 μg/dl of haemoglobin (green colour) or to 5×10^6 r.b.c./l (green dots).

NOTE: The best method for examining urine for the presence of erythrocytes is microscopy.

A high concentration of ascorbic acid will inhibit, by reduction, a weak positive reaction.

Faeces

Occult blood (p. 243)

(a) **Okokit (Hughes and Hughes)**. This is a tablet test based on a peroxidase reaction with guaiacum as the indicator. Make a smear of faeces on the test paper. Put a tablet on the smear, then put 3 drops of diluent reagent on the tablet. A blue colour appearing at about 5 minutes indicates a positive reaction. The test is relatively insensitive and does not respond to the pigments present in a normal mixed diet, or to iron tablets.

NOTE: Excess dietary ascorbic acid may mask a weak positive reaction.

(b) **i. Haemoccult (Smith Kline Instruments)/ii. Fecatest (Labsystems Oy)**. These are similar tests, with guaiacum as the indicator impregnated into the test card. Make a thin smear of faeces on the test card – this can be done by the patient. Add to the smear 2 drops of reagent. A blue colour appearing within 30–60 seconds indicates a positive reaction.

(c) **Peroheme 40 (BDH Chemicals)**. This is a similar test with 2,6-dichlorophenolindophenol as the indicator. Make a smear of faeces on the test paper. Add to the smear 1 drop each of reagents 1 and 2. A red-pink colour appearing within 2 minutes indicates a positive reaction. This test is more sensitive, and a diet free of meat and green vegetables for 3 days is advised; iron does not interfere.

Blood

Glucose (p. 58)

(a) **i. BM-Test-Glycemie (Boehringer) / ii. BM-Test-Glycemie 20–800 (Boehringer)**. These are specific strip tests for use with fresh capillary blood, designed to be read by eye, for semiquantitative estimation, against the maker's colour chart. The instructions for use of the strips need to be followed exactly.

Ranges: i. 3–45 mmol/l (60–800 mg/dl)/ii. 1–45 mmol/l (20–800 mg/dl).

(b) Dextrostix (Ames). This is a similar test for use with fresh capillary or venous blood (avoid fluoride as preservative!). The colour changes may be roughly matched by eye against the maker's colour chart, but should be used with a reflectance meter to give a semiquantitative measure of blood glucose. The manufacturer's instructions for the particular reflectance meter must be followed exactly.

Range: 0–14+ mmol/l (0–250+ mg/dl).

(e) i. Reflotest-Glucose (Boehringer) / ii. Reflotest-Hypoglycemie (Boehringer). These are similar tests for use with fresh capillary blood or venous blood/plasma/serum, and are designed to be used only with a reflectance meter.

Ranges: i. 4–20 mmol/l (70–350 mg/dl)/ii. 0.5–8.5 mmol/l (10–150 mg/dl).

INDEX

A

Abetalipoproteinaemia, 86
Accuracy, in clinical chemistry, 8
Acetate, 51, 72
Acetest, 272
Acetoacetate, metabolism (*see also* Ketosis), 79
Acetoacetic acid, urinary, *see* Ketonuria
Acetone, plasma, *see* Ketosis
  urinary, *see* Ketonuria
Acetylcholinesterase, 121
  prenatal diagnosis and, 165
Acetyl coenzyme A, 56, 79
  ketosis and, 79–81
β-*N*-Acetylglucosaminidase, 218
Achlorhydria, 231
  tests for, 230–2
Acid, *see* under individual acids
  definition, 42
Acid phosphatases, 178–9
  Gaucher's disease and, 88
  plasma, reference values, 179
    raised, causes of, 179
  prostatic disease and, 179
Acid-base balance, *see* pH, Acidosis, Alkalosis
Acidaemia, definition (*see also* Acidosis), 46
Acidosis, 45, 48–51
  compensatory mechanisms for, 46–8
  decalcification and, 185
  diagnosis of, 51–2
  intestinal secretion losses and, 238
  ketosis and, 51
    diabetic, 63
  lactic, 71–2
  metabolic, 49–50
  renal disease and (*see also* Renal tubular acidosis), 223, 224, 225
  respiratory, 49
  symptoms of, 48
  treatment of, 52–3
  uraemia and, 224
  uric acid and, 99
Acromegaly, 144–5
ACTH, *see* Adrenocorticotrophic hormone
Acute phase proteins, 112
Acute tubular necrosis, *see* Renal failure, acute
Addis count, 218
Addisonian crisis, 159
Addison's disease, 158–9
  carbohydrate metabolism in, 66, 69
  hyperkalaemia and, 37
  pituitary, 141
  sodium loss in, 30

tests for, 159–60
urea retention in, 96
Adenosine triphosphate (ATP), 55
Adenylate cyclase, and hormones, 137
Adipose tissue, distribution, 21
  metabolism, 79
Adrenal cortex (*see also* Adrenocorticotrophic hormone and under individual hormones), 153–61
  androgenic hormones, 155
  corticosteroids, 153–5
    glucocorticoid activity, 154
    mineralocorticoid activity, 154–5
  function tests (*see also* under individual tests), 159–61
  hyperactivity (*see also* under specific diseases), 156–8
  hypoactivity (*see also* Addison's disease), 158–9
Adrenal medulla, 169–70
Adrenalectomy, 155
Adrenaline: carbohydrate metabolism and, 58
  phaeochromocytoma and, 169
Adrenocorticotrophic hormone (ACTH) (*see also* Adrenal cortex), 138–9, 152–3
  Addison's disease and, 158–9
  Cushing's syndrome and, 156–7
  hypopituitarism and, 140–1
  plasma, 156
  response tests, 159–60
Adrenogenital syndrome, 157
Afibrinogenaemia, 111
Agammaglobulinaemia, *see* Hypogammaglobulinaemia
Age, and reference values, 12
Alanine transaminase, plasma:
  in liver disease, 198
  reference values, 198
Albumin: CSF, 249
  hepatic synthesis of, 188
  liver disease and, 196
  metabolism, 106–7
  plasma (*see also* Proteins, plasma), 106
    alterations of, 107–8
    reference values, 106
Albuminuria, *see* Proteinuria
Albustix, 271
Albym-Test, 271
Alcohol: carbohydrate metabolism and, 66, 6
  Cushing's syndrome and, 156
  gout and, 97
  lactic acidosis and, 72
  liver disease and, 87